Sahaja Yoga

Heal and Integrate your Subtle Energy System

by

Saraswati Raman

ISBN 978-1-965679-09-8 (Paperback)
ISBN 978-1-965679-10-4 (Ebook)

This book is dedicated to
Adi Shakti, residing in the hearts of all Seekers of Truth.

Contents

PART II
The Mystery of Music

PART III
Incarnations – Steps to Momentum in Human Evolution

Prologue

It was a rainy day after the Krishna Janmashtami celebrations. The year was 1987. On a beautiful, soulful evening of discourses, Bhajans and aarti at the temple, I had just retired to my room after a light dinner. The day was not over yet for me. It was the beginning of a study in Vedanta that I had undertaken and as usual, I was writing notes reflecting on the insights of the day. It was not unusual for deep thinking and contemplation occurring, virtually experientially, as I wrote away into my diary. Many of these writing would bring revelations that often ushered me into a silence and stillness and I was much in awe at their magnificence.

A little later, on that night, I had gone into meditation, with the oil lamp burning and it might have been quite some time, for, when my eyes opened, I was lying sideways in the seat of meditation. A glance at the watch and it was 1:30 at night. I sat up, but strangely, I could not feel any sensations in my hands, and I couldn't recollect my whereabouts. I felt strangely lost and did not know where I was. I felt disconnected from my mind and feelings and felt only my body move, I remember coming out on to the balcony and being perplexed at the surroundings. I sat down on the floor and looked blankly not knowing what was happening. It was then, after a few moments, that I felt a certain consciousness coming back from the head into my body and suddenly the sensations of my hands and face returned. My eyes brightened and tears welled. I smiled at my own recognition of myself and slept through the rest of the night.

But what happened strangely after that night, when my soul seemed to have gone on a nocturnal journey after that deep meditation, was that, I had become strangely disjointed. That is, when the consciousness or soul had returned into my body, it seemed to have upset the balance of the subtle system. I became very absent minded; I would suddenly stand staring intensely at the living kingdom coming alive on a tree, or dodge at the ants and insects coming in the way as I walked the narrow paths or stand lost in thought before the Shiva or Ganapati idols at the temple. Sometimes, I would go along with the sound of the temple bells as it tapered away into silence or get lost into the meanings of the Sanskrit Slokas that seemed to unfold a huge thought process. Although, I did realize that something strange was happening to me which was beyond my control, I went along with my parents to the psychotherapist who after prolonged questioning and discussions diagnosed me with Schizophrenia, a disease which indicated a chemical disorder in the brain. I was put on medication, three types of medicines, Trinicalm Plus, Tankodep2, and Depsodiaz, three dozes a day totaling to about 12 tablets a day of different colors and combinations.

During the next few weeks, I slept for hours on end during the days and nights without any awareness of the time of the day or night. I would wake up at odd hours, eat only puffed rice and generally in a drowsy state. I would meditate for hours at a stretch. I was unable to bring myself to do anything concrete. A liquid flowed continuously from my Sahasrar and through my gullet into my stomach. It kept flowing and flowing for a couple of days. I didn't know what it was. I saw visions of the evolution of life from the oceans, the fishes, the birds, the animals and lots of trees and nature continuously. I needed assistance of someone (invariably it used to be my mother or sister) to even cross the road while going to the doctor or to the temple.

The revelations that I was going through during my waking hours were so exciting and so stunning, that I was drawn into the vortex of timelessness and went through the various processes of evolution, of the transition of the living kingdom from the waters, to the birds into flight, the animal kingdom on the terrestrial land of the distant lands, the lovely inhabitations of the living forests, the gentle growth of the roots of the trees and blossoming of the flowers in slow motion as it were, the rising and the setting Sun, I was just lapping it up. This was inter-twined with hours and hours of sleep, drowsiness as an aftermath of medicines, only to wake up again into a state of half wakefulness, and half dream state of evolutionary visions. This went on for about 3 months, when the Doctor felt that I was better off occupied and so it would be advisable for me to return to my office where I worked. So, after the long leave I went back to work reluctantly and not knowing how I would cope.

With difficulty, as days passed, I got into the routine of work and Bombay life. The medicines that I was consuming had become food for me, and my body had become addicted and adjusted to it. A couple of years later, some incidents had triggered a serious outburst following which my parents took me to another neurologist recommended by the earlier psychotherapist and was given ECT treatments a couple of times. The medicines were also revised and I was once again living a life inconsequentially, numbed to a life devoid of emotions, pain and dreams. The days came in and they went out. My office routine continued, with nothing to celebrate, nothing to grieve, nothing to talk about. I had become a zombie. But with no distractions of any kind, my concentration power was immense and I could concentrate and put focused attention on difficult problems and calculations and successfully solve it. I would engage in hours and hours of work without getting disturbed or diverted and this led to success on my work front. Nobody even guessed that there could be some serious mental illness in me.

The breakthrough in this monotony came when a dialogue with an office colleague, discussing my early days in spirituality triggered a recollection that revealed the waste that my life had become. He suggested that I attend a meditation session at one of the centers in Thane. That one session shook up something in me and after that I started attending every center that was holding meditation sessions on every day of the week. The self motivated discipline and regular meditation increased an awareness which made me realize the addiction, slavery and dependency on medicines and their consequent side effects, which I had been taking for Schizophrenia over the years.

The Sahaja Yoga meditation that I practiced involved the activation of chakras and energy centers and channels of my body which energized me increasingly, every day. I used meditation, contemplation and continuous vigilance over my recurring habits and tendencies and corrected them as an ongoing process to become the personality that I wanted to be. Repeatedly I would go into a vicious circle of making the same mistakes and habituated responses to situations and suffering the same results and actions from people. Every time I repeated the mistake, I became more and more aware, earlier than usual. Then, I was able to detect earlier but I would still react and later realize. But then a stage came when I became aware much earlier and even before I made the response; so I had time to modify my response according to my beliefs and value system. This I feel is what each one of us is facing and somehow do not have the technique to correct ourselves and we go through life in regrets.

Conventional drug therapy treats the patient as a passive recipient, leading to suppression of nerves and the neuro-transmitters, the interceptors that carried messages between nerves and thoughts are cruelly cut, leading to suppression of emotions, feelings, love, beauty, courage, bravery and the very desire to soar into the heavens. Of course drugs are themselves invasive and perceived by the immune system as foreign substances which are toxic and so have to be coped up with. Many drugs render the immune system inoperative or greatly weakened.

Sahaja Yoga as Alternative Medicine is still in its nescient stage. The fact that doctorates have been awarded, theses on the application of Sahaja Yoga for treatments of diseases like bronchial asthma, stress, blood pressure, heart ailments, anorexia, angina and epilepsy etc. have been accepted at hospitals goes to show that Sahaja yoga as an Alternative Therapy is being accepted as a truly effective method of treatment. Medical breakthrough has been documented in Australia in the cure and treatment of AIDs cases by suing Sahaja Yoga techniques.

Sahaja Yoga technique is spontaneous and effortless which can be practiced by anybody irrespective of their background, religious beliefs or way of life.

The technique is simple- it is a way of activating a mechanism- the Kundalini which is the divine energy that lies dormant in the Sacrum bone at the base of the spine. This mechanism is the moving force of our enlightenment and is a living force, which seeks self-organization, self- regeneration and ascent. Through self-organization which is its innate ability to heal, it renews balances and recycles and brings about an ascent in one's abilities. Ascent is its ability to transcend the mind and body and to attain collective consciousness.

Sahaja Yoga is a process of meditation wherein the sacred feminine energy called the Kundalini seated in the triangular sacrum bone becomes awakened and ascends through the seven subtle energy centers called as chakras existing within every human being. This process is that of Self- Realization, where the Kundalini after being awakened, pierces the seven chakras, passes through the central channel or the Sushumna Nadi and emerges at the top of the head in the fontanel bone area, and is felt as a gentle cool breeze.

Sahaja Yoga method of meditation brings a breakthrough in the evolution of human awareness. The mysterious Kundalini energy accomplishes this and facilitates the blossoming of hitherto hidden, lost or forgotten qualities within us of pure innocence, spontaneity, creativity, security, compassion, collectivity, forgiveness and integration. Thus the transformation takes place within us. By this process a person becomes moral, united, integrated and balanced.

When the Kundalini power passes through each chakra or psychic centre, the person will have complete control over the corresponding sense organs controlled by these chakras. Thus through her awakening, an individual will become a completely balanced person, physically, mentally, emotionally and spirituality. So this feminine energy which is actually one's true mother makes a person absolutely integrated and fit to achieve his purpose in life.

Through the practice of Sahaja Yoga, our awareness gains a new dimension where absolute truth can be felt tangibly – on our central nervous system. As a result of this happening our spiritual ascent takes place effortlessly and physical, mental and emotional balance is achieved as a byproduct of this growth of our awareness. We then realize that we are not this body, mind, ego, conditionings, emotions or intellect, but something of an eternal nature which is always residing in our heart in a pure, undisturbed state as the Self, or the Spirit. The Spirit is the source of true knowledge, peace and joy.

Long –term Sahaja Yoga meditation practitioners experience a better quality of life and functional health than others. Perhaps, most importantly is the observation that there appears to be a relatively robust and consistent relationship between the meditative experience of mental silence and health, especially mental health. There is evidence that meditation can have short and long-term effects on both function and structural brain plasticity in addition to its already recognized ability to cause relaxation and reduce stress. Until 2006, the US National Center for Complementary and Alternative Medicine (NCCAM) defined meditation as an "a conscious mental process that induces a set of integrated physiological changes termed the relaxation response". Remarkably, however, in 2006 the NCCAM reviewed its definition of meditation describing a new central feature. "In meditation, a person learns to focus his attention and suspend the stream of thoughts that normally occupy the mind." The fundamental change is in emphasis from the physiology of rest (a Westernized understanding of meditation) to the experience of "suspension of thought activity" (a more classical eastern idea of meditation).

L Aftanas and S Golosheykin have shown that the practice of Sahaja Yoga Meditation, and the experience of mental silence, is strongly reflected in both brain electrophysiology and mood. A study by the same group demonstrated reduced emotional reactivity in long-term meditators' compared to controls which was reflected in psychological, physiological and electrophysiological reactivity to standardize stressful stimuli presented in a video film. This provides evidence for the notion of "emotional detachment" and hence enhanced emotional stability and resilience to stressful events.

A smaller intervention study by Morgan over just 6 weeks showed a significant reduction in anxiety, depression and related symptoms in patients with major depression compared to controls which appears to reflect the clinical relevance of Aftanas's findings. This has broader implications particularly as understandings of the relationship between neuroplasticity and meditation emerge. Lazar studied a group of Buddhist meditators and found that meditators compared to controls had significantly increased cortical thickness in right middle and superior frontal cortex and insula suggesting that meditation is associated with delaying of the usually age- related thinning of right frontolimbic brain regions. Hence it is quite possible that long-term meditation may facilitate both electrophysiological and structural changes in brain function that may explain why the population of long-term meditators manifested an apparent advantage as compared to the background population particularly in mental health scores.

While we acknowledge that cross-sectional studies are prone to a number of confounders, the implications for population mental health are nevertheless worth considering. Given that neuropsychiatric disorders such as depression and substance abuse are increasing in incidence as well as their impact and that there are few long-term curative options for many of these conditions, there is merit in exploring the role of preventative strategies such as meditation. The findings of this study warrant further examination of meditative practices as a conceptually innovative preventative and therapeutic option for public mental health. The meditation technique assessed in this study is low/zero cost and to date has not been associated with any adverse effects; hence further exploration of this approach in enhancing general well being, quality of life, and mental health would seem to be highly worthwhile.

Taking my own case, Sahaja Yoga mediation, helped me not only to fully put an end to medicines, in the year 2004, three years after I started Sahaja Yoga Meditation during which period I continued with taking the prescribed medicines. I was not only able to better my performance at work resulting in two promotions thereafter, but also acquire my dream qualifications of BAMS and MD in Alternative Medicine as also an MBA in Banking Finance and Hospital Management. I was also inspired to take up a certification course in Image Management as an independent consultant. All this increased my confidence, and was instrumental in me being selected as a trainer at the Staff Training College of the Bank where I worked, training over 9000 people through 450 training programs.

To conclude, I may say, that one should be awake to the Presence when the Divine comes calling, then with a little bit of effort, perseverance and a positive attitude, even Schizophrenia like illnesses can be handled effectively.

Acknowledgements

Every experience is learning, and my first and foremost acknowledgement of gratitude goes to that life process itself that has taught me the nuances that has culminated in the writing of this book. Many have been my teachers in this journey of life and my heart and soul bows down to them.

I would like to thank my mother Smt. Vijayalakshmi Raman who had more faith in me than I had in myself. It was she who instilled in me the immense courage and faith since childhood, which has now helped me in standing rock solid even amidst all adversities. How much can I express my gratitude to my father, C N Raman, who taught me that every time I faltered, when times were trying and everything seemed all uphill, it is in such times when you feel all low and lost, that you should never quit.

I am very thankful to my no-nonsense sister, Savitri, who was and is a wall of support in times of indecision. I will forever need the support of my cool, enigmatic, and understanding brother Ganesh, whom I know will always be there for me.

I thank A D Nikam who introduced me to Sahaja Yoga and mentored me for several years during the practice of Sahaja Yoga techniques.

I thank the many fellow travelers who have all in no small measure contributed to the learning of the living process that is Sahaja Yoga. I would like to particularly mention the names of Mr. Parag Raje, Mr. Arun Apte, Mrs. Chandrika Nair, Mrs. Pramila Rao and many others.

This book is dedicated to Adi Shakti,
residing in the hearts of all Seekers of Truth,
liberation and ultimate fulfillment in life.

PART I

Chapter 1

What is Sahaja Yoga?

Sahaja yoga is a process of meditation wherein the sacred feminine energy called the Kundalini seated in the triangular sacrum bone becomes awakened and ascends through the seven subtle energy centers called as chakras, existing within every human being, and the individual Spirit becomes one with the universal Spirit. This is a process of Self Realization through the central channel or the Sushumna Nadi where the Kundalini after being awakened pierces the seven chakras and emerges at the top of the head in the fontanel bone area and is felt as a gentle cool breeze.

Sahaja Yoga method of meditation brings a breakthrough in the evolution of human awareness. The mysterious Kundalini energy accomplishes this and facilitates the blossoming of hitherto hidden, lost or forgotten qualities within us of pure innocence, spontaneity, creativity, security, compassion, collectivity, forgiveness and integration. Thus the transformation takes place within us. By this process a person becomes moral, united, integrated and balanced. As Shri Mataji says, "Sahaja yoga is different from other yoga because it begins with Self Realization ".

Through the practice of Sahaja Yoga, our awareness gains a new dimension where absolute truth can be felt tangibly – on our central nervous system. As a result of this happening, our spiritual ascent takes place effortlessly and physical, mental and emotional balance is achieved as a byproduct of this growth of our awareness.

We then realize that we are not this body, mind, ego, conditionings, emotions or intellect, but something of an eternal nature which is always residing in our heart in a pure, undisturbed state as the Self or the Spirit. The Spirit is the source of true knowledge, peace and joy. Self Realization is the actualization of this connection with our Spirit, which as Shri Mataji advocates, is the birthright of every human being.

When the Kundalini power passes through each chakra, or psychic centre, the person will have complete control over the corresponding sense organs controlled by these chakras. Thus through her awakening an individual will become a completely balanced person, physically, mentally, emotionally and spiritually. So this feminine energy which is actually one's true mother makes a person absolutely integrated and fit to achieve his purpose in life.

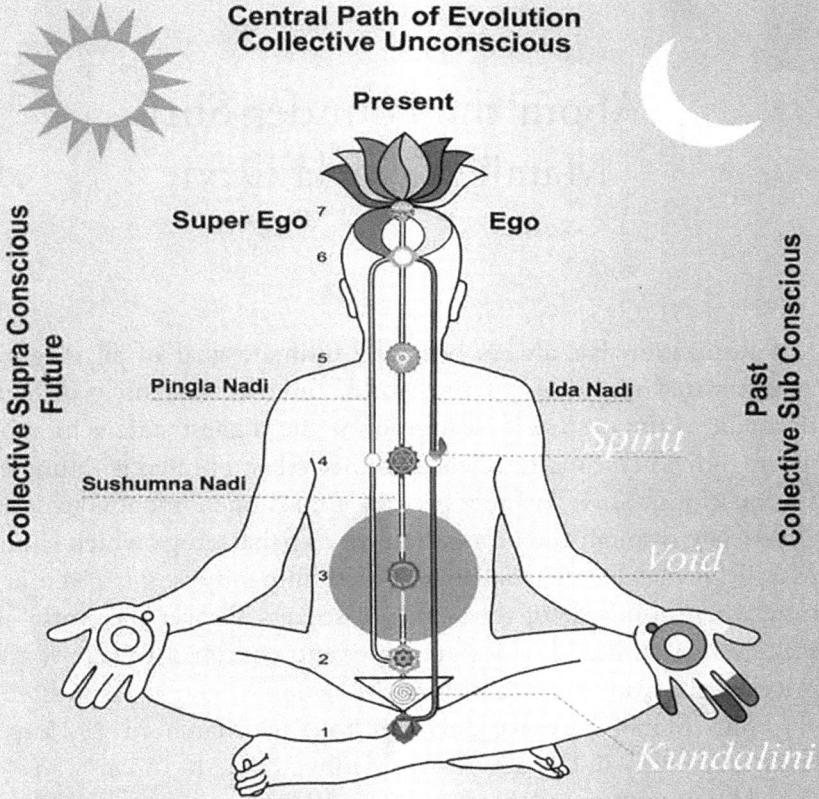

Subtle System

Central Path of Evolution
Collective Unconscious

Present

Super Ego ⁷

Ego

Collective Supra Conscious
Future

Pingla Nadi

Ida Nadi

Spirit

Sushumna Nadi

Past
Collective Sub Conscious

Void

Kundalini

1	2	3	4	5	6	7
Mooladhara	Swadisthan	Nabhi	Anahat	Vishuddhi	Agnya	Sahastrar
innocence	creativity	evolution	security	collectivity	forgiveness	integration

Chapter 2

About the Founder-Shri Mataji Nirmala Devi

Self Realization has always been the ultimate goal of all religions and spiritual traditions of the world, but was extremely difficult to attain in the past. Self Realization is the highest state achievable where individual consciousness is connected and united with universal consciousness. It has now become a mass phenomenon achieved effortlessly through the process known as Sahaja Yoga which is Shri Mataji Nirmal Devi's invaluable gift to humanity- a gift given at a time when hundreds of thousands of seekers all over the world are seeking the truth and hence are ready and equipped to receive this priceless gift from Adi Shakti Herself.

Shri Mataji Nirmala Devi was born on March 21 1923 to a Christian family in Chindwara, in Madhya Pradesh, India.

Her parents were Prasad and Cornelia Salve, direct descendants of the royal Shalivahana dynasty. Seeing the beauty of this child who was born with a spotless brilliance they called her Nirmala, which means "Immaculate". Later on she came to be known by the multitudes by the name of Shri Mataji Nirmala Devi – the revered Mother who was born with her complete Self Realization and knew from a very young age that she had a unique gift which had to be made available to all mankind.

Her parents played a key role in India's Liberation Movement from under the British rule. Her father, a close associate of Mahatma Gandhi, was a member of the Constituent Assembly of India and helped write free India's first constitution. He was a renowned scholar, a master of 14 languages and translated the Koran in Marathi. Her mother was the first woman in India to receive the Honors Degree in Mathematics.

As a child, Shri Mataji lived with her parents in the ashram of Mahatma Gandhi. Gandhi saw the wisdom of this child and used to appreciate her immensely, affectionately calling her Nepali due to the Nepali features of her face. Shri Mataji's involvement in the freedom struggle is extremely remarkable. She was courageous and played a daring role as a youth leader of this campaign. She was even arrested and put into jail along with others during the 1942 Quit India Movement.

Shri Mataji was born with a complete understanding of the human nervous system and its energetic counterparts. In order to become acquainted with the scientific terminology associated with these subjects, she studied medicine and psychology at the Christian Medical College in Lahore.

Shortly before India achieved independence she married Sir. C. P. Srivastava, one of India's most dedicated civil servants, who were knighted by the Queen of England, and who served as Joint Secretary to the Prime Minister's office of the late Shri Lal Bahadur Shastri. Later he was elected for 16 consecutive years as the Secretary General of the United Nations International Maritime Organization.

As Sri C. P. Srivastava moved in fame from the Indian history to the worldly scene, Shri Mataji, after fulfilling her familial duty of bringing up her two daughters, embarked on her spiritual mission

On 5th of May 1970, on a lonely beach of Nargol (about 150 kms From Mumbai) a divine spiritual experience filled her whole being and suddenly she found an answer to her question. She discovered a historical process of en-masse Self Realization through which thousands of people could get this connection to their Spirit and thereby achieve their inner transformation.

Mataji made this experiment of awakening the spiritual power of every human being, which the Hindus call Kundalini, the Muslims as the Ruh and which the Bible describes as the Holy Ghost. She tried it first on the people near to her and noticed they were transformed physically, mentally and spiritually. Slowly she found out that only this process had the potential solution for all human problems and therefore decided to spread it on an en-masse level.

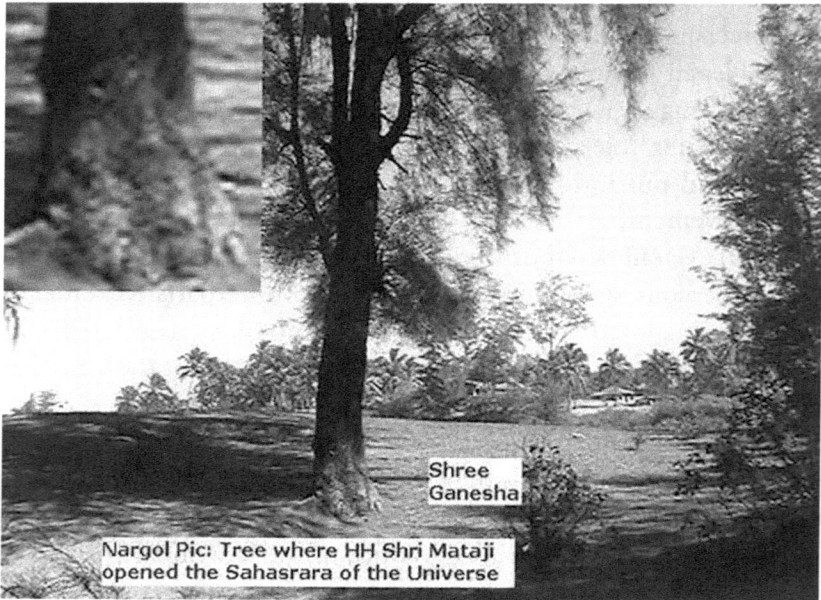

Shree Ganesha

Nargol Pic: Tree where HH Shri Mataji opened the Sahasrara of the Universe

She invested her own time and money to talk to people and give them the key to their own spiritual power. Those few people who felt this spiritual power flowing like a cool breeze over their whole body; especially over the palms of their hands and on top of their heads around the fontanel bone area; were quite astonished. It worked. Under the instructions of Shri Mataji they tried giving this power to others, which really gave them the faith that this was the true spiritual experience that was being prophesized in every religion.

Since 1970, Shri Mataji Nirmala Devi traveled all around the world teaching the techniques of Sahaja Yoga, absolutely free of cost, maintaining and insisting that one cannot pay for your enlightenment. Shri Mataji dedicated her life to triggering the spiritual ascent of mankind through Self Realization, reclaiming the role of women in the spiritual evolution and guiding humanity to correct today's moral dilemmas.

Large number of people, without distinction of race, religion, age or social status has acknowledged the value of her teachings by establishing Sahaja Yoga centers in over 85 countries. These people who live a normal family life, tap into their inner spiritual power through daily Sahaja Yoga meditation and have achieved a complete balance in their lives on the physical, emotional, mental and spiritual level, through their direct and tangible experience on the central nervous system.

Our beloved Mother Shri Mataji Nirmala Devi, who gave us the secret knowledge of Kundalini, taught us how to experience the cool breeze that establishes our connection with the all pervading Cosmic power and encouraged us to experiment with the Nirmal Vidya that has transformed the way we understand things confronting us. As she says, when the drop becomes the ocean, it is the ocean that is going to nourish us, strengthen us and guide us but this can happen only when the connection between the drop and the ocean is fully established by dissolving into the greatness of the ocean, so also it is only the sincere desire of a Sahaja yogi to be collective that can bring about this expansion of his being.

Coming from a drop status, we still continue to be engulfed by the past memories of the limitations of a drop. But the sharpness of attention developed through thoughtless awareness and doubtless awareness will enable us to closely observe our patterned responses and behavior and with patience we can attempt to change the counterproductive patterns and cultivate more pleasant and finer qualities.

Becoming increasingly sensitive to others and understanding them, by not being judgmental, being tolerant and responding based on an insight about our own shortcomings will lighten the load of suppressed emotion that we have been carrying with us over the years. A letting go of the emotional guard that once adorned our faces will allow us to express our finer qualities and true feelings in a more genuine way. With a greater awareness as to what is working against our higher nature, we can work at neutralizing them and focus on enhancing and nurturing the human element in our relationships and life in all its aspects.

This understanding of what Sahaja yoga has brought about in us can be carried forward to its next level so as to make it a part of our everyday life; can happen only if we are sincere in our efforts.

What does it mean to have large heartedness? Shri Mataji says that the heart has seven auras just like the brain which actually control the thinking pattern of the brain. The brain has two institutions- that of conditioning and ego. When a person becomes too egoistic, the auras of the brain get pressed and the heart is unable to influence the thinking process. With diminished usage, the auras of the heart become smaller and smaller, and ultimately disappear to make a person stone hearted. The heart is sensitive while the brain is not. When the heart is boiled in the heat of brain waves, it starts hating people, making us say harsh, hurting and sarcastic words to them. Conditionings of the brain make a person sly and perverted. Conditioning and ego boosts the brain and freezes the heart thereby making us forget how to be reassuring, protecting and nourishing to others.

With self-realization and Kundalini awakening, the Kundalini moves upwards to touch the Brahmarandra which is the seat of the heart. And when that happens, all the hurt that we have endured and suffered over the ages, get dissolved and disappears. After this the heart starts functioning. We should then work on enlarging the heart's auras to engulf as many Sahaja yogis as possible. This will ultimately bring about large heartedness where we can place our Mother, surrender to her and worship her.

Chapter 3

The Subtle Systems of the Human body

The Three Channels

Anatomists describe two nervous systems in the human body – the cerebro- spinal and the sympathetic system. The cerebro-spinal begins with the brain, continues down the spinal cord, and ramifies to all parts of the body through the ganglia from which nerves issue between every two successive vertebrae.

The sympathetic system consists of two cords which run almost the whole length of the spine, situated a little forward of its axis and to the right and left respectively. From the ganglia of these two cords, sympathetic cords proceed to form the network systems called the plexuses from which in turn, as from relay stations, emerge smaller terminal ganglia and nerves. In addition we have a third group called the vagus nerves, which arise in the medulla oblongata and descend independently far into the body, mingling constantly with the nerves and plexuses of the other systems.

Human beings cannot avoid these two influences. Each person carries two channels of energy, which reproduce the two great biological rhythms on the individual level. These are the *Rajo guna* or *Yang,* and the *Tamo guna* or *Yin,* which, together, correspond, in medical terms, to the sympathetic nervous system.

The Left Channel

Tamo guna, which is also known as the Ida Nadi, or simply the "left channel", begins below the sacrum bone and ends in the right hemisphere of the brain. This corresponds to the left sympathetic nervous system, which Shri Mataji calls the "superego".

It constitutes the feminine, lunar side of the personality. The Anima, as defined by Jung, is its reflection at the psychological level. This left channel controls our desire and emotions, and integrates all our previous experiences. It is responsible for remembering all the information acquired by education, information which is stored in the various strata of consciousness. This channel ensures, for instance, that a child who has suffered burning will not go too close to the flame of a candle again. It acts as a sort of "brake" on the personality.

It is this channel which prevents action that does not comply with the canons of morality, or with the conditioning acquired during life, particularly childhood. When an individual bends too much towards this side of the personality, inhibitions to action will outweigh the capacity to act. He or she will become lethargic, introverted, listless and even fearful. The main effect of alcohol and narcotic drugs is to swing the psyche towards this side of our nature. If a correction is not applied, the imbalance intensifies and can culminate in psychiatric disorders such as depression or schizophrenia. Self-destructive tendencies can increase and somatic diseases such as angina pectoris or cancer develop.

On the other hand, if this channel functions in a normal and balanced way, the individual avoids depressive states and is joyful in all circumstances. This is usually true of children who have had the benefit of a normal, innocent and happy childhood.

The Right Channel

Rajo guna or Pingala Nadi controls the masculine side of the personality. It begins at the level of the Swadishtan chakra, situated in the region of the right kidney, and ends in the left cerebral hemisphere, which Shri Mataji calls the "ego". It corresponds to the right-side sympathetic nervous system, and, for simplicity, we will refer to it as the "right channel".

This is the channel of action and creativity on both the actual and the intellectual levels. This is Jung's Animus. The right channel made it possible for humankind to free itself from the constraints of nature and climate. It allowed mankind to organize societies and, by developing technical abilities, they founded the first civilizations. It is this channel that allows Man to project himself into the future, and to invent.

Where the left channel is the brake on human nature, the right channel is its accelerator. The right channel is essential because it allows humankind to take individual responsibility. In a way it is the "steering wheel" of the personality which makes it possible to undertake a course towards a destination. However we can only use this steering wheel if the learning and experience acquired through the left channel continue to give the information we need to avoid dangers, and about the changes of direction the weather conditions demand.

An overactive right channel leads to excessive development of the ego, causing domination and the misuse of power. Aggression, destruction, wars and conquests all stem directly from the right channel activity. An unbalanced left side leads to self-destruction, while imbalances on the right, with their ego consequences, lead to the destruction of others. The right and left channels are the dual poles of the personality which, when in balance, allow the individual to lead a life of harmony.

Sushumna, the Middle Path

The Kundalini rises along the central channel, known in Sanskrit as the *Sushumna Nadi*. *"In Sushumna, the breath leads the pure man into a pure world,"* says the *Prashna Upanishad1*. The *Yogatattwa Upanishad* confirms that: *"The Breath rises in the Sushumna up to the crown of the head."2* Through Self-Realization, the balance between the right and the left channels is restored and inner harmony re-established. This is the first purifying work of the Kundalini.

Sushumna is the Middle Way the Buddha spoke of. It is the way of balance between the right and the left channels, the way of evolution. Human beings are normally slaves to their mental activity. Thoughts arise from two sources: the right hemisphere of the brain, the superego (an extension of the left channel) which recalls past events, or the left hemisphere of the brain, the ego (the prolongation of the right channel) which projects into the future.

During realization, the Kundalini absorbs the ego and the superego. Thoughts fade away. There is no past, no future. All that remains is reality, that is, the present. And in the present the Spirit, shining in the heart, penetrates into the consciousness of the individual. The Spirit alone *IS*. Kundalini and the Self are one.

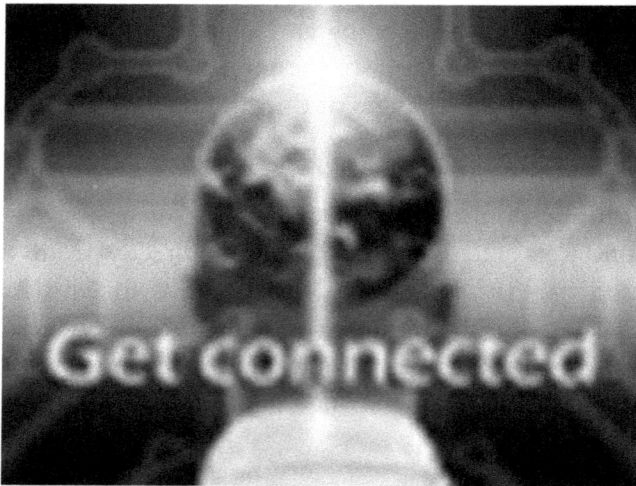

Chapter 4

Sahaja Meditation or DHYAN— Mooladhar to Sahasrar—a journey of exploration

Let us begin with a prayer to the Adi Shakti to guide us through this process - a journey in which her guidance and leading by our little finger, like a mother to her little child can alone lead us from the path of darkness to light - from the path of ignorance to wisdom.

First, place the right hand over the left heart, and say this with affirmation," I am pure Atman. I am of the nature of shuddha Chaitanya. It is formless and is of the nature of absolute knowledge, i.e. Existence knowing by itself, of itself, it is of pure love, it is of peace, it is bliss. It is NItya shuddha Mukta Chaitanya and Gyan swarup. It is the essence of Chaitanya. It is the pure Shiva tatwa.

Then place your hand on the forehead, with palm on the Agnya chakra. Here you say, " Shree Mataji please forgive all of us, we human beings in our ignorance have assumed mind to be the controller of everything and in this process have accumulated a lot of impressions over a period of millions of years, which have formed a huge residue of subconscious. Based on this subconscious we formulate thoughts which lead a huge baggage, a huge accumulation of future projections, imaginations into the future leading to a huge mountain of super conscious. Being irretrievably trapped in this we are continuously making mistakes knowingly and unknowingly. Please forgive us mother. Hame kshama keejiye maa."

en place your hand on the back Agnya and say the mantra, "Twamewa Sakshat Shree Mahaganesh Sakshat Shree Adi Shakti Mataji Shree Nirmala Devyai Namo Namah; Twamewa Sakshat Shree Mahalaxmi Sakshat Shree Adi Shakti Mataji Shree Nirmala Devyai Namo Namah." Shree Mataji, whatever I may have said knowingly or unknowingly which may have hurt anyone or caused harm to anyone please forgive me"

Then place the hand half on the left neck, the fingers placed lightly over the spine on the back of the neck and the neck itself turned slightly on the right. Sincerely pray, the words coming from the heart center as it were," I am the pure Atman; hence I am not guilty of anything. I am pure. If at all I have done or said anything wrong then it is because of the distortions of my mind based on past wrong tendencies or unknown past ignorance. I shall be alert, and vigilant, so that with the power of my attention I will check any wrong thought that will come up in a similar future situation. Mataji, please give me the courage to do so."

Thus the entire charkas from neck upwards get cleared and become very vibrant and pure.

Then place the right hand facing Shree Mataji, and the left hand on the void, all fingers spread out and thumbs facing the center heart. Here say," Twamewa Sakshat Shree Adi Guru Dattatreya Sakshat (5 times) Shree Adi Shakti Mataji Shree Nirmala Devyai Namo Namah." Then put your left hand in front of Shree Mataji and place your right hand on the Nabhi and say," Twamewa Sakshat Shree Adi Guru Dattatreya Sakshat(5 times) Shree Adi Shakti Mataji Shree Nirmala Devyai Name Namah." While saying this remember Shree Mataji's words that all the 10 gurus who were incarnations of Dattatreya had come at different points of time to set right the things that were wrong at that point of time and all of them had worked together in unison to bring about the evolution of the Virat as a whole.

Then put your right hand in front, and left hand on the liver and say," Twamewa Sakshat Shree Rajarajeshwari Sakshat (3 times)

Shree Adi Shakti Mataji Shree Nirmala Devyai Namah. While saying this remember that Shree Rajarajeshwari is responsible for making us work according to each one's Dharma in other words each organ will perform its own dharma. When the chakra gets cleared vibrations cool or hot will come in the palm of the right hand.

Next put your left hand in front and place the right hand on the left side of the abdomen and say," Twamewa Sakshat Shree Gruh Laxmi Sakshat Shree Adi Shakti Mataji Shree Nirmala Devyai Namo Namah." At this time remember the qualities of hospitality of any householder. When the chakra is cleared the cool breeze will flow on the left hand.

We should thereafter raise the Kundalini and take Bandhan. Only at this time the path is clear for the Kundalini to rise and tie up in knots on the Sahasrar.

We pray silently to Mataji to guide us in our Dhyan.

We begin by putting our attention on Mooladhar chakra and say the Ganesh Mantra. We could visualize the four petals representing the four qualities of Ganesh tatwa. Then check the balancing by putting the attention on the central channel and the flow of vibrations on both the palms of both the hands. Then come to the Mooladhar i.e. The triangular bone in which is located Gauri Kundalini. Say the Gauri Kundalini Mantra. You can immediately feel Mother Kundalini rise. Immediately bring the attention to the Nabhi chakra on the spine and say the Laxmi Narayana Mantra. Don't dwell for too long on each chakra. Because when Kundalini is rising on a cleared passage dwelling for long on each chakra may even damage the chakra. You can see that the chakra is activated and one should move along. Only check the balancing of central Nadi and the vibrations on both hands. If necessary saying the first of the three Maha mantra leads to immediate balancing. Please check this out for yourself before accepting. It does happen.

Then Kundalini comes down to the Swadishtan chakra where you say the Brahma Deva Saraswati Mantra. One could also say Hazrat Ali Fatima Mantra for additional effect. Check the balancing. The Kundalini travels in a circular way on both sides equally and meets just below the central heart chakra. There with attention on the front side say the Adi Guru Dattatreya mantra. Check the balancing.

Then go to the Anahat chakra. There say," Twamewa Sakshat Shri Jagadamba Sakshat or Shree Durga Sakshat as many times as you like preferable 12 or 16 times as by that time the lotus there actually starts opening fully. You will become courageous and self confident.

If any catch is there on the left heart you can say the Shiva Parvati mantra and if necessary i.e. if catch or slight discomfort is there on the right side say Sita Rama mantra. Come once again on the center heart and then move up to the Vishuddhi chakra. Here say Radhe Krishna mantra. Repeat it as many times as you feel necessary to actually feel the Kundalini move on its own effortlessly upwards.

Then put your complete attention on three inches above the bone on the spine at the Vishuddhi chakra i.e. On the point of the medulla oblongata which you can feel as a very luminous or energetic point within you skull above the throat which is the back Agnya, we say the mantra, "Maha Ganesh Sakshat, Shree Maha Laxmi Sakshat Shree Adi Shakti Mataji Shree Nirmala Devyai Namo Namah." When you say this with complete attention you will feel as if a bulb is lit up at that point. This is the ego of the Virat. It starts feeling very light inside the head. Then take your attention equally from both sides stretching from the hollow of the ears to the socket of the eyes to ultimately join at the point of the Hamsa chakra in between the two eyes. There say Hamsa chakra devta mantra followed by Mahasaraswati Mantra.

As you say it move your attention from the physical Hamsa chakra to coincide or reach near as far as possible near the illumined medulla oblongata point. Once you do this your muddled head becomes clear and literally wise - the Viveka Buddhi starts getting illumined. Over a period of time this even strengthens the optic nerves to relieve you of the need to wear any spectacles in future.

The next chakra is the Agnya chakra. This is a very subtle chakra as the space here to be crossed is very narrow. Our attention has to become very strong to pin point at the right area. We should try to focus from the Hamsa chakra upwards and you can actually be guided gently by Kundalini herself up the narrow bridge through the Agnya chakra.

Here it is sufficient if you say the beeja mantra ksham as it is as powerful almost as powerful as Yeshu Maria Mata Mantra. When you have crossed the point somewhere inside the head at a point behind where we put the bindhi, we are then faced with the 11 forces of the Ekadashi Rudra. Until you say the Ekadashi Rudra Devata Sakshat mantra you can actually see the 11 forces guarding protectively the boundaries of Sahasrar.

Then we should recall the twins Gautama Buddha and Mahavir, the erstwhile Luv and Kush of Rama era, and guide them as they move and cross at a point above the Agnya chakra inside the skull Buddha from right to left and Mahavir from left to right while saying the Mantra. The moment you finish it you will immediately feel a few dew drops like sensation on the Sahasrar which is said to be the feet of Adi Shakti being gently descending on top of the head at the Sahasrar.

There only you can do is surrender. Surrender absolutely at the feet of the Maha Shakti, the Para Shakti, the Adi Shakti, the universal mother where you have to simply BE. You have to do nothing. Just feel yourself like a cell in the body of the Mother. It is only here that you can actually experience Innocence, the Ganesh tatwa in totality.

Just experience it. Enjoy it. You can just simply stay there. You can also ask anything you want of your Mother. She will only give it to you. It depends on your wisdom to use mother's exclusive attention to ask wisely. Whatever you ask will be granted. Will you ask for material things? You can. She will not deny you. But it will only make you want to ask for more. Ask for thoughtless awareness. You will get it. You will want more of it. You could ask for Atma Saltshaker and you will feel it descending upon you from above flowing through the Vishuddhi and go to the heart giving you a gentle pleasure. Then it goes down to Nabhi giving you a sense of absolute satisfaction and contentment. Then it rises up again and settles down in the heart - in unison with the Shiva tatwa.

Lastly, don't forget to thank your mother for having given what you have asked for. For what is a heart that has no gratitude for the invaluable treasure that has been just showered upon you with no expectations?

Thank her. Bow down your head and humbly prostrate.

Then once again rise up the Kundalini, take Bandhan and slowly wake up and come back into the world - the familiar world that you know. Slowly rub your eyes and the soles of your feet before you get up. Jai Shree Mataji.

Chapter 5

How to Develop Vibratory Awareness in Sahaja Yoga?

Sahaja Yoga is all about the use of vibratory awareness. Through this we begin to feel the effects of our behavior and that of the environment on our subtle instrument. Through vibratory awareness we can diagnose problems at a very early stage and then use various Sahaja techniques to bring the spiritual body back in to balance and clear any obstructions that may develop.

Another great benefit of Sahaja Yoga is that we can help each other in a very real and tangible way. By developing our vibratory awareness we can diagnose the condition of each other's chakras (energy centers) and then take steps to remove any blockages, and restore the system back to health and normality.

WORKING ON EACH OTHER

When we work on each other we can discern this new vibratory awareness much more quickly and we begin to clearly experience the flow of vibrations either in the hands or around the body. This is because the flow of vibrations increases substantially and this has the effect of helping the Kundalini to rise higher and with greater force; it also takes us deeper into meditation. Some people find it difficult at first to experience thoughtlessness for longer than few moments. Working on each other makes us go spontaneously into it.

Another marvel of working on each other is that as we work on and clear each other's chakras, we also clear our own. For example if you start to work on someone and find there is a catch (i.e. an obstruction) on the Nabhi chakra and you give it a bandhan and some vibrations, this will also start to clear and open your own Nabhi centre. It can be a source of great joy to experience these different vibrations flowing through you as you work on different centers.

Furthermore if you find you have got a particular blockage on one of the centers, e.g. Vishuddhi, it is easier to clear by asking someone with a good Vishuddhi to work on you. This is because as they will have stronger Vishuddhi vibrations flowing through them, it will be easier for them to clear this centre for you.

PROCEDURE

1. Go into meditation
2. Put a bandhan on yourself and raise Kundalini
3. Put a bandhan on person receiving vibrations and raise their Kundalini
4. Bring their mechanism into balance.
5. Diagnose which chakra(s) needs working on
6. Put bandhan on ailing chakra(s) and give it vibrations
7. When cool, finish by putting on bandhan and raising Kundalini

A STEP BY STEP GUIDE

For the purposes of clarity we refer to the two parties as one giving vibrations and the other as receiving vibrations.

1. Go into meditation

Before we start working on anyone it is important to go into meditation first ourselves. We can do this by putting our attention on the top of our head and try to find that silence within. Ideally we should be in thoughtless awareness all the time when we are working on others as this will maximize the flow of vibrations and keeps us clear.

2. Put a bandhan on yourself and raise Kundalini

    Stand behind the person you will be working on, put a bandhan and raise your Kundalini. Putting on a bandhan will protect our instrument, bring us into balance, bring our attention inside and help us get into a meditative state.

3. Put a bandhan on the person receiving vibrations and raise his Kundalini

    Putting a bandhan on them will protect their instrument, bring them into balance, bring their attention inside and help them get into a meditative state.

4. Bring their mechanism into balance.

    Put your right hand above their head and see if you feel anything. You may feel some coolness above i.e. over their head or maybe some heat if things are working out. If Kundalini is not coming through, you can raise their Kundalini again to increase the flow.

    Then put both your hands towards the photograph of Shree Mataji and determine what you feel on your own instrument. Next put your attention on the person receiving vibrations and put your right hands towards them. See if you feel anything different. We do this so as to separate our own catches from those of the person whom we are working on. It may be difficult at first but with practice you will find that this new vibratory awareness will start developing rather quickly.

    It is often necessary to bring the instrument of the person receiving vibrations into balance first. When you put your hands towards some people you may experience a difference in the flow of vibrations in each hand. You may find, for example, coolness on the right and warmth or heaviness on the left, if the person tends to use his left side channel (Ida Nadi) too much. To bring this into balance raise the right and bring down the left until you feel an even flow in both hands.

Conversely you may feel warmth or tingling on the right hand and little or nothing in the left. This is often the case with people who predominantly use their right side but prefer not to use their emotional side very much. To bring this into balance raise the left and bring down the right. Such people are often over active - doing this will make them feel much more relaxed and peaceful.

5. Diagnose which chakra(s) needs working on

When you have brought their instrument into balance again put your attention on the person to see what you feel. This time focus on the fingers and see if you can find out which chakra needs to be worked on; it may take several seconds to get a clear indication.

During the early stages when we are developing this skill we may feel very uncertain about exactly what we feel and it is very tempting to just ask another Sahaja Yogi who may have greater sensitivity; this does have some merits. To develop our own sensitivity it is important that we start to operate on what we actually experience ourselves. In the beginning when our sensitivity is developing we may find it difficult to separate our own catches from those of the person receiving vibrations, but with a little practice it does become easier.

Another way of diagnosis is to run your right hand over the chakras of the person receiving vibrations to see if you feel any areas giving off heat. Feeling these changes in temperature is often one of the first experiences of vibratory awareness for many people.

Some people find that at first they do not feel much on their hands but more on the body. This is especially the case if your left Vishuddhi is not very clear as this interferes with the sensitivity of the hands. You may find that you feel other people's catches on your own body when you put your attention on them. Or alternatively some people can feel where the Kundalini is stopping and thereby ascertain where the catches are directly by using the attention. Use whichever works for you best to begin with, after a while you will be able to use all of these methods.

6. Put bandhan on ailing chakra(s) and give it vibrations

When you have worked out which chakra needs to be worked on then put a bandhan on it. This is always a clock-wise motion from the front and anti clockwise from behind as this is the way in which the chakra is actually spinning on the horizontal plane.

Then give it some vibrations. This you do by taking vibrations from the photograph of Shree Mataji or even from the cosmic energy with the left hand and giving them to the chakra with the right hand. After a while the experi-ence of vibrations flowing into the left and out of the right will be quite clear.

In between clearing each chakra, it is helpful to raise Kundalini again a few times to push any blockages that may have been loosened up and can be brought out through Sahasrar chakra.

In addition to this you can use other methods such as candle treatment, mantras and draining the left or right side.

We can put a bandhan on a chakra with the candle or just hold the candle flame near the problem area and it will burn off any obstructions. After a while you can actually feel it sucking the bhada (catch) and clearing the obstruction. It is also very useful for clearing the whole left side, which you can do by moving the candle flame up and down the Ida Nadi (left side).

The left channel can be cleared and drained off of all impurities, heat or excess negativity by placing the right hand on the earth until you feel the clear vibrations on the left palm placed on the lap. Similarly the right channel can be cleared by lifting the left hand up towards the sky to drain the right side. In addition to draining the left and right channels, this action also clears the chakras that are obstructed on either the left or right side.

7. Finish by putting on bandans and raising Kundalini

When the person you are working on has their Kundalini established in Sahasrar and their vibrations are flowing then you can bring the session to a close by raising their Kundalini three times and putting a bandhan on them.

When you have done this raise your own Kundalini and put a bandhan on yourself. It is usually a good idea to sit and meditate quietly for a few minutes after working on someone to settle yourself down and ensure that you stay in the centre.

WHAT TO DO IF YOU ARE NOT SENSING THE VIBRATIONS?

Some of us take a little longer than others before we start feeling things very clearly on our hands. To develop our sensitivity it is very helpful to foot soak daily. However until we do clearly feel the vibrations we can adopt another more systematic approach.

Follow steps 1, 2, and 3 above and then systematically put bandhan on and give vibrations to all the chakras starting with Mooladhar. This in itself will start to clear both the person receiving vibrations and yourself and will also make you more sensitive. Both of you will also start feeling the qualities of the chakras as you work on them in turn, and they start to open.

For example you will both experience:

Mooladhar	Greater support for the Kundalini and a sense of innocence will be restored
Kundalini	More strands of the Kundalini will rise
Swadishtan	Strange thoughts will stop and our creativity will increase
nabhi	Greater peace and satisfaction

Void	Greater sense of stability
heart	Deeper experience of security, love and joy
Vishuddhi	Weight lifted from the shoulders, less guilt, more sweetness
Agnya	Less thinking and more forgiveness
Sahasrar	Silence, integration and bliss

After trying the above a few times and also being attentive to what you feel on your fingers, you will soon start feeling the vibrations on your hands.

ISSUES TO BEAR IN MIND

When we work on people we also have to exercise sensitivity of another kind. For example when we work on someone; they are in meditation; so we should try not to disturb them unnecessarily by trying to have a conversation with them, telling what to do, or asking sensitive questions. We can always have a friendly chat afterwards. Similarly when we find catches on the person receiving vibrations it is better to just try and clear them; as during this process we act as channels for the Divine energy to flow.

There is often a temptation to start healing those we know who may be very ill. We should Endeavour to make our own instrument strong, as during the early stages of our Self Realization, our own instrument is often a little vulnerable and we have yet to learn how to keep ourselves clear. If there is someone you want to help it would be better to bring them to a meeting where they can get their Self Realization and then let them work it out using Sahaja Yoga methods.

Self Realization works out best in a collective situation where we all help each other. Sahaja Yoga is more than just a body of knowledge. Through vibratory awareness we start to experience life in a new way and by regularly getting involved in a workshop each week we can hasten the development of this new awareness and deepen our connection with the Spirit.

Besides Sahaja Yoga it is such a relaxing, pleasant and enjoyable experience for both the person giving vibrations and the person receiving it, so let us experiment and enjoy.

Chapter 6

Divine Discrimination

Our worth is determined not according to the power we possess but according to how we use that power. Within all of us lie several self-serving aspects of nature that was a part of the evolutionary process that each of us have undergone and some of these qualities may be either active or may be lying dormant waiting for the right conditions for self-expression. If these tendencies are of the lower aspects of nature it will only create conflicts and spread it to others, just like the ripples created by pebbles thrown into a pond have the effect of reaching the other side of the shore.

On the other hand, love which manifests in the form of care, concern, helping those in need, not out of any sense of duty, hope or reward but of a heartfelt desire to do so, has the power of connecting and allowing life to flow in joy.

Changing a pattern of behavior will call our intense working of the witness attitude. Witness attitude or sakshi Bhava which can be developed through regular practice of Sahaja meditation, will enable us to observe our own responses to situations which are triggered off on account of age old patterns of neuro-muscular responses that have created particular pathways over long years of time some of which may even span several lifetimes. These pathways will continue to prompt the same pattern of behavior. Watching our response as and when the situations arise, and repeatedly correcting our reactions to negative stimulus will weaken the pathways and ultimately a time will come when due to the reconfiguration of the response patterns we will be once and for all be free from the crippling patterns of negative behavior.

One might ask how can one modify the habitual dislike of a person who arouses nothing but irritation and start liking him. Mother says, put a sankocha like that of Shri Rama. While talking to each other educate yourself, train yourself to say things that are sweet and nice which will make the other person feel that this person is properly brought up in the Sahaja yoga tradition.

Instead of criticizing or passing judgments about the other person look for something admirable in him or her. This will modify the switching arrangement in your neural pathway. This, if done in a witness state and done repeatedly, will bring awareness in your observation which will change the pattern of behavior.

Divine discrimination is the blessing of a clean and pure Agnya chakra developed out of a sense of forgiveness of behaviors both of others and ourselves arising out of human weaknesses and conditionings. Conditionings that are accumulated through our experiences not only of this life time but over several life times, which are all are recorded in our subtle system, and communicated to the Kundalini energy, color our responses when manifested at the Agnya chakra. That is why we respond in different ways to the same situation or differently at various times.

The root chakra, the energy center at the base of the spine or the Mooladhar sends messages based on these recordings to the subconscious that gets reflected in our responses. The Mooladhar chakra which is placed in the pelvic plexus is connected to the left and the right sympathetic nervous system. Keeping this chakra pure and chaste through right behavior and conduct, we can develop the right Viveka or discrimination.

While meditating the Kundalini rises through the Sushumna Nadi in a Realized person provided both the right and the left sympathetic nervous system or the Ida Nadi and the Pingala Nadi are in balance. This can be checked by feeling if the flow of breath through both the nostrils is even or not, which is normal during sunrise and sunset. At other times, when the left nostril is blocked and you are breathing through the right nostril, while meditating, the Shakti rises through the right channel, the Sun channel, and the seeker might experience heat or burning around the neck.

Again, as Shree Mataji says, if any effort is put in by obstinate abstinence or by indulgence, the excitement of the sympathetic activity starts, putting a pressure on the subject's attention causing it to move on the Ida or the Pingala Nadi. This causes terrible heat in the body and one may suffer from restlessness. Instead of rising to the thoughtless awareness in meditation, the seeker may enter into the past or the sub-conscious or may become clairvoyant. People may experience such heat if you try to focus your eyes on the Agnya chakra. It would be better to focus on the Sahasrar chakra or on the space between the two nostrils where they separate in the respiratory system, as it helps to bring back the body in balance.

Hence it is important that while meditating one should be in a balanced state. If we are trying to strain the left or right sympathetic systems, it will ultimately break the connection with the central path of the parasympathetic. Licentious behavior and its justification through perverted intelligential arguments cannot help us in our evolution but will only expedite destruction of the human personality.

Shree Mataji explains that the argument is always put forward that if you inhibit your desires a phenomenon of conditioning takes place. But one must realize that if you indulge in your desires too much, your ego gets conditioned too. The unfortunate part is that the awareness of ego conditioning is not evident. In such cases the ego becomes so colossal that the harm caused by the ego conditioning is not evident, and it is even greater than the super-ego conditioning commonly known as sub-conscious suppression. The middle-path is the fulcrum which rests on wisdom.

Knowledge of abnormal people cannot guide the destiny of normal human beings. Licentiousness makes man depraved and weak personalities and he finds himself ill-equipped to fulfill the program of evolution that is built-in in him. In conclusion, Shree Mataji says that for a seeker of Sahaja yoga it is necessary to become like a child to enter the kingdom of heaven i.e. the Sahasrar. He must lead a life of temperance, piety and virtue, with respect of familiar and filial relations. Judgment, relying on the artificial behavior of modern times does not depict the deep significance of divine love.

Speaking on the sanctity of marriage and the wonderful benediction that it showers, Shree Mataji says, that at this juncture of Kaliyuga, what is necessary is to provide the spiritual parenthood for the many great souls who are waiting to be re-born to ascend into higher stages of evolution. Hence to move from the four stages of awareness into the fifth dimension we should develop divine discrimination to lead of life of balanced activity, neither of indulgence nor of total abstinence leading to a personality devoid of love and compassion.

The Mooladhar chakra emits electromagnetic vibrations which with the tetravalent valency balances the positive or the negative valences of the other elements thereby firmly keeping the personality grounded. If this chakra gets disturbed, a person's discrimination gets affected and is easily influenced by passing fancies and perverted tendencies.

Hence the secret to develop divine discrimination is to maintain the sanctity, innocence and chastity of the Mooladhar chakra that guides the Sahaja yogi as a magnet to its goal.

Chapter 7

Likes and dislikes

The beauty and excellence that we see in people, children, creatures, plants, nature, music and even inanimate objects like carpets, are reflections of aspects of our own nature that we acknowledge as beautiful. Flowers, gardens, music, art architecture and other works of beauty, art or excellence that we create, or simply appreciate are all reflections of the beauty or excellence in our own nature.

When we like or dislike what others do or what they stand for, this touches on aspects of our own nature which we are either happy to acknowledge or prefer to ignore. The greater our identification with them, the more intense is our response. When we quarrel with someone, we only try to put across our point of view without listening to someone else's. We become biased and prejudiced in our opinions. This leads to friction and may even get to a point where people don't talk to each other and want to have anything to do with each other.

When we are in a group talking to each other or discussing any common subject, we should respect the other individual's viewpoint and give him a chance to express it without interruption, and then perhaps he will give you the same opportunity. Nothing brings a person of a sound mind to the point of violence more quickly than the feeling that you are not listening to him. Listening indicates respect. Listening makes the other person feel important. Let the person to whom we are talking know that we can appreciate the way he feels.

We can settle earlier misunderstandings or ill feeling by saying, "You must have felt very upset and irritated when the last time you asked me to help you, and I did not. It might have made you feel that I couldn't care less." Or "If the situation was reversed, I would feel the same like you."

We find that we often communicate better with a person who will listen to us without judging. We all need to have at least one person with whom we can open our hearts without having to fear about anything. We all need to be that person who will accept others as they are. Many times there is no need for a listener to express any opinion. Just to be able to be there so that others can share their feelings with a sympathetic human being is enough.

I read a beautiful chapter in Gods and God men of India, a book written by Khushwant Singh, wherein he narrates an interview with God. I reproduce it here.

I dreamed I had an interview with God. "Come in," God said, "So you would like to interview me?"

"If you have the time," I said. God smiled and said, "My time is eternity and is enough to do everything; what questions do you have in mind to ask me?"

"What surprises you most about mankind?" I asked.

God answered: "That they get bored with being children; are in rush to grow up, and then long to be children again. That they lose their health to make money and then lose their money to restore their health; That by thinking anxiously about their future, they forget the present, such that they live neither for the present nor for the future. That they live as if they will never die and die as if they have never lived..."

God's hands shook and we were silent for a while. Then I asked..."As a parent, what are some of life's lessons you want your children to learn?"

God replied with a smile, "To learn that they cannot make anyone love them: what they can do is to let themselves be loved. To learn that what is most valuable is not what they have in their lives, but who they have in their lives to learn that it is not good to compare themselves to others.

"All will be judged individually on their own merits, not as a group on a comparison basis! To learn that a rich person is not the one who has the most, but is one who needs the least. To learn that it only takes a few seconds to open profound wounds in persons we love and that it takes many years to heal them.

"To learn that there are persons who love them dearly, but simply do not know how to express or show their feelings. To learn that money can buy everything but happiness. To learn that two people can look at the same thing and see it totally differently; to learn that a true friend is someone who knows everything about them…. and likes them anyway. To learn that it is not always enough that they are forgiven by others, but that they have to forgive themselves.

I sat there for a while enjoying the moment. I thanked Him for His time and for all that He has done for me and my family. He replied: "I'm here twenty-four hours a day. All you have to do is to ask for me and I'll answer."

In Her talk at Rahuri in 1987, Shree Mataji's parting words were," You have to be giving like the sun….You carry the sun with you. And you should spread love and warmth and let them feel that the Sun has been brought from India by you….. You are yogis, you are not ordinary people, and you are Yogis. You represent that category of people who are known for their righteousness, for their compassion, and love. So I wish you all best of love, enjoy your journey, enjoy everything and pass this joy that you have achieved here to other people, to other Sahaja Yogis and to other people who are not even Sahaja Yogis.

Chapter 8

Giving and Generosity

Giving has the greatest joy and pleasure. As Sahaja yogis all joy giving qualities are within us which we should discover. The more we give to others the more Life will give to us. This involves forgetting our own welfare and being more thoughtful about the needs of others.

After being enlightened in Sahaja yoga we could give our time and devote our energies for the emancipation of human beings by helping them come up in life. Instead of finding faults with them or condemning them we could help them in a positive way by helping them to stabilize themselves in their meditation. We can be channels for the flow of unlimited love which has the power to bind all those who give it to each other. Love is a force that can transform people in a way as to accommodate more people, have a tolerant attitude of the limitations of the other and help them to find their strengths.

The generous appreciation of the loveliness of the good qualities in others, the real caring about the happiness and welfare of others the giving of ourselves and our belongings to those who need it all can be cultivated and made to grow in us. Instead of repressing the feelings and passions within us, if we give it an expression by having a sincere desire for the better, for the lovelier things in life, not only for ourselves, but for all life around us then it is easier to grow in spirituality.

As it is said, blessed are those who ask nothing of the universe, but only give. The great sage Patanjali said that when all desire to possess ceases, then all things flow to a man's feet. Shri Mataji has said several times, that generosity is the only way you can express your love to others. All your material wealth and everything have no meaning unless you show generosity for other people, but one should do it silently. All the great saints, the Sadhguru who were born in India were monuments of generosity. Generosity also means to give our time, attention and care to another person. When we fully accept another person by offering forgiveness and tolerance with a generous heart has a tremendous power of healing wounds, feeling of loneliness, fear and insecurity.

Serving another person food before ourselves, helping someone cross the road, assisting a person how to reach a certain place when he feels lost, being willing to listen to a person in distress, allowing others to sit, or pass by are all acts of generosity which involves our attention, loving kindness and sensitivity to a great extent. It is not heroic actions that define generosity but the simple willingness to give and care.

Just being present for someone is one of the greatest acts of generosity and benevolence that one can do for someone. As Shree Mataji said at the Sahasrar Puja at Austria in 1985, When you surrender, you enjoy not only your absoluteness, but you also enjoy seeing that Absoluteness in others. Then in that state of Niranand your compassion becomes like an ocean to encompass all, and you are willing to give and share with one and all that comes in the sphere of influence.

Chapter 9

Forgiveness

It has been written in all scriptures that one should forgive. Forgiveness is the Divine power under whose vibrations the explosive agitations of anger, guilt and hatred are neutralized. Forgiveness is the strength of the mighty. In today's world where goodness is more often than not, met with opposition, forgiving is the means with which we can release emotionally those who we feel have committed a wrong against us.

When we are treated badly, if instead of condemning the offender, we forgive them freely, then we wipe the slate of our consciousness clean. When we forgive someone, we find that some pockets of tension that may have been built somewhere within the body gets released and we find ourselves at peace with ourselves. In the same way, one should also forgive oneself for offences we may have committed so that we can get rid oneself emotionally of the anger that may have built within ourselves.

Why is it sometimes so difficult to forgive and forget; that is, to let go off completely? This is because the human ego demands punishment or vindication for the injustice or wrong done. Feeling "right" by maintaining resentment against others may be more important than forgiving them and enjoying harmony, inner peace and improved health.

Insisting on your lawful rights may be more important than the possible benefits of conceding and letting go. This may even mean that there is some satisfaction in maintaining the circumstances as strained as they are. But forgiving is a Divine virtue, hence forgiving someone, will actually make us free of all baggage. Forgiveness involves forgetting, letting go and moving on.

Forgiveness breaks the chain of cause and effect. When someone treats us badly or says something insulting, our response to that action based on anger and resentment builds a wall and affects our relationships. Very often it is not that someone can harm us without our consent, but it is the kind of response based on our pre-conclusions that makes all the difference. It is the consequence of whatever choice we make. This causes more damage than solve problems.

As it is said, to err is human but to forgive is divine, every human being makes mistakes so it is better to forgive a person, even before expecting the other person to ask for forgiveness, and focus instead on our own mistakes and make efforts in removing them.

Whenever we are ill we need to introspect and see whom we have not forgiven. Forgiving means give up and letting go of things. It has nothing to do with going and telling the person who we feel that we have wronged or who has treated us badly that we have forgiven him or her. It has nothing to do with condoning a certain behavior or action that they have done to us in the past. We do not even have to know how to forgive. All we need to know is to be willing to forgive.

We all know how painful it is when we have to undergo the pain and have nobody to understand us. Then we must realize that they who need to be forgiven most, what pain they may be undergoing. We need to understand that what they did at that point of time when they did it, was what best they in their wisdom knew had to be done, the best that they could do with their understanding, awareness and knowledge that they had at that time.

We need to choose to release the past, the burden and baggage of the past by forgiving everyone including ourselves. We need to affirm and say, "I forgive anyone whom I may have hurt by not behaving the way I should have behaved, or the way you wanted me to behave, or the way you wanted me to do it. I forgive you and I set you free." By saying this we become free. And this freedom begins the healing process and we are set on our path for greater enfoldment and expression of our true natural self.

Forgiving opens up our Agnya chakra and allows the Kundalini to pass upwards to the Sahasrar and unite with the cosmic energy. Therefore it is essential that we forgive for expediting our own ascent.

Chapter 10

Trust

When others trust us, they hand us the power that they would not have otherwise given to someone. When someone trusts us, it is our responsibility to see that we do not betray that trust. It is a trust that we shall not harm one another or deceive one another.

When we pass unjust judgments on others, it is because we want to show that we are superior to them in some way. The more inferior we make them appear in our eyes or in the eyes of others the more superior we feel, more so if that person is a socially or politically important or powerful person.

We often tend to look for the bad points in other people, regarding their behavior or something what they said, so that we can brand them as useless, or cheap or worthless without considering the circumstances or the situation that have influenced them. It could be that their loneliness, their personal loss or family circumstances that have led to it. Coming to conclusions in this way and labeling them as that kind of man or that kind of woman will only distance ourselves from them and cause disharmony.

We betray the trust of many good people who may be dissimilar to us in many ways but yet their natures may be no less noble than our own.

Don't close your heart even when your feelings have been hurt. For contraction causes its own pain. How others behave towards us is not under our control but how we treat ourselves and we behave towards ourselves when our feelings are hurt is entirely in our hands. We are hurt only when we expect something from another.

Quite often we fall a victim to the same expectations even after experiences of earlier failures. This is what hope does to us. Misplaced hope will always cause havoc with the heart until realization. Silent observation and acceptance of our repeated careless responses and misplaced expectations will one day shake our benumbed brain out of its complacency and make us sit up and have a hard look at how we have been reacting. And suddenly all things will click in place.

Divinity works through us in strange ways but our acceptance will make the path a lot easier and lighter.

Our Growth is our own responsibility

We must realize that every being is here to develop his own evolution according to the dictates of his soul and his Soul alone, and that none of us must do anything except encourage others in that development.

As we grow in Sahaja yoga, it is our growth, our stability, the balance of disposition and the peace and joy that we radiate that will hasten the development of those around us and also attract more people to Sahaja Yoga. Very often, if we try to convert or bring other family members, it can cause much misunderstanding.

If someone in the family is following some other path, if we try to put a pressure on that individual into accepting our beliefs, it may not actually work out for that person. Each person must unfold, as each flower, in his or her own time. You cannot force a bud or a seed to become a flower or blossom overnight.

Spirituality is very individual. While we need not and cannot hide and meditate, we should follow our spiritual discipline without making the other family members feel guilty or uncomfortable that they are not doing the same. Otherwise it will only cause resentment.

Shri Mataji has time and again mentioned about the freedom to pursue and bloom in our own freedom and freedom to be wise in our choice. Very often the children who are forced to follow will react by doing exactly the opposite. The best way to attract people and change people is by example, by our own exemplary behavior, by our progress and steady growth, by not thinking that we are superior or trying to show off our spiritual endeavors, but by expressing the kindness, thoughtfulness, love and understanding in very gentle ways, ways that touches people and inspires them to want to know more about the practices that enable you to behave and perform in such an exemplary way.

Chapter 11

Guilt

A sense of guilt at some point of time or the other has caught every one of us. Guilt always looks for punishment and punishment brings pain. When we find a sense of guilt engulfing us, what we should try to do is find out whether it is a factual guilt or you are just feeling guilty without any valid justification for it. This can be done only through a detached, honest and objective analysis and reasoning.

We should check whether we have actually breached any of society's codes or failed to observe any duty or simply because others say that you are guilty. If it is the latter, then they may be expressing opinions that they have themselves adopted from others or it could be factual. If it is factual, then the way to get rid of this guilt is by eliminating the self-destructive messages that we have been feeding ourselves.

If we have set up some or the other mechanisms for ourselves that are designed to deprive ourselves they should be eliminated so that we are free to enjoy our true worth, then lead a more fulfilled, respectful and happier life.

This in turn will open the way for the development of the highest aspects of our nature and the fullest expression of our inner beauty and love.

A person who is habituated to feeling guilty will often be found saying, " I knew such a bad thing was going to happen, and you won't be there to help", or "I just thought as much, just when the deadline was approaching, you would go on leave.". Such a person is often the self-pitying kind and would almost invariably draw us into a conversation of how hopeless things are.

Almost always we are pulled off balance, and our energy is drawn into their guilt feeling by creating a doubt on our part. And as soon our energy is drawn into their field of experience, they immediately get a boost of energy and feel more secure.

Guilt and self-pity is also a kind of conditioning which a person has developed over a period of time to meet his need for sympathy or nurturing that he has lacked since childhood or for a long time. When we lend our sympathies to such a person who has been helplessly trapped unknowingly in the vicious circle of self-validating guilt, we are indirectly energizing the very sentiments and further pushing him into the intimidating traps.

Of course, there will be cases where we should feel concern or sympathy for someone in a difficult situation, but we are not really helping a person by lending our energies that are only boosting a person's guilt trip. When we really and truly practice Sahaja yoga meditation, we develop that state of clarity when in an instant we can recognize self-pity or a genuine difficult situation.

When in the light of our full awareness we respond in a way so as to present to the person who is on a guilt trip, his unconsciousness will be beaten up to awakening. This can be done with very gentle and polite words such as, "The way you are putting, and it feels to me as if I am supposed to feel guilty for it." Or one could say, "I don't feel that I have done anything wrong at all."

Of course, in such situations we must really have all the courage to say so, because while we are honestly trying to sort out the situation, the other person's reaction would invariably be, "I knew I couldn't count on you for help" On most occasions, the person with the guilt would invariably feel insulted and angry.

In such cases, an enlightened Sahaja yogi is like a mentor to another and is trying to help other to become aware of the state of unconsciousness in which he is in. For this, he has to keep providing the energy and keep the conversation or dialogue going even though he may be at the receiving end of all abuses or insults, as a result of the anger and outburst of the victim of guilt. But eventually, the very act of listening to the outburst will make that person aware of the guilt trip on which he has been riding.

His behavior comes within the light of his own awareness and that light itself is enough to wash away the pain of guilt that he has been harboring all along.

And when he basks in the light of that wisdom, the lightness of feeling that engulfs him as a result of the lifting of a lifetime of guilt will make him truly feel a huge sense of gratitude of having been there for him.

This is the role a Sahaja yogi has to play dispassionately, in helping one another grow into full bloom, into a fresh new perspective that is refreshingly more nourishing.

Chapter 12

Criticism

How often we have observed people talk ill about others. Talking about the bad qualities of others, gossip and spreading discomforts of our own brothers and sisters begets those very qualities to multiply in us.

Jesus said to one of his disciples, "If one of your brethren was asleep and the wind had blown off his garment, what would you do?"

He answered, "We would cover him."

He said, "No, you would rather expose him further."

They cried, "God forbid that we should act in such a way!"

Jesus said, "But it is the same when you hear a word against your brother and carry it to others!"

Shri Mataji says, don't accept anything bad. Once you start believing a person as bad, a fortress is built and you don't believe anything else. This can be broken open only through Sahaja yoga, when the Brahmarandra, which is the seat of the heart, is opened by the rising Kundalini. By raising the Kundalini again and again and making the Brahmarandra wider and wider, the heart will take charge of the brain.

The world is like a mirror. Most of the problems we have with people are reflections of the problems we have with ourselves. We don't have to go out and change everyone else. When we gently change some of our own ideas, our relationships improve automatically.

Criticism is destructive. It is the fastest way to create resentment and destroy a relationship. The immediate reaction to criticism is to justify, to blame. It is very easy to say others are wrong but we must realize that we can only correct where we are wrong so what should be easier and more logical is to correct ourselves than to correct others.

If we find faults with one another, if we criticize one another, we are only reducing the energy in the channels which is the power of Sahaja Yoga.

Sahaja yoga is a collective phenomenon; it can work best when all the channels work together in harmony. When collectivity is disturbed through criticism, problems develop in the Vishuddhi whose effect is seen at the Sahasrar where there is an integration of all energies, all powers. All the centers are in the brain, in the Sahasrar.

When the brain becomes affected and this goes beyond a certain level, the Heart chakra gets affected. This combination of Vishuddhi, Sahasrar and Heart chakra can be a very deadly combination and if either left or right Agnya joins in, Shri Mataji warns, you develop the Ekadashi Rudra.

Thus criticism in any manner either others of ourselves, locks us in the very same pattern or conditioning that we are trying to come out of. Criticizing has become a habit with most of us and it has never worked. Let us come out of it and see what happens. Understanding and being gentle with ourselves will help us to come out of it. We have to accept ourselves as we are.

Self-acceptance and self approval will help us change the pattern and make us more loving towards ourselves and thereby to each other as our Mother has always wanted us to be. Only when compassion starts flowing from us that our channels will become empty to receive more compassion and love from our Mother.

Ekadashi Rudra–place near Rahuri in Maharashtra-visited by Shri Mataji

Chapter 13

Creating Positive Patterns of Thought and Behavior

When the brain becomes enlightened through regular practice of Sahaja yoga meditation and becoming established in thoughtless awareness and doubtless awareness we can very easily recognize in a witness state our patterns of behavior and consciously make an effort to change into desirable patterns of behavior. In order to be able to do this one must first recognize and acknowledge fearlessly, the lower and the higher, the good and the bad qualities in us. And then slowly, every time the lower aspect of us comes to the front and expresses or tries to express it, the same should be replaced by the higher aspect. It is difficult, no doubt, but it can be done, by persistent efforts, day in and day out. It requires tremendous patience and solid desire to transform into a beautiful human being.

Now, what is it that prevents us from expressing the higher and more sublime qualities is the limiting pattern that we ourselves have cultivated to survive in difficult times, or to attract love or respect that we desired desperately to have.

Let us look at the following behavior patterns:

1. I have to appear to be rich, strong and intelligent; otherwise I will not have the respect and adoration from people.

2. If I am not respected or admired, I feel unimportant and worthless.

3. I want to appear superior and saintly so as to gain the approval and acceptance of the society.

4. I prefer to be aggressive, critical, rebellious and stubborn as otherwise I feel vulnerable, powerless and controlled.

5. I want to be possessive as otherwise I feel rejected and neglected.

6. I prefer to be unemotional and unavailable as then it gives me a sense of importance and pride of appearing to be busy and in control.

7. I have to appear miserable, angry, helpless, lonely or unwell, if I have to attract sympathy and love.

8. I like to appear independent and desirable as it gives me security, admiration and a sense of being powerful.

9. If I appear to be wise and right, I can attract trust, security and submission of people. Being obeyed, accepted and looked up to is more important to me than being compassionate, caring, loving and responsible.

10. A paternal or a maternal or a dominating demeanor makes me feel included and loved and this is more important to me than being natural, dignified, sincere and honest.

11. I try to conform to what is normal in the society as I do not want to be unloved, excluded, unwanted or rejected if I try to be different.

When we observe these patterns what we need to do is prevent ourselves from expressing it the next time. Our brain is a highly sensitive and sophisticated instrument. It is easy to lower the standards of integrity by mentally justifying that if we do not behave that way people will take advantage of us. It is easy to succumb to patterns of paralyzing behavior. We need to constantly remind ourselves that we have to cultivate the higher aspects as this will give us greater fulfillment in life. The change has to happen slowly. Hasten slowly as it is said. Perseverance is the key word. If at any point of time we find ourselves saying or doing something we had decided to throw out of our system, do not be angry or annoyed with yourself. Forgive your-self. Make a greater resolve not to repeat the next time that happens.

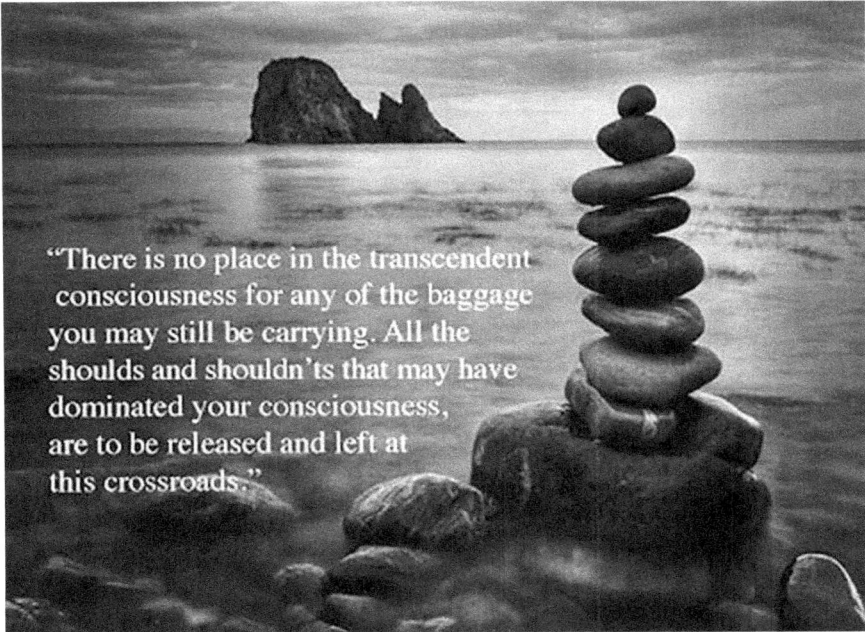

"There is no place in the transcendent consciousness for any of the baggage you may still be carrying. All the shoulds and shouldn'ts that may have dominated your consciousness, are to be released and left at this crossroads."

In due course of time, the realigned pattern of behavior will start showing results. The limiting or crippling behavior patterns will fade and disappear and there will come a time when we ourselves will wonder, whether we were like that. The gradual change will bring out the finest qualities and the innermost beauty will shine in exuberance.

Love manifests in our courtesies towards all, particularly those who we do not know. When we do something for others, it may be because subconsciously it may be the same thing what we wish to be done to us in similar situations.

It can be seen in our identification with others even those with whom we are in conflict, seeing in their behavior, their hopes, fears and needs and recognizing them to be no different from our own. It rejoices in wishing the welfare of others just as it would have been if it was for our own fulfillment.

In the course of a conversation, listen to the other person respectfully. Irritated people are usually surprised when you ask, "Is there anything else you want to tell me?" They are so used to listening the other person asking them to shut up, that when you ask them so beautifully, all their aggression will evaporate and will start behaving very sweetly.

Often the problem is not that we don't care, but we do not know how to show or express that we do care. One way would be to give our total attention when someone is talking to us. It is listening with a sense of deep receptivity. When we are deeply receptive, then in that mindful stillness, in the absence of formulation of response, in the absence of an impatience to interject when the other person is speaking, there is more than a mere exchange of words. In those moments are possibilities of connection at a deeper level, moments that can be charged with awareness, moments that can give us a chance to select the words that we speak, words that are nice, sweet words, not words that would wound.

The awareness holds the potential to be a source of connectedness that can build bonds of love with all people who come in contact with us. Our communication is non-judgmental, non-reactive but holds a cultivated restraint.

Chapter 14

Intuition and Vibratory Awareness

The discretion of the Ida Nadi is intuition. If we develop that discretion within through our meditative powers, we develop intuition. Intuition is nothing but taking the help of the Ganas, who are surrounding all Sahaja yogis. If we learn to take help from the Ganas without much difficulty we tend to say the right thing. The whole of Sahaja Yoga, Shri Mataji says, say fifty percent at least out of that, is based on intuition.

What is intuition? How does it work?

Intuition is a perception beyond the physical senses that assists us in all fronts. It is the new awareness that arises once the Kundalini is awakened, and the whole central nervous system is enlightened, which allows us to feel what is happening to the chakras of ourselves and those of others. If we can accept that every atom possesses a form of consciousness, then when atoms of like consciousness come together and coalesce, there comes into existence a body of energy which expresses a definite vibratory pattern. These energy patterns are present in the form of the seven major chakras in the human being.

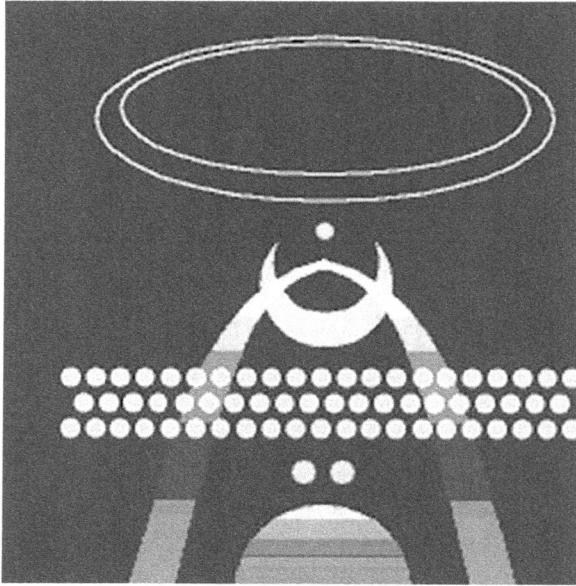

Each major chakra is associated with a different frequency and quality of energy. But consciousness as an energy field is something that is extra sensory and is able to operate beyond the limitations of space and time. Collective consciousness is the ability that emerges when we are able to raise our awareness above the level of individual egos and merge our energy fields and be able to work interactively with others.

For example when Gene Rodenberry imagined a future where Star Trek's Spock was able to meld his mind with others, we find that more of us are able to intuitively read others' thoughts and emotions and also able to think and create together without having to consciously communicate through our five senses.

We have to reach that absolute point where we can jump into collective consciousness. It is beyond thinking and can be felt on the fingers. They are the signal that comes from the Absolute and that has to be decoded through Nirmal Vidya that Shri Mataji has so lovingly been teaching us all these years.

The Kundalini records and decodes all that information and tells us from time to time what is right and what is wrong. It is in the fullest of awareness that we come to know, not only about others but about the whole.

When the Kundalini rises, our attention or awareness is filled with enlightenment. In that state of consciousness, our subtle system has the ability to understand itself, control it and be connected to the all pervading vibratory fields. Hence even when we are not thinking, by merely being thoughtlessly aware, our operating system can feel on the finger tips and hands the cool breeze about the energy centers of others and will be able to control the relationship with others.

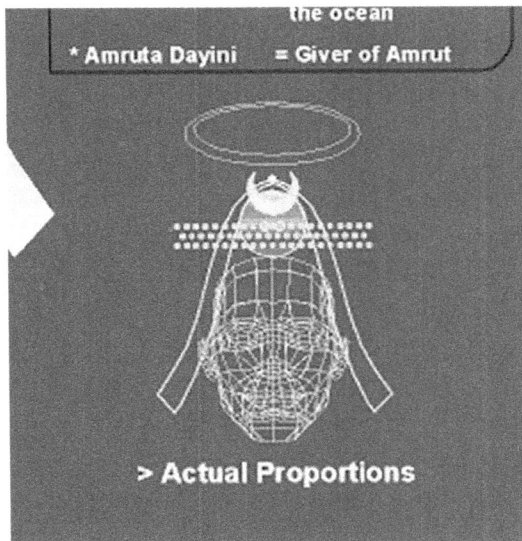

This consciousness which is present in each and every person, in the form of vibrations, on being awakened can be used intelligently to improve our present situation and in general help the whole mankind to go to a higher level.

WHAT WE CAN DO WITH VIBRATIONS?

(Source - www.valaya.co.uk)

Vibrations are a very useful extra sense. It is the element of the Sahasrar Chakra, the centre of integration whose nature is Absolute

Truth. By feeling Vibrations we can know the truth in many ways. We can know the state of our own being, whether we are getting sucked into any illusions or troubled by thoughts, worries or even desires.

We can check the Vibrations of anyone alive or dead, anywhere in the world, and we can work on them by giving bandhan. Strong cool vibrations indicate that the person is or were a realized soul. We can check the Vibrations of anything, such as books, films, artifacts etc... It is not necessary to read a book or see a film or painting to get an idea of its Vibrations and hence the sort of effect it might have on us.

We can even ascertain the Vibrational outcome of any decision that we may be going to take. By asking to be shown the Vibrations of different outcomes one can get a clearer idea of what are good decisions spiritually. For example if one was having a difficult time at work, one might ask the questions: Should I stay working here? , and Would it be better to leave?,

One of these alternatives might feel cooler on the hands, with less catches; we might also feel our attention rise up to Sahasrar and enter a state of thoughtlessness for one and come down to Agnya or lower for the other. One may also feel the Spirit in the heart jump with joy for one alternative, and another way of sensing is to put attention on the Void (abdomen); a good decision will feel comfortable, calm and grounded, and a worse one fluttery.

We can use vibrations to check the truth of any concept or thought, to find out whether they are genuine or not. For example, one can ask questions like: Is there God?, Who is Shri Mataji?, Can we save people from the grip of materialism?, A flow of cool Vibrations and a state of thoughtlessness and bliss as the attention rises to Sahasrar indicates Truth. We can also ask to be shown the truth of any facts (2+2=4 has vibrations, 2+2=7 not so much) or situations (Was this person responsible for this act?)

However, we should be careful while checking the Vibrations of things or situations where in we are emotionally involved, as we can be fooled. In such situations it is probably wise to ask a disinterested person to check for us. A way of checking things without any bias is to write the alternatives on pieces of paper, mix them up so we don't know which is which, and test the Vibrations of the different pieces of paper.

Chapter 15

Purity of Dedication to your Goal

The great Sufi saint Rumi, says that Love is the factor that will carry a man, in fact all humanity to fulfillment. "Mankind has an unfulfilled desire and he struggles to fulfill it through all kinds of enterprises and ambitions. But it is only in love that he can find fulfillment." But love itself is something which goes hand in hand with enlightenment. Both increase together.

Enlightenment of the brain gives us all the subtle understanding of the all pervading cosmic power. After Kundalini awakening one often experiences blissful happenings, miraculous coincidences and situations that appeared so difficult before being done in such a facile manner. It often makes us wonder, what is it that has made these things happen? How is it that I got this blessing? How could these transformations take place? When the brain starts understanding these wonderful happenings, it starts trusting the heart.

When the brain starts trusting the heart, devotion arises within us and it becomes totally surrendered to the Brahmarandra which is the seat of the heart. Now it is the liver that is controlled by the Swadishtan chakra that supplies energy or fuel to the brain to think. But when the brain becomes surrendered to the heart, all thinking comes from the Swadishtan which is the seat of all creativity. Hence all work done by the brain becomes enlightened work. The brain which is enlightened and connected to the all pervading power, when it works on creative ideas, it achieves results. Thus an enlightened person has the power to achieve anything.

An enlightened person, whose Kundalini is awakened and linked to the cosmic power around, he becomes an instrument of Divine force. Thus, when the Atma tatwa is awakened, the light of wisdom shines forth through the intellect and his mind emits a fragrance of love unblemished by the egoistic desires. Such a person is accommodative and can truly influence the collective consciousness.

The Sahasrar chakra is the final development of the subtle system within humans, enabling to rise, in every sense, above the world of mental activity and emotional concepts. The collective consciousness which arises when the Kundalini energy rises through the Sahasrar chakra allows direct perception of reality on the central nervous system. We can know ourselves as pure spirit, pure joy, pure attention and pure truth. Vibratory awareness allows our perception to transcend the senses and go to the essence of all creation.

Shree Mataji speaks of the 14 stages of reaching the Sahasrar chakra in her speech on the Maha Sahasrar Puja on 5th May, 1983, excerpt of which are given below.

"Fourteen years ago (or we could say already thirteen years have passed and now the fourteenth year has started) this great work of opening the Sahasrar was accomplished in this world. I have told you about this many times on every Sahasrar day; as to what had happened, how it was done and what its importance is. But the fourteenth birthday is very important because man lives at fourteen levels and the day he crosses over the fourteenth level, he becomes a complete Sahaja Yogi. Therefore, today Sahaja Yoga has also become Sahaja Yogi.

God has created fourteen levels within us. If you simply count them, then you know that there are seven Chakras within us. Besides these, there are two more Chakras, about which you do not talk much-they are the chakra of Moon (Lalita,) & chakra of Sun (Shri). Then there is "Hamsa" Chakra. Thus there are three more-seven plus three make ten. Then-there are four chakras above the Sahasrar. And about these chakras also, I have told you-ARDHA-BINDU, BINDU, VALAYA and PRADAKSHINA. These are the four.

After coming to Sahaja Yoga and after your Sahasrar has opened, you have to pass though these four chakras, ARDHA-BINDU, BINDU, VALAYA and PRADAKSHINA. After passing through these four chakras only, you can say that you have become a Sahaja Yogi. And if you see from another angle, we have to cross fourteen stages in reaching up to Sahasrar; if you divide them then there are seven chakras situated on Ida Nadi (Channel) and seven on Pingala Nadi.

When man makes his ascent, he does not do so in straight direction. He comes first to left then goes to right, then again to left and then again to right. And when Kundalini ascends, it also does so, dividing herself into these two. The reason for it can be understood if I take the example of two ropes. These two ropes together, side by side-in the process of going up or coming down cross over twice. When Kundalini ascends, you see on the chakra whether the left in caught or the right is caught. Although Kundalini is only one, but on every chakra you see both the things-thus you know whether left is caught or the right. Thus, within us, if each chakra is divided into these two-left and right---then seven two's are, fourteen; similarly within us first of all fourteen stages have to be crossed before reaching the Sahasrar. And if you understand this-that these seven, and seven above-this way also a path of fourteen is created.

Therefore this thing 'fourteen' is very important in Kundalini Shastra (Science). We should fully understand that we become entitled to the Blessings of Sahaja Yoga only after rising above these fourteen stages. We should unceasingly march forward and (as we imbibe it) get completely 'dyed' in it.

Rajana, Birajana-these words I have said to you many times earlier, also; but today, specially, we should understand that on Sahasrar day what is Rajana (to reign, to be the master), what is Birajana (to assume).

Now, you are sitting, you look at these trees. This is the tree of Shriphala. Coconut is called Shriphala. This grows along the sea-coast. The best fruit grows at the sea coast-the reason being that it is the 'Dharma' of the sea. Wherever there is dharma, only there, the

Shriphala blossoms. Where there is no dharma, Shriphala will not grow there.

All things are contained in the sea. All sorts of-cleanliness, dirt; everything is inside it. This water is also full of salt. Christ had said that 'You are the salt of the earth'. Means, you can enter into everything. You can impart taste to everything. The 'prana-Shakti' (Life-force) that we take in, if we don't have salt within us, then even that pranashakti cannot work. It is a catalyst. And this salt-it fully organises for us to live, to live in this world, to live in the 'prapancha' (illusionary world).

But when this thing rises towards God (Paramatman), then it leaves all the salt below -everything is left. And when the light of the sun falls on these trees, the sap of the whole tree is sucked upwards – through its leaves because evaporation takes place-then, this water flows upwards through the trunk;--leaving 'everything'. It crosses those fourteen things and on reaching the top, is formed Shriphala. You are that same Shriphala.

Also Shriphala is made up in a strange way; there is no 'phala' (fruit) in the world like the Shriphala. No part of it (tree) goes waste. You can see that the Shriphala is also like human being's Sahasrar. Like the hair we have, the same way Shriphala also has hair. You are protected by them. And inside this-like we have cranial bones- inside the Shriphala too there's a hard kind of a covering on the outside. After that inside us--- grey matter and white matter-two such things are inside us. In the Shriphala, too, you see-white matter and grey matter, and inside that is water, which is the cerebrospinal fluid inside us. Inside that (Shriphala) also there is water-that is the limbic area.

Our brain is the fruit of the whole of our evolution. Through this brain we have got all kinds of powers. With this is collected all the wealth that has been received by us. Now, the Atma (Spirit) resides inside this heart and after Sahaja-Yoga its light spreads within us in seven layers, from both sides that can happen only when one's Sahasrar is open.

Till now, we have been doing the same job with our brain -ego and super-ego-- But after realization, we work with the help of our Atma. Atma, before realization resides within the heart,--absolutely separate-as a 'Kshetragya' (witness of the field). It is separate from us. It is not in our Chitta. After realization, it comes into our Chitta, first which you know, is in the Void. After that, its light comes into the truth, because as the brain gets enlightened we know the truth. "Know". Doesn't mean that we know through the intellect, but know in reality (Sakshat) that this is the truth'. After that its light is seen in the heart. The heart becomes profound, heart starts expanding, starts becoming vast, and its power of love starts increasing. That's why-'Sacchidananda-Sat, Chitta and Anand (Truth, attention and bliss (joy).

Truth within our brain, Chitta, within our dharma; and joy within our Atma-start getting enlightened. Its light spreads gradually at first. It's a subtle thing, and in the gross set-up we live in, it becomes difficult to catch hold of that subtle. Gradually that hold also develops, after that you start to grow, to progress. With the opening of a single curtain of Sahasrar, the Kundalini comes up. But its light does not start spreading all around just then. The Kundalini has just come up and you have saluted the seat of Sadashiva. Within you, the light of Atma has started flowing hazily. But it has not yet fully blossomed in this brain.

Now, the surprising thing is that if you want to spread it through your brain, you cannot. You know well, that when you work too much with your intellect, heart-failure occurs. And when you work too much with your heart, the brain fails. There exists a relationship between them. It's a very deep relationship. And because of this deep relationship, when you get your realisation their relationship has to become deeper. The moment it gets completely integrated, your (Chitta) attention becomes completely Parameshwar-Swarup, (one with supreme God).

But how are the dissolution of ego and super-ego affected? If you beat down the ego, the super-ego comes up, if you beat down the super-ego, the ego comes up. How to win over the super-ego and the ego? There's only one door for that-Agnya chakra. By working on the Agnya-chakra the two, get completely dissolved, And as soon as they get dissolved, the heart and brain first establish a complete concord. "It is this oneness that we have to achieve."

So, your heart becomes the Sahasrar and your Sahasrar, the heart. What you think is in your heart; and whatever is in your heart, that only you think. When your state becomes like this, then, any kind of doubts, any kind of disbelief, any kind of fear-no such thing remains. When both the things become one you try to understand this point-which the brain, through which you think, makes your Manas understand, and takes care of it; that brain it becomes your Mana. When such a state comes, then you become the complete Master (Guru). Such a state we should definitely achieve.

Definitely, you have become Shriphala. But I always talk of what is ahead. Have you seen how people climb the coconut tree? He ties a rope around himself and keeps hooking that rope higher and with its help, he climbs. In the same way, as we climb, our own rope has always to be kept hooked higher. Only then your climbing is very quick. But mostly we keep hooking the rope lower. While coming down, you do not even need to hook the rope. You just loosen it a bit and-zoom -you will come down! That arrangement is already made-for coming down. It is to climb up, for which arrangement has to be made. So, to become something, hard work has to be put in.

Therefore 'Always set your sight higher' now even to see this fruit (Shriphala), you have to take your sight up. Even their sight is set upwards, because without keeping their sight upwards,-they know- that 'neither can they get Surya or get this work done, nor can they, become Shriphala.

Your Sahasrar is also like this very Shriphala-is extremely dear to Mother; and this very Sahasrar should be surrendered to Her. And the One, who is sitting there, 'is the 'fruit' of 'all' things. The roots of this tree, fixed in the soil below, they are also borne out from it. Its trunk, its hard work, its evolution - all' this in the end becomes that fruit. Everything is inherent in that fruit. You put that fruit in the soil and again the whole of this thing will be borne out.

In the whole world, whatever work of God has taken place, the form of its fruit is our Mahayoga of today! So you should feel blessed and becoming like this "Shriphala", you should be surrendered in offering. It is only removed from the tree when it is mature-otherwise it is useless. If it is removed from the tree and offered, thereafter the

Puja is considered accomplished. So, to understand Sahaja Yoga;--in a very great symbolic- form verily (Sakshat) Shriphala itself is standing before you.

In the same way you also have Shriphala. Fully mature it. There is only one way to mature it, that you have concord with your heart. There is no difference between the heart and the brain. From the heart we desire and from the brain it is fulfilled. When both the things become one, only then will you be fully benefited. You have got it for a very much higher purpose and keep it at that higher level and only on attaining that accomplished wonderful unique state you can consider yourself blessed.

Look at these trees. The breeze is flowing in the opposite direction. Actually the trees should be bent towards this side. But in which direction are the trees bowing down? Have you ever marked that all the trees are facing in that direction? Why? The breeze is coming from that direction and pushing them, even then, why are the trees bending towards the same side? Because they know that 'It' (Sea) is the one who is the Giver of everything. Being reverent and extremely humble, they are bowing to it. The dharma which is inside us, when it gets fully awakened, starts fully manifesting, only then will the Shriphala inside us be so sweet, beautiful and nourishing. And then the world will get to know from your life itself- 'what you are'-and not from anything else.

To accept any kind of compromise, to loosen hold on you in any matter, does not behove a Sahaja Yogi. A person, who is a Sahaja Yogi, should bravely make his path and move forward. Look at the way these trees hold such a heavy fruit so high. In the same way you have to hold your head high and while holding it high, remember that the head should be respectfully bowed towards the sea-the sea, which is the sign of dharma. It has to be reverently and humbly bowed (;) towards the Dharma.

Finally, the brain, or the Sahasrar should radiate love .We should only consider whether-"Whatever I am doing, is it in love? Is everything, my talking and all my activities being done in love?" And if you are really doing that then you have accomplished and acquired that thing, about which I have been speaking, namely "that concord" which should be achieved. Then that concord has been established within you.

There is only one Shakti (power) which we may call 'Love' and it is only 'Love' that shapes all things to become beautiful, shapely and fully organised. (Anant Ashirvad) to you all.

Chapter 16

Stress Management through Sahaja Yoga

Man today finds himself in a very unique situation of having to respond and tackle a variety of complex situations day in and day out for which he finds even his multi-dimensional personality inadequate. Ours is a restless age- an age where rapid changes in technology are causing a breakdown of old values and fragmenting our personality. The result of this is tremendous psychological disturbances, stress and tension. Happiness seems to be eluding us and we are constantly seeking answers. In the name of religion people of different countries and communities are waging a war amongst themselves.

Self-realization is the only way you can get the light in.

Sahaja Yoga is a simple technique of self-realization, wherein the dormant energy, which is inborn within you, is awakened and connected with the all-pervading cosmic energy. It is an empirically verifiable scientific method that explains how the very desire for becoming united with the Absolute is built within us as Kundalini.

What is Stress?

Stress is anything that causes fear, anxiety, worry, apprehensions, anger and even excitement when we face difficult situations in daily life, whether mental or emotional. Continuous efforts to cope with such situations have adverse effects on human systems for want of relief from mental and emotional strains and it leads to diseases.

According to Dr. Vernon Coleman, who after discussions with several doctors from various regions, has come to the conclusion that 90-95% of the illnesses can be blamed totally or mainly on psychological forces, 98% headaches are stress or pressure-related, a vast majority of indigestions are due to stress etc.

Some stress is good and even found necessary to feel stimulated, to keep away from boredom and depression and to achieve improved performance. A sense of high achievements and high self-esteem enables a person to cope with higher and higher levels of stress till the optimum level or stress threshold is reached.

What is Stress threshold?

Stress threshold is the point where any more pressure will become counterproductive. It is the point where more pressure will lead to fall in productivity and contentment. This point differs from person to person, depending upon one's ability to cope with the pressure.

Some people can sustain higher levels of pressure; some thrive on stress while some suffer enormously even under modest amounts of stress. There are fairly fixed stress threshold levels for activity and inactivity. At one end there is inactivity that we can cope with and at the other end, it is activity that we can cope with. If the range between them is narrow one is stress-prone.

When Stress is harmful?

By itself stress never causes a problem. It is the way one responds to stress which leads to problems. The response is generally in three stages:

Alarm - In the face of a challenge or a threat, the nervous system is highly stimulated, heart rate increases, muscles become tense, and breathing becomes fast. The body system is now ready to fight or flee.

Resistance - If the cause producing the stress continues the body chemistry adjust to that situation (i.e. steady flow of adrenal and other glands secretion and in order to keep the body at a more easily maintained level of arousal during the time needed to fight or get away.

Exhaustion - If the challenge continues for a long time, the resources for arousal and resistance are used. They are involuntary physical responses to stress for which built-in mechanisms exists in the human body. Even imagining or thinking about an upcoming situation may trigger these.

So long as the problem is solved and we are able to rest, even the acute effects of stress are not dangerous to a healthy person. Due to repeated occurrences of emergencies, the person has to pass through the stages of alarm and resistance time and again in the accumulated pressures causing exhaustion, diseases or emotional problems, leading to fall in performance levels, productivity and strained relations within the family and at workplace.

Sometimes, however, a person may even get withdrawn into a depression. These are chronic effects of stress, which are the signals that life style or work habits should be adjusted before worse problems emerge. That is the importance of effective stress management.

Stress Management

A number of ways have been evolved over the years to tackle stress. Many resort to drinking, smoking, and drugs etc., which are harmful. Relaxation techniques have been found to be more effective than others and meditation is the best relaxation technique. In Sahaja yoga, the regular practice of meditation, after the self-realization, can bring necessary additional change as the person is evolved leading to a balanced outlook toward events and situations he has to face in daily life.

Stress Management through Sahaja Yoga -

Sahaja yoga meditation brings about equilibrium between the sympathetic and Para-sympathetic nervous system response in the process knocking down the sympathetic dominance usually seen in stressful situations, and thereby helps prevent stress disorders.

The technique is simple- it is a way of activating a mechanism- the Kundalini- which is the divine energy that lies dormant at the base of the spine. This mechanism is the moving force of our enlightenment and is a living force, which seeks self-organization, self-regeneration and ascent.

Through self-organization it sustains and protects the human system. Self-regeneration is its innate ability to heal, renew, balance and recycle. And, ascent is its ability to transcend the mind and body and to attain collective consciousness.

One who practices Sahaja Yoga meditation, finds himself move into a different dimension which enables him to harness the unused sectors of the brain. Once this happens, a new supply of energy is available to us. The actual experiences of people moving into this level of functioning are a feeling of total inner silence, complete health and well-being. There is thoughtless awareness and the person feels a cool breeze of vibrations on the head and on the palms of the hands.

Recent research conducted on varied groups of individual Sahaja Yoga meditators has revealed that the practice of Sahaja Yoga is accompanied by decrease in tension, anxiety, depression, neuroticism and hypertension. With meditation there is an experience of inner peace and harmony and one moves in the direction of greater self-control, self-awareness, actualizing one's potential and thus moves towards happiness.

Electrical Brain Activity-

Electroencephalograph (EEG) reports indicate the following changes in the brain activity during Sahaja Yoga meditation:

1. At the initial stage, on commencing meditation, the alpha brain wave pattern increases, which creates a sense of relaxed awareness
2. As the meditation progresses the brain activity shifts to long chains of low voltage theta activity signifying deep physiological relaxation as is attained during deep sleep states.
3. And, during a very deep meditation state, the EEG pattern again changes and this time bursts of high efficiency beta peaks occur.

It appears from all these studies conducted that the human nervous system begins to function in an entirely different way after the Sahaja Yoga meditation practice. Some other dramatic changes clearly reported are:

1. Oxygen consumption decreases within 5 minutes of starting the meditation.
2. Heart rate and respiration rate also decrease.
3. Blood lactate concentration, which is associated with high states of anxiety, also reduces.
4. Adrenalin, which correlates with high blood pressure, drops.
5. The galvanic skin response is a measure of the activity of the sweat glands. This is related to the sympathetic nervous system that regulates the level of tension or relaxation. The Sahaja Yoga practice increases skin resistance thereby significantly reducing tension.

Dr. D Chug at the Lady Harding Hospital, New Delhi, has conducted these experimental studies.

Chapter 17

Managerial Transformation
By Sahaja Yoga

Management is an exceedingly complex art. It is at times mathematics, at times poetry, but always in a balanced sense. Management means dealing with people. It is the responsibility of the managers to get the maximum out of the people for the maximum productivity for which the managers have to understand human nature and behavior. So the first step towards management will be to know what the qualities of a good manager are and then how to transform the human beings for the best results of the Organization.

Quality of a Good Manager:

- He by nature is not resistant to organizational needs and normally considers work as a natural activity.
- He is ready and eager to assume responsibility.
- He has no favorites.
- He is not rude, irritable, hard-driving and a rough manager; on the other hand he believes that good relations increase productivity.
- He has no immoral behavior to his colleagues of opposite sex.
- He is creative.

- He is lovable.
- He is not adverse to change in an organization

Man's desires are unlimited. As soon as one is fulfilled, another appears in its place. Once a need is satisfied it no longer becomes a motivator of action and behavior. When the physiological needs of man such as food, clothing and shelter are reasonably satisfied, his next need is safety that means security of employment and freedom of arbitrary management actions.

When physiological and security needs are satisfied, his social needs become important. He wants to have a feeling of belonging, a sense of being part of a social group or community. The next need of man after all this is his need for achievement – the gratification of ego and self- importance. In this way the desires keep increasing to aggrandizement and accumulation. There is a lack of satisfaction which ultimately will have behavioral consequences.

Learning does not believe.

The Japanese believe that continuous training can lead to continuous improvement in performance. Therefore, in most Japanese Companies, everyone from Sweeper to a Managing Director attends training classes throughout their career. This approach is also known as the Zen approach, as opposed to the Chinese approach, which is known as Confucius approach. According to the Zen approach, the purpose of training is continuous improvement in the performance of whatever one does- no matter what one's work is, everyone can improve on his or her career by continuous training.

The Confucius approach, on the other hand, holds that the aim of training is to qualify the trainee for a more important job, in other words, the training is for promotion. The Confucius approach emphasizes attention to status, wages and other benefits, rather than the excellence of work.

Today management experts are talking and lecturing on TQM (Total Quality Management), Zero Defect Management etc. The mantra of continuous improvement like other TQM Principles sounds wonderful. But it is not easy to implement.

So, while the management commitment to continuous improvement may be unflinching, it is often unable to translate the noble intention into action. It may be noticed that these are all a mental approach. These management experts are overlooking the fundamental fact that humans being cannot be transformed into better humans only by learning and training.

Then a human mind is exposed to certain knowledge or behavioral attitude only through the mental approach, the process of learning and training, up to a certain point is absorbed but after that it coils back. It generates reactions in his mind, body and life style. Thus after some time, the manager and executives may not be able to contribute their best by training alone

TRANSFORMATION IS AN INSIDE JOB:

According to the Meta Science of Sahaja Yoga, as revealed by H Mataji Nirmala Devi, there exists a subtle system in each human being, consisting of various energy centers called chakras and nadis or nervous system which control our physical, mental and spiritual activities. They manifest in gross body outside the spinal cord and neural plexuses and control functions of respective parts of the human body.

The nadis can be further classified as the central nervous system and the autonomous nervous system. The autonomic nervous system consists of the parasympathetic and sympathetic nervous system. The sympathetic nervous system is further subdivided into left and right. The LSNS (left sympathetic nervous system) which is also called Ida Nadi or moon channel represents the power of desire in individual. It brings our attention to memories of the past.

The energy flow in the Nadi is blocked by conditioning, superstitions, guilt feelings, too much self-pity, sexual perversion and pornography. Movement in this side gives rise to reactions, which are stored in a balloon like structure on the right side of the brain known as superego. As long as this channel is active there is a human desire to remain alive.

RSNS (right sympathetic nervous system) represents our power of actions. It is also known as Pingala Nadi or sun channel. It makes us to think, work, plan and organize for the future events. The reactions generated due to all these actions are stored in a balloon like structure at the end of this channel at the left side of the brain and is known as ego.

While we may have control over sympathetic nervous system, it consumes a lot of our energy.

Thus the managers or people who are using LSNS too much are people who

- Often think of the past, are very emotional, avoid meeting people and are introverts.
- They cannot face criticism.
- Such managers are by nature indolent and work little, lack ambition, and dislike responsibilities.
- They are inherently self centered and indifferent to organizational needs.
- They prefer to be led.
- They are by nature resistant to change.
- They are gullible and ready dupe of the charlatans and the demagogue.
- They sit in the corner of the office and try to hide themselves.
- Efforts of the management fail to obtain the desired improvement
- In these types of people as there is no harmony, it results in poor performance.
- In other words, these groups of people are dealt with management by control and this does not yield optimum result.

The managers or people who are using their RSNS are:

- Always very aggressive.

- They like to dominate over others and make employees or colleague's life miserable.
- If they are leaders or head of the departments, they do not delegate anything so as to keep the credit of any success for themselves only.
- They become barrier for effective communications, as proper two -way communication means explanations, question, criticism both up and down and not only one way.
- They are invariably hard taskmasters and workaholics and may not be able to get best from the people working under them.
- They carry work home.
- They do not believe in team effort.
- These people are always rushing around and looking busy.
- They appraise their subordinates usually looking at their faults.
- They are mostly self centered and may not be prepared to take decisions with the organization's interest in mind.

When the Kundalini energy or the energy of the super cosmic force lying just below the spinal cord in the triangular bone known as sacrum bone, is awakened during the process of Self-Realization, it rises through the central channel piercing the six chakras on her way. After she pierces the fontanels bone area, one feels cool breeze or vibration in his or her palm and on top of the head. This brings forth a new dimension in the human personality of a collective at the same time a very compassionate and peaceful person.

This brings about a transformation in the individual and he begins to exhibit the beautiful qualities inherent in every chakra which gets reflected in his everyday activities in the office or managerial sphere as well. It may sound fantastic but it has happened to people from all walks of life around the walks life around the world- to scientists, physicians, engineers, professors, and common man. To experience Sahaja yoga one should open one's mind and heart to receive the blessings.

Energy Centers and their impact on our behavior:

1. The first chakra, which is Mooladhar, gives us qualities of moral values like innocence, purity, wisdom and auspiciousness.
2. The second chakra, the Swadishtan chakra gives us the power of creativity.
3. The third chakra known as Nabhi grants us satisfaction, peace, generosity, welfares and determines our relationship with our spouse. It also controls our success in business and prosperity with honesty.
4. The fourth chakra known as Anahat chakra gives us security, power of pure love and determines our relationship with our parents.
5. The fifth chakra known as Vishuddhi chakra determines our personality how we talk sweetly, aggressively or diplomatically and how pure is our relationship with opposite sex.
6. The sixth known as Agnya chakra gives us the power to forgive others.
7. The seventh chakra known as Sahasrar chakra is the integration of all chakras. Here all the qualities represented in the physical, mental, emotional and spiritual aspects of the human being gets integrated and he begins to pour forth the divinity in him in all his actions.

Chapter 18

Sahaja Yoga and Treatment of Diseases

Sahaja Yoga as rediscovered by Shri Mataji Nirmala Devi aims at achieving holistic health care for people. The science focuses on awakening the dormant primordial energy (the Kundalini), whereby a flow of subtle cool cosmic vibrations in the body is achieved which nourishes and rejuvenates each and every cell of the body. As late Dr Umesh Rai, director of International Sahaja Yoga Research and Health Centre at Vashi Navi Mumbai had discovered, "As a result of meditation, which is the basic aim of Sahaja, the body manufactures certain fluids which have curative powers, which help in overcoming the most severe of ailments."

Dr Rai has researched at the Lady Hardinge Medical College and Associated Hospitals, New Delhi, on the role of Sahaja Yoga in the treatment of psychosomatic diseases.

He maintains that while with the advancement of the medical sciences, infectious diseases have been wiped out and heart and kidney transplants are quite successful, scientists have yet to find an answer for the treatment of psychosomatic diseases which are on the increase in the developed as well as the developing countries. Some such diseases are hypertension, migraine, bronchial asthma, epilepsy and others.

"The doctor of today practicing modern allopathic medicine has entered a stage of superspeciality whereby they assign separate parts of the body to be treated by a specialist. Due to this approach doctors are not able to view disease as a disturbance to the whole organism. They treat a particular part of the body without taking into consideration the psychological and social aspects of the patients illness", says Rai. "One could be physically fit, but emotional problems or social isolation could make a person very sick."

He advises recourse to the ancient Indian scriptures like the Patanjali's Yoga Sutra that mentioned yoga as the most essential technique to keep the body and mind healthy. This is true even today but there is a need for integration that is not merely the inner but covers external life as well. "For yoga to be more relevant today, it needs to touch both the physical and mental aspects of health, which is encapsulated in the Sahaja Yoga. This science borders on all that which one is born with," says he.

It is based on our subtle nervous system. When the dormant primordial energy present as three and a half coils in the triangular sacrum bone gets activated on doing Sahaja Yoga, it ascends and activates one's six subtle chakras and piercing through Brahmarandra, it unites with the all pervading cosmic energy." And with this actualization in the limbic area of the brain, subtle cool vibrations start flowing from both palms and the top of the head and in this vibratory awareness, one can feel what chakras are blocked, and can also work out their correction to cure different diseases.

To verify some of the claims of Sahaja Yoga, a systematic research study was organized in the physiology and medicine department of Lady Hardinge Medical College and Associated Hospitals in New Delhi. The research projects studied were psychological effects of Kundalini awakening by Sahaja Yoga and the effect of Sahaja practice on psychosomatic diseases like hypertension and bronchial asthma.

Says Ellerbe, the most important aspect of this science is to achieve a state of thoughtlessness which is the most difficult of things to achieve. But once you get your mind free, you gradually begin to feel a calm stillness within," says she.

The International Sahaja Yoga centre at CBD Belapur founded and started by Shree Mataji Nirmala Devi is a unique centre of its kind in the world, where treatment is done by vibratory awareness, developed by Sahaja yoga meditation. Besides Indians, people from

United States, UK, Switzerland, Belgium, Austria, New Zealand, Australia and several other countries of the world are admitted and treated for various health conditions. Today this centre has more international visitors than Indians.

Narrating about a rare recovery of a patient, S S Agarwal from Delhi Dr. Rai in his interview with the Indian express said, "His was a case of chronic renal failure, for which doctors had ruled out all treatment, except ongoing dialysis. By applying Sahaja yoga, we aroused his Kundalini energy (which is a dormant energy at the base of the spine) and directed it towards the kidney to clear his blocked chakras." Today, Agarwal's medical reports indicate near normalcy.

Etienne Loyson, a 62 year old architect from Belgium, is just spell-bound, "Earlier I had high blood pressure. Doctors abroad had suggested taking several tablets ongoing as the only treatment method. But today, with Sahaja yoga treatment and the blessing of Shree Mataji Nirmala Devi, I am full of energy. I have stopped all medicines and I feel I am just 30 years old."

Katherine Reid from England (who suffered from irritable bowels syndrome) is a happy woman today, in contrast to her life previously when she had to take several medicines prior to her arrival in Navi Mumbai. "I feel much better having stopped my medication completely. My health has improved by about eighty per cent." Anna Kargaity, a Canadian who suffered from depressive psychosis is full of smiles today. "I now have a positive outlook towards life, being able to develop my own personality and express my feelings", she says. Similar benefits were highlighted by Belinda from Australia, Kumar from Canada, Bryan from USA and others.

On being asked as to why so many foreigners are coming to India, when advanced medicines are available with doctors of modern medicine all over the world, Dr. Rai added, "The doctors abroad don't have a treatment for the psyche of human being, except giving tranquillizers, sedatives and anti- depressant drugs. These are not only harmful, but also habit-forming. In view of this, Sahaja yoga, which can control the psyche of human being by meditation, has become very popular to the treatment and prevention of psychosomatic diseases like bronchial asthma, migraine, irritable bowel syndrome, infertility, multiple sclerosis and sodalities, to name a few. It is all due to the blessings of Shree Mataji Nirmala Devi, who founded Sahaja Yoga centre, and has enlightened thousands of people all over the world."

Sahaja yoga is a cognitive therapy as well as curative breakthrough:

- It enables the individuals to intervene on the central nervous system and the state of their centers and channels of energy (chakras).
- It gives access to a subtle form of energy, Kundalini. This energy can be accessed through almost effortless, natural techniques to bring balance and health in one's mind, body, and emotions.
- It raises the human awareness to a new dimension of collective consciousness which enables the individual to feel the energetic state of another person and help in improving it.

Some of the research confirmed benefits of Sahaja yoga:

1. Sahaja Yoga has achieved tremendous success in treatment of innumerable chronic fatal diseases. Recent medical investigations reveals that individuals suffering from hypertension, cancer, chronic asthma, epilepsy, diabetes, arthritis and heart ailments have recovered completely after practicing Sahaja Yoga meditation.
2. Another astounding medical breakthrough documented from Australia is the cure and treatment of AIDS cases by using Sahaja Yoga techniques.
3. The healing effects of Sahaja Yoga have encouraged doctors and others in the caring professions to develop centers where Sahaja Yoga techniques could be applied to patients suffering from a variety of ailments.
4. In fact, Dr. Valentina Gostera, who works as a pediatrician in general hospital in the Soviet Union, was able to give her

two patients a new lease of life. One was a child with an 11-inch liver, where all diagnostic and surgical recommendations made by a team of doctors did not yield results.

5. Finally she treated the child on the principles of Sahaja Yoga and the liver started to heal gradually. After a few weeks, the liver shrunk back to its normal size. The same doctor at a party treated another case of fatal asthma, where the man who collapsed after an asthma attack, began to feel an easing of the symptoms. He had been suffering asthma for the past 45 years and now he has fully recovered.

6. Also, Dr. Chug's pioneering work presents experimental evidence to show the beneficial effects of Sahaja Yoga on essential hypertension and bronchial asthma. Hyper tension being due to excess of right- sided activity, Sahaja yoga practice corrects this imbalance in the neural communication. Similarly, asthma is said to be due to constriction in the cardiac center on the right side. Thus relieving this constriction causing asthma leads to instantaneous relief.

7. Further, diabetes, cancer of the blood, kidney troubles and heart attacks, according to Sahaja yoga being disorders as a result of excess mental activity, and skin disorder, anorexia, angina and epilepsy being caused due to a tendency to dwell on the past or indulge in depression, therapy would essentially be directed to rectify these imbalances and to attain peace within.

How does meditation bring about these effects?

Sahaja yoga meditation triggers a process within the autonomic nervous system, a complex set of nerves that governs the function of all the organs of our body. Imbalance within this system is the cause of both physical and psychological illness. The process of meditation rebalances this system thereby allowing our natural healing processes to revitalize and rejuvenate diseased organs.

The ancient yoga tradition triggers the inner healing process in terms of seven subtle energy centers that exist within our body.

Each of these centers governs a specific set of organs, and aspects of our psychology and spirituality. Imbalanced function of these centers results in abnormal function of any aspect of our being (physical, mental or spiritual) that relates to the imbalanced centre.

Meditation through the specific process that involves the awakening of the innate, nurturing energy, the "Kundalini" causes it to rise from its position in the sacrum bone and pierce through each of the chakras, causing each of them to come into a state of balance and alignment. The chakras are rejuvenated and nourished by the kundalini's ascent. As the Kundalini reaches the brain and the chakras within it, mental tensions are neutralized. An inner state of mental calm is established. This inner silence becomes a source of inner peace that neutralizes the stresses of daily life, enhancing creativity, productivity and self-satisfaction.

BRAIN WAVES

In order to try and understand what it is about the Sahaja Yoga meditation that makes it special some sophisticated brain imaging technology was used. A pilot study of advanced Sahaja yoga meditators using a QEEG (quantitative electro encephelo gram) has yielded some very interesting results. This method is able to produce two-dimensional maps of the electrical changes in the brain as the meditator enters into the state of meditation.

The study was conducted in Australia on a small group of meditators who were each asked to meditate while wearing a QEEG head cap designed to pick up the tiny electrical signals produced by the brain. They were instructed to sit quietly for some time, then to commence meditation and signal when they had definitely entered into the meditative state called "thoughtless awareness". The findings were fascinating: all three of the meditators displayed widespread changes in brainwave activity that became more intense as they meditated.

Widespread, intense "alpha wave" activity occurred initially. Alpha wave activity is associated with relaxation and is thought to be a beneficial state. The remarkable thing, however, is that as the meditators signaled that they had entered into the state of mental silence, or "thoughtless awareness", another form of brain wave activity emerged which involved "theta waves" focused specifically in the front and top of the brain in the midline. Precisely at the time that the theta activity became prominent, the meditators reported that they experienced a state of complete mental silence and "oneness" with the present moment, a state which characterizes the Sahaja yoga meditative experience.

There are several remarkable features about this pilot study which warrant further investigation.

First, very few meditation techniques have shown this kind of consistent change in the theta range suggesting that the technique may have a unique effect on the brain. We were only able to find one other study, out of several dozen published in the scientific literature, that showed changes of this nature. This study involved a group of Japanese Zen monks.

Practitioners of Sahaja yoga often claim to feel the chakras (energy centers) within the head open up as the meditative experience intensifies. They assert that it is this experience which is the essence of true meditation and that very few other meditation techniques enable the subject to repeatedly access this experience.

Second, it is very significant that the changes observed in the brain images occurred at the moment the meditators reported experiencing the meditative state. This suggests that the QEEG method may make it possible to directly study mystical states of consciousness! The fact that these changes occurred within minutes rather than hours or longer suggests a relatively effortless or spontaneous process (as suggested by the name of the technique - "Sahaja" is Sanskrit for "effortless").

Third, the focus of theta activity at the front of the head and top of the head, both in the midline, suggest that structures deep within the brain, possibly the limbic system, are being activated. The limbic system is responsible for many aspects of our subjective experiences, such as emotion and mood, so it is no surprise that meditation, which is traditionally associated with blissful states, might involve this part of the brain.

Finally, in speculation, the two areas of theta activity coincidentally correspond to the two main chakras in the brain, according to yogic tradition. The forehead chakra called "Agnya" or "third eye" is located in the centre of the forehead while the chakra at the top of the head, is called "Sahasrar" or "crown chakra" and is traditionally associated with the limbic system.

The research has shown promising results for the treatment of asthma, headache, menopause and depression.

Frontal Midline Theta: log(power) during meditation

Subject 1, 5.6 Hz

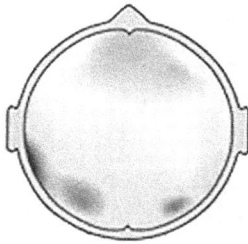

Subject 1, 7.6 Hz

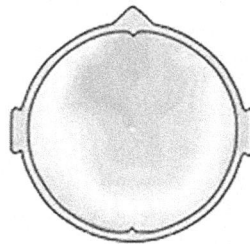

Subject 2 (deep), 6 Hz

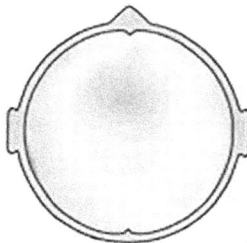

Subject 3, 5.6 Hz

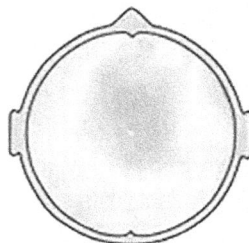

"What a great thing it would be if we in our busy lives could restore into ourselves each day for at least a couple of hours and prepare our minds to listen to the voice of the great silence.

The divine radio is always singing if we could only make ourselves ready to listen to it, but it is impossible to listen without silence."

Mahatma Gandhi

Meditation is an eastern tool that offers western health practitioners a new way of looking at health. While, for most of us, focusing on the absolute present moment is virtually impossible, it is this razor's edge of "thoughtless awareness" that the easterner seeks to cultivate and sustain in meditation. The vast inner silence of the thoughtless state leaves the mind uncluttered. By existing in that "space-between-the thoughts" one is neither enslaved to one's past nor confined to a predetermined future. The inner silence of meditation thus creates a naturally stress-free inner environment.

Is it possible for humans to live in the present moment? Yes, it is, and most of us encounter living examples of it regularly! Observe closely the next small child you encounter. They have no worried lines on their faces, are almost always playing and enjoying themselves, and rarely complain about bills, jobs, chores, etc.

If one happens to have an unpleasant experience it is quickly forgotten and life goes on. They are naturally balanced, living-in- the present, stress-free beings. Who has seen a toddler hold a grudge, worry about the next meal or even think about what they did yesterday or will do tomorrow? They are so focused on the present moment that they are entirely spontaneous, unpretentious and usually very happy. They are in a constant state of effortless meditation.

Living in the moment is not, however, a regression to immaturity. It is an evolutionary step in which we return to our childlike innocence and simplicity but in full awareness of ourselves, our place in society and our moral role and responsibility. How does one tap into and sustain a connection with the present moment? How does one escape the brainstorm of mental stress that we all experience? It is possible through the "Sahaja yoga effect." Sahaja yoga meditation appears to offer a method by which each of us can tame the brainstorm, realize a state of peace and tranquility and begin to heal our body, mind and spirit.

Chapter 19

CEIB Technology

The technology of a complex energy and information balance (the CEIB technology) based on Sahaja Yoga, which implements the concept of vibratory awareness was offered by Mrs Nirmala Srivastava at the IX All-Russia Scientific and Practical Conference "Health, Peace, Morals, Culture, East-West" to the President, the Government and the Federal Assembly at **Moscow, june 9-10, 1998,** and called it the Nirmala CEIB technology. It has been successfully applied in health treatments at several medical institutions of St.-Petersburg, as well as in the Research and Rehabilitation Center in Bombay, India.

The concept of vibratory awareness is a universal key to self-cognition and environment-cognition, as well as harmonization of their interaction. Fundamental research works conducted by modern scientists confirm that the human being does not only have a protein-nucleic nature, but a field nature as well (energy-informatics fields). Any information existing in the Universe can be percepted by human sub-consciousness. Vibratory awareness helps using the knowledge received at the level of sub-consciousness and implementing it in the protein-nucleic form of life.

Applied aspects of the vibratory awareness concept reveal themselves in the process of the reserve energy activation of the creative principle (SECP), or the 'Kundalini energy phenomenon" according to the ancient oriental terminology. The reserve energy activation of the creative principle manifests first of all at the level of the main aspects of our brain: the informational, the modular (i.e. energy aspect), and the programming aspect.

At the D.O. Otto Obstetrics and Gynecology Institute (TGI) of the Russian Academy of Medical Science, the Nirmala CEIB technology has been successfully applied in the prenatal and postnatal periods without side-effects influencing the mother's and child's health... The studied technology included patients' organism's functional condition (OFC) control before and after the energy-information balance treatment; such control was conducted under the criteria of modified Akabane testing.

It is worth to mentioning that the GI of the Russian Academy of Medical Sciences would normally apply the Nirmala CEIB technology in the cases when conventional methods of treatment did not bring the expected positive results. In some of the cases, the CEIB treatments were successfully applied in life threatening situations, for instance, bleeding during childbirth, in surgery and others. Simultaneously, OFC was controlled according to clinical analysis results. More than 90% of the patients taking CEIB treatment demonstrated significant improvement and returning to normal health condition.

A large group of patients successfully participated in the Nirmala CEIB technology treatment course at the TGI and comprised of pregnant women suffering from hard toxicosis, diabetes mellitus, bronchial asthma, threat of pregnancy interruption at different stages, heart, liver and kidney diseases, tumor of the womb, benign tumor, ovary hyper stimulation syndrome, as well as hematological diseases and acute hemorrhage. In 1996 the infants suffering from hemolytic disease were treated as well.

Persistent remission and increasing health level were found in the following cases after applying the Nirmala CEIB technology alone:

- ovary hyper stimulation syndrome (one month after the disease occurred);
- asthmatic attacks at early stage (a patient in a post -operation period);

- drug-induced allergy;
- post-natal loss of reflex on urination;
- Healing vesicle sheath fistula, as well as fistula in abdominal cavity.

An on -going preventive course of the Nirmala CEIB technology treatments, used by blood donors at the TG Blood Transfusion Department, resulted in a high level of life safety of donors and recipients: no case of post- transfusion hepatitis among recipients has been registered at the Institute in the period of 7 years 1990-1996.

This wide experience continues to be developed at the Dr. U.K. Rae Research and Rehabilitation Center in Navi Mumbai, India, where the work is conducted by high-category well-known physicians.

The vibratory awareness technology helped doctors successfully treat their patients without speaking their language and without the usual informational exchange between a patient and a doctor. The following diseases were successfully treated by the Nirmala CEIB technology in the above mentioned Center:

- liver cancer;
- epilepsy;
- ischemic heart disease;
- hypertension;
- lung cancer with metastasis in mediastinal space;
- tongue cancer with metastasis in the sub mandibular lymph nodes;
- myocardiopathy;
- cerebral palsy;
- Down's syndrome;
- skin hyper pigmentation;
- malaria;
- Bronchial asthma with neurodermitis, etc.

As a result of work with the seriously ill children in the above mentioned center, it became clear, that the cause of the many health problems of these children lies in the parents' problems. That is why it is advisable in such cases to conduct the energy-informational correction of children along with that of their parents. After the correction course, such family usually acquires not only physical but also spiritual health.

Especially fast results were achieved while treating children and their parents at the same time. For example while treating a 5 year old child suffering from cerebral palsy, hyper tonus of the limbs disappeared after 3 weeks of treatment. A 5 year old girl with Down's syndrome started walking on the second day of Nirmala CEIB technology application. A child with psoriasis had a remission after two weeks of the treatment. After a month of treatment, the skin on a patient with hyper pigmentation became lighter and 3 months later the pigmentation almost fully disappeared. A patient with bronchial asthma and neurodermitis lowered her usage of the inhalator containing hormones from 7 times a day to twice a day after 4 weeks of the treatment. The manifestations of the neurodermitis existing since her childhood have disappeared.

In 1997-1998, 32 patients were treated using this technology, including 10 children. In the meantime, 27 of their relatives have mastered the Nirmala CEIB technology and actively assisted in the treatment process.

The studied group included patients with the following heavy diseases:

- a state after total resection of thyroid (the patient suffered from cancer);
- lung cancer; melanoma with glaucoma crisis;
- larynx papilloma;
- depression;
- ischemic heart disease;
- cirrhosis of liver;
- epilepsy;
- bronchial asthma;
- neurodermitis;
- obesity in the second degree,

- dysplasia of cervical spine (a 12 year old child after a birth trauma);
- von Willebrand's disease in a heavy form;

Good results of the treatment of the larynx papilloma should be noted. Since 1996, 4 surgeries had been conducted in order to remove the papilloma. Three Nirmala CEIB technology sessions were carried out with 4-day intervals, after which the patient practiced the technology on his own. After one month of treatment his voice appeared and an on-going remission is being observed in the course of the year.

A female patient with melanoma had glaucoma crisis removed after one hour of the first treatment day. One month later she was successfully operated for the eye enucleating. She was dismissed from the hospital on the 6th day after the operation. On the 7th day the patients got an artificial eye inserted. Blood pressure, which used to be 180/120 mm, and blood sugar (the patient had diabetes millennium) came to normal. In her appreciation letter the patient wrote that the sullen, gloomy feeling no longer existed and stimulus to life is back, "even friends of mine, who knew about my illness, are surprised about how cheerful I am..."

A 4.5 year old girl weighing 11 kg, who used to suffer from a neurodermitis, is recovered after 2, 5 months of regular treatment conducted with her and her close relatives. An on-going remission is being observed in the course of the year. The girl gained 3 kg since then.

Periodically we observe a group of patients suffering from the von Willebrand's disease at the Republican Hemophilia Treatment Center. In 1994-1995 treatment sessions were conducted systematically ones a week in the course of 9 months. Three patients of the group are demonstrating the on-going remission in the course of over 3 years, even though they only practice Nirmala CEIB technology from time to time and do it on their own. Worth mentioning is that, in cases of highly spiritual patients, the activated reserve energy of the creative principle continues the process of patient's harmonizing on the physical and spiritual level without the patients' special efforts.

Figure 1 demonstrates the results of an OFC express testing of the patient T.: the original condition and condition after Nirmala CEIB technology course several serious diseases disappeared.

In order to analyze results of applying the Nirmala CEIB technology, we also use self-estimation reports prepared by our patients.

The patient G. had a total resection of the thyroid with following side diseases: Ischemic heart disease, duodenal ulcer, gastric ulcer, hypertension (second degree), migraine; there were 7 surgeries in her anamnesis with the last surgery performed on June 7, 1997. One month later, the patient started the Nirmala CEIB technology practice.

"The process of the recovery goes fast, yet very subtle and gently at the same time sometimes I even don't recognize it. Now I feel happy, depression and fear of death are gone. I don't keep my attention on the disease, as if I have never had it. I sleep well. Feeling of anxiety has disappeared and I've become more calm, wise and patient. Also, I've got a feeling of self-esteem. I wish people good and want to help them."

"People come to me to talk about their problems and troubles. I try to help them as much as possible, giving them advice on how to recover physically and spiritually. I used to have a frequent strong headache, which could not be relieved by any medicine. Now the migraine has completely disappeared nasal bleedings are over."

"Blood pressure is 140/90 mm, and it used to be 260/120 mm. The ulcer doesn't bother me anymore. The tiredness is gone now. I feed vitality and joy. My hair doesn't fall out any more, it has become thicker. There is a shine in my eyes. Everybody says that I look younger than I really am."

Chapter 20

Healing the Left Side

Diseases of the left side are caused due to lethargy and originate from the subconscious. Low blood pressure, cancer, tumor, epilepsy, schizophrenia, viral diseases, multiple sclerosis, meningitis, Parkinson's disease, arthritis, rheumatism, slip disc, spondilytis, TB, asthma(left heart) anemia, sciatica, polio and osteomyelitis, muscular and skeleton dystrophy (lethargic heart), childlessness (left Swadishtan), infections, neurosis, depressions, are all diseases of the left side.

Indulging too much in ruminating about the past and being engrossed in the subconscious, results in strengthening the Superego, and leads to a lethargic temperament that causes clots in the blood. False Gurus, hypnosis, alcohol, drugs (heroin, opium, hashish, marijuana), black and white magic, communicating with evil spirits, occultism, sex magic, homosexuality, perversion, tantrism, masochism, psychoanalysis - all cause mental disturbances.

Other manifestation of the subconscious illnesses are slyness, frightened behavior, talking too little, nervousness, lack of self confidence, shy of public, miserliness, excessive thinking of the past, all of which result in going deeper into the subconscious.

Cold Left Side

Left sided people are those, who are docile, who bear up the lot of others, cry and weep much and are on the losers end. They have

92

problems because their organs, like the heart, liver, intestines, have all become very lethargic.

Besides, they might also have some sort of bhada (catch) in them, in the sense they are possessed by someone. Of course some are possessed on the right side also. But left side possessions are peculiar, because they give you pain in the body. Right sided person does not get any pain himself, he gives pain to others, he is sarcastic, aggressive, he troubles others but left sided people have pain themselves.

Method to see which chakras are affected on your left hand:

Give yourself a bandhan raise the Kundalini and using a burning candle, move it with your right hand below the outstretched left hand, slightly touching your left hand with the flame. Do not move too quickly or too slowly, lest you burn yourself. You can make 11 or 21 rounds of movement. Turn the left hand and look where the soot is on your hand. This indicates the chakra that has the damage or affliction which needs to be cleared. If you do it every day, you can clearly see for yourself, how negativity works out.

Treatment of Left Side Problems

If you have less or no vibrations on your left hand, then there is an "overuse", imbalance or damage in the left side. There are several ways of correcting this imbalance:

1. Raising the vibrations from the right side and lowering on the left side, beginning from the right waist to the left as is done in bandhan but on the reverse side. This is similar to taking Chaitanya or vibrations from the balanced side and giving it to the exhausted side.
2. Left side is to be cleared by light. Place a lighted lamp in front of the photograph of Shri Mataji; put the left hand towards the photograph and right hand on Mother Earth. The left hand gets the light, and the light passes through,

and the right hand which is on Mother Earth, sucks all the negative forces. When you do this you will know when you are cleared out when the vibrations start flowing on the left palm. You can also feel the vibrations flow into Mother Earth through the palm of the right hand.

3. After having cleared the left side, we have to do the salt water treatment. Before beginning the treatment, get a tub of Luke warm water; add a fistful of salt to it. Stir it well. Also get a mug of clean water for wash after you have finished. After having got this ready, sit with both hands towards the photograph and put both feet in the tub of salt water. You must allow the vibrations to clear you out. Sit with eyes open for 5 to 10 minutes. Do not sit for too long. Get up, wash the feet with the clean water and throw out the salt water properly in a disposer. This should be followed by meditation. Doing this every day for about 10 minutes has a very good effect on the left parasympathetic nervous system.

4. With left hand towards the photograph and the right hand holding a burning candle or camphor, slowly raise it up and down on your left side, in order to warm up the frozen left side.

5. Stop daydreaming, and indulging in the past. Be dynamic and not lethargic.

6. Warm up the left side with a protein diet. When there is a problem on the left side, it means that it is frozen, and we have to try to defrost and warm it up again.

7. Use the Mantra "Om Twamewa Sakshat, Shri Mahakali, Bhadrakali, Kalikali, Sakshat Shri Adi Shakti Mataji, Shri Nirmala Devyai Namah Namaha".

8. Don't leave the house without giving yourself a bandhan. Attention must be within all the time. Wobbling eyes fritters away the attention. Fixing the attention, makes it focused and you feel very relaxed and relieved.

Some left sided diseases and their treatments

1. **Allergies**

   Allergy is an extreme reaction of the body due to intolerance to changes in the environment, food or atmospheric conditions. Left sided people are often afflicted by all kinds of allergies through their lethargic liver. Allergies are also caused when the body has to adjust to extreme effects of switching over from cold to hot things, like taking a bath in cold water and then hot water or taking coffee and then immediately drinking cold water. The system cannot adjust to these sudden changes.

   The spleen, which is in the area of the left Nabhi, is both a speedometer and an adjuster. When there is a sudden change, it causes a problem since it has to suddenly provide its energies to either increase or decrease the flow of the red blood corpuscles. This drives the spleen crazy and causes allergies.

   When a child has an allergy, its left Nabhi will catch. A child is naturally influenced by its mother, so by curing the left Nabhi of the mother it is possible to get the child rid of a catching left Nabhi. This can be done with the help of a little flame. Put your right hand on the left Nabhi of the child and your left hand towards the flame of a candle, and the child will be cured.

   Cow's or buffalo's milk aggravate conditions of allergies and eczema. But if the animal is smaller than you, like for e.g. a goat – the milk will not cause any harm. That was the reason why Mahatma Gandhi used to take goat's milk instead of the milk of a cow or a buffalo.

2. **Angina Pectoris**

   Angina Pectoris is caused due to the narrowing or hardening of the arteries on account of their getting clogged due to a clot due to which the supply of blood to the heart is restricted. It is caused due to a strain on the heart and in such conditions, even a slight excitement or extra activity provokes a heart pain, causing the person to slow down his activities. This leads to a lethargic heart.

People who take to all kinds of mantras or those who smoke cigarettes and chew tobacco spoil their left Vishuddhi. This makes the pumping of the heart difficult and it becomes tired. Due to extreme left Vishuddhi caused due to tension and worry and wrong life style contributes to the constricted arteries, high blood pressure and increase work for the heart. This makes the heart a very lethargic heart and ultimately leads you to angina. Saying the following affirmation: "Mother, you are my beej (seed) mantra, you are the Mantrika", will provide some relief.

Again with the right hand on the left Vishuddhi with fingers touching the spinal cord on the back of the neck and your head turned to your right, say, "I am NOT guilty at all, I am the pure Atman and I forgive everyone, Lord", will help clear the Vishuddhi chakra. Use light and fire to clear the left side with Ajwain along the left side across the back.

3. **Articaria**

Articaria is also a psychosomatic illness. When your liver is lethargic, it becomes vulnerable to disease and the person is not using much of his energies. Sauna helps in its activation and revival. This is also the root of blood cancer with people who are hectic.

Use gheru (worm eaten wood or the powder of worm eaten wood), rub it on a stone to extract a paste and take with honey. This is good for the elderly as well as it consists of soluble calcium. This paste has to be applied locally as well as all over the body. Then cover the body with a black cloth or soft tissue paper helps in giving heat to those parts.

4. **Asthma**

Asthma is mostly a left sided psychosomatic disease, where the lungs become lethargic. It sometimes can be right sided in people who are dry and dominating. In some cases the dryness of the peritoneum, could also be due to despair and a resigned attitude due to loss of someone dear like one's father, or even if he is totally unhappy about himself. It can also be a combination of any of the above. What is needed in such situations is to establish our sense of security. This can be achieved by placing an ice bag on the liver for 15-20 minutes twice a day. Sometimes the dryness may be due to sapping of energy on account of possession by a dead person or relative. The spirit of the dead person sucks up all the energy and is literally feeding on you.

In such cases, go into a meditative state, and bringing the dead person into conscious awareness, tell them that you are a realized soul and that you are perfectly well. Ask them to go and take their rebirth, and fulfill the purpose of their existence. Request them to assume a body by being born again so that they can get their Self-Realization. Asthmatic patients should not eat food that contains fat. Massaging the head with oil will be cooling and provide relief.

5. **Cirrhosis of the liver**

Liver which is situated on the right side of the abdomen just under the diaphragm is a vast chemical laboratory producing bile, cholesterol, lecithin, and blood albumin which is vital to the removal of tissue wastes, prothrombin essential to the clotting of blood and numerous other enzymes. It inactivates unnecessary hormones, breaks proteins into sugar and fat, synthesizes amino acids used in building tissues, and detoxifies drugs, poisons and toxins from bacterial infections. When there is cirrhosis of the liver, there is progressive degeneration of the liver structure and functions, and gradually the liver contracts in size and becomes hard and leathery.

A person with an infected liver is constantly complaining, finding faults with others, angry, very prejudiced and is very unbalanced. Cooling of the liver with ice packs, dietary regulation through liver diet, given at the end of this chapter will be very helpful in keeping the liver in optimum condition.

6. **Depression**

A person is depressed because he is constantly dwelling on the past as a result of which his entire left side is affected and frequently slips into the subconscious. Regrets of the past and a melancholic attitude further deplete the energy. Such a person to get back into balance should stop all lethargic attitudes and become focused on some kind of activity. The treatments that could be used to come off the grips of the subconscious powers are the matka treatment, shoe-beating, candle/camphor treatments, the modalities of which are mentioned elsewhere in this book.

7. **Diarrhea**

Diarrhea, commonly known as loose motions, is a condition where a person passes watery or loose unformed stools, which may be even acute or chronic. The chief cause of diarrhea is eating of extremely imbalanced food or overeating or eating wrong foods, putrefaction of the intestinal tract, fermentation due to incomplete digestion or excessive dosage of laxatives.

There is an imbalance as far as proteins are concerned due to which their muscles are weak. Hence these people also suffer from cold. Shri Mataji has suggested a simple method i.e. to boil fennel seeds and mint together in water and add a little sugar or candy sugar to it. Taking this compound twice or thrice a day will stop the diarrhea.

8. **Diabetes**

You get diabetes due to imbalance in the left Nabhi and Swadishtan. Now diabetes is not caused as a result of lethargic ways of the pancreas but it is actually (the) over-active pancreas that becomes lethargic. Pancreas is responsible for converting sugar into digestible parts or glucose or glycogen. This is done by the endocrines of the pancreas. This activity regulates the sugar level in the blood. The liver also has the function of supplying energy to the brain for thinking. When we think too much or are involved in too much brain activity most of the energy from the liver is utilized by the brain. Then what happens is that the sugar is consumed faster than it is manufactured, as a result of which the liver becomes over-active.

When the liver becomes overactive it is sucked up which is compensated by pouring of glycogen by the pancreas. Due to this over-activity, it becomes unable to produce insulin that regulates the sugar level in the blood and the person is diagnosed as diabetic. A lethargic liver causes diabetes, but the lethargy is due to over activity.

One of the functions of insulin is to increase the uptake of sugar by the liver. But when the liver has limited energy to secrete insulin, it needs to be artificially injected in. But in Sahaja Yoga we have a cure for this without injecting anything externally. You can cure diabetes by raising the vibrations from the left side and then bringing it down to the right side. When you raise, there is an awakening of the energy and then it starts working.

When it starts pumping energy due to the activation of the Swadishtan which is now in connection with the divine power due to awakening of the Kundalini energy the liver starts working out. But supposing the liver is in such a bad shape, that the individual Kundalini energy is insufficient, we need to tell Adi Shakti to play her part; this we do by raising the energy from the right side to the left side. She awakens it first. Adi Shakti works it out.

First you try to raise it with your own self, with your own hand, your own Kundalini, from the left to the right. But still it may not rise. If it is a bad case, then you have to rise from the right to the left. Like cases like infantile diabetes.

The question is often asked why children get diabetes.

Shri Mataji had clarified in one of her talks that children carry the blood of their parents and if the parents have been diabetic the blood that carries the pattern and message is passed on to the children. Every cell in the human body carries a complete pattern or structure and it is the principle of a cell to duplicate or produce more of it. It is molded by the kind of a personality you have. The mother's blood goes into the child's blood thereby carrying the same pattern there and that blood is then circulated.

If the mother is diabetic the child will also be diabetic. If the father is diabetic the son will also be diabetic. Women normally woman don't get diabetes, but if the women are very manly like politicians or housewives who plan too much about their household – what to cook and how to entice the husband etc. Such women are prone to be diabetic.

Diabetes is the action of the right side, affected by the left side. Right side being vulnerable, like when you think too much and pay no attention and remain in your habits, then a fear element to your vulnerability. Just like a hard working man, when he thinks too much, all his fat cells are used for the brain making the left side drained and vulnerable. Being afraid of something and then feeling guilty about it also tends to assist diabetes.

Correction and cure of this condition is the reciting of Hazrat Ali- Fatima mantra for energizing the left Swadishtan and Nabhi. Left Nabhi gets first affected, by having fear of wife or worries for her, or for any other family member. This fear and consequent vulnerability can be cured by clearing your Agnya chakra. Train yourself not to think too much by going into a state of thoughtless awareness. Take more salt as it neutralizes the action of sugar secretion, because it has got water of crystallization. Use ice on right Swadishtan and Nabhi. Avoid sugar, after proper tests, if necessary."

In Her advice to mothers in Sydney in March 1983, Shri Mataji very clearly affirmed, "See how I told you that when you are diagnosed for diabetes, the blood sugar comes in not because of sugar but because of thinking too much."

Dwelling on the subject of diabetes, Shri Mataji further went on to clarify how a diabetic normally tends to lose his or her eye sight. Speaking at Delhi on 3rd February 1983, she said, that when the Swadishtan Chakra goes out of order. It is represented here at the back [of the head], which is 'around' this back Agnya. So when you have diabetes or anything like that, people start becoming blind … You have seen many diabetic people get this blindness.

So first of all cure your diabetes by curing your Swadishtan. And also you can use an ice around your Swadishtan at the back … If it is Swadishtan you have to use the water [ice] but if it is 'just' the possession, then you have to use – without diabetes, if it is a possession – then you have to just use the light. That is how we cure our Agnya Chakra." (Talk on the Agnya Chakra, Delhi 3/2/83, Nirmala Yoga no.18)

"Now diabetes you do not develop by taking too much sugar – take it from Me. In India if you go to a village, you'll see that he takes sugar in such a manner that in the cup the spoon must stand at right angles, otherwise he won't take it. But he never gets diabetes. The reason is he doesn't think of tomorrow - he just works hard, eats his food and sleeps off, nicely. He doesn't take sleeping pills either. So this diabetes comes by over thinking and can be easily cured if you can take to Sahaja Yoga." (Talk at Worchester Hall, UK 1/8/89, www.irelandyoga.org/talks)

"If a pregnant woman is over thinking then the child may have diabetes."

9. **Drugs**

If you take cannabis you are definitely dragged into Ida Nadi and the ego recedes for the time being. All drugs take you away from your awareness. My experience about the druggist and chemist has been a painful one. Those who come were very slow. They have been very weak and vulnerable to left-sided attacks. I am sorry for the druggist. They have to use their will to accept the challenge and give up their slavery to drugs. (Letter to Jeremy, 1982, printed in Nirmala Yoga no.12)

Now, drugs hit you on the left-Nabhi or on the right. The ones that hit you on the left-Nabhi can take you very deep, down. And you can be sometimes so aggressive, despite the fact that you have taken a left-sided one. It is surprising. Just, you see, suddenly you get stunned. That person can become mad. Anything can happen to a person who takes drugs. (Advice on the treatment of virus infections, Pune, 1/12/87)

10. Epillepsy

Epilepsy is caused by the extreme movement of the attention to the extreme left. Collective subconscious is the state into which you go. This happens when you develop some fear or fright, being a weak person on the left side. Also when you happen to be involved into an accident or sudden fight or jerk.

The cure is to bring attention to the centre. To do this first bring it to the right, by saying Gayatri Mantra. Then shift to the centre by taking Shri Brahmadeva Saraswati Mantra. On moving to the right you start feeling vibrations .Stop at this point. Do not say any more Gayatri Mantra because you must not go too much on the right. Too much on the right means the frequency of vibrations starts decreasing. It needs proper adjustment from one side to the other.

It is important that you must get the vibrations. If not then repeatedly raise the Kundalini till you feel vibrations. Another best way is to put the left hand towards the photograph and the right hand is to be pressed on Mother Earth. Take Shri Mahakali Mantra, so that the vibrations start flowing. Use candle, from the back on the left. Candle treatment, shoe beating, matka treatment and foot-soak are the treatments recommended.

11. Infection

Infections are left sided diseases caused by bacteria or viruses. Treatment of the left side and the affected chakras is by use of vibrated water and vibrated soap. Vibrated ghee is also very good.

12. Fat

Question: Why has God created this Ego and Super-Ego within us?

Answer: From our stomach, the Med, the fat, rises into our brain, passing through all these centers, evolving to be the cells of the brain. Even brain is the Med, fat cells, what you call as Mendu. So for the Med to become the Mendu, it has to evolve, to achieve a certain amount of charges of awareness, of human awareness. (Q&A, Bharatiya Vidya Bhavan [Delhi], 22/3/77. Printed in The Life Eternal 1980)

Intake- For left side, if people eat Fat it is bad because the fat is stored and it is not available for circulation. For thin people their fat is available, so they can eat fat. But for fat people, they should only put fat in their nose, oil in the ears, etc. For fat people oil massage on the head is very good. These people can massage with Golden Amla hair oil. It cools them down. (Shivaratri 1987)

And, health-wise for those in the central channel, they are more on the fatter side, I should say, because they have gas in their body, lot of gas. The Prana Shakti is in the centre. The Prana enters into Sushumna. That creates the gaseous body. The gaseous body is not heavy, it's very light. They walk very fast, they are active. But to look at, they look plump, normally. If they are not they try to be plump. (Sickness and its cure, New Delhi, 9/2/83, Nirmala Yoga no.25)

13. Fever

Fever is caused to those whose liver is out or who has over worked his liver. He gets heated up. It can be corrected by putting ice on the liver. Malarial fevers are right sided, i.e. mosquito bites. Bacterial fevers are left sided. These are mainly due to certain food such as fungus, like mushrooms, stale food, etc. (Shivaratri 1987)

14. Flu

Flu, first of all, this is again left side, they have got a very good medicine in India - Basil leaves. Take lots of Basil leaves and make a concoction, boil it up in a pot, make it absolutely like an essence. Take it out quite thick, put tea and water in it, just make it the way you want to make it like a tea, with milk or whichever way you want it, less milk, sugar, because the taste may not be so good, and then you drink it. Before that you have to prepare some Ajwain smoke, inhale Ajwain smoke afterwards, you do it for three days, you will be alright, cleared out. (Rahuri Q&A 13/4/86)

15. Fungus

One of the worst things is fungus. It is from the left side. Again, the attack is on the left side; it is all from the dead. And you have to use the left side towards the photograph and the right hand to the places wherever you have the fungus. You may take it out that way. But do not eat cheese. All the Sahaja Yogis should not eat the fungus cheese that is the blue one, the crust one. All fungus must be avoided and also mushrooms if possible. (Rahuri Q&A 13/4/86)

16. Lack of Memory

Lack of memory is caused by overactive right side. Put the left to right 108 times and take the mantra: "Ya Devi sarvabhuteshu, Smruti rupena samstitha, namastasyai, namastasyai, namastasyai, Namo Namah".

Cirrhosis is nothing else but left side problem, is a lethargic liver, and gives you allergies. For Cirrhosis, left hand towards the photograph and right hand on the Mother Earth, putting hot water bottle on the stomach. Or even giving bandhan to your liver with the light is alright. (Rahuri Q&A 13/4/86)

Why do we call this liver, because of liver we live? Liver is very important in Sahaja Yoga. I know that in medicine we don t know much about liver. It is absolutely curable in Sahaja Yoga. Liver is the one which sucks up all the poisons and throws it into the blood.

Such a man who is always thinking, all his energy is going to the brain and other organs are neglected. First thing that is affected is liver. Now bad liver because it cannot throw its heat which is the poison of the body, so what happens is that heat starts rising. If it rises to the right side it goes to the right heart chakra which controls the lungs. Such a person can get asthma. Then it goes down to the kidney, with this heat kidney coagulates and you need dialysis and if not you die, but you die bankrupt.

17. Lumbago

For lumbago, you give Ajwain water. For muscular lumbago use Ajwain for intake and gheru (for application only). In lumbago, the bone gets twisted, therefore, use vibrated kerosene oil mixed with some other oil. In a few days it gets alright. (Shivaratri 1987)

18. **Malaria**

Fever is caused to those whose liver is out or who has over worked his liver. He gets heated up. It can be corrected by putting ice on the liver. Malarial fevers are right sided, i.e. mosquito bites. Bacterial fevers are left sided.

19. **Meningitis**

It is a left side bacterial disease, see BACTERIAL DISEASE.

20. **Menopause**

Menopausal symptoms often feature or are worsened by psychological and psychosomatic factors. As there is limited research into the potential role of psychological interventions, especially meditation, for the treatment of these symptoms the current study adopted an AB case series design with a follow-up phase. Fourteen women who were experiencing hot flashes and other menopausal symptoms and receiving no treatment for them attended meditation classes twice weekly for 8 weeks and practiced daily at home. A mental silence orientated technique of meditation called Sahaja Yoga was taught.

Substantial improvements in all measures occurred at post treatment. Changes in vasomotor symptoms, especially hot flashes, were most prominent as a significant decrease. All other symptom measures improved substantially from baseline to post-treatment, non-parametric analysis indicating that most of these changes were significant. These findings tentatively suggest that menopausal symptoms, especially vasomotor symptoms, and particularly hot flashes, might be substantially improved by using meditation."

Abstract to: Ramesh Manocha, Barbara Semmar, Deborah Black (2007) 'A Pilot Study of a Mental Silence Form of Meditation for Women in Perimenopause', Journal of Clinical Psychology in Medical Settings 14(3):266-273

21. Menopausal flushes

[a pilot study using SY meditation] -The results were very impressive with all women experiencing improvement in their condition. In fact 9 out of the 10 women reported at least 50% reductions in the frequency of their hot flushes. Six of these women had a 65- 70% improvement in their hot flushes which, after eight weeks of meditation treatment, is comparable to that seen in conventional hormone replacement therapy!

(Dr.R.Manocha. Researching meditation: clinical applications in healthcare. Diversity (Australian Complementary Health Association) June 2001; 2(5):2-10)

22. Mennstrual problems

If somebody is not having a child, and then she has a left Swadishtan problem. Same problem is also true for heavy periods. When there is too much stimulation in the Parasympathetic, in the sacral region, there is too much flow resulting in heavy bleeding. Other results are diarrhea and excessive urination.

Cure: Use of Gayatri mantra, initially. But it must also be backed by some medicines. You can give Ajwain smoke (even for surgery patients). (Shivaratri 1987)

23. Mental Problems

Apart from that [i.e. diseases of the physical side] we have the mental troubles with people. Like a left sided person will have a mental problem, like he will be a sly person, he will be a frightened person, he would not be talking to others, he would be nervous, he would not have self-confidence, and he will be running away from public. And also then, he comes schizophrenic that he hibernates sort of thing in the house, becomes like a cabbage. That kind of a lunatic he becomes. (Sickness and its cure, New Delhi, 9/2/83, Nirmala Yoga no.25)

Americans have got into problems of very serious nature, of very horrible diseases which I have predicted. Two of them, one which comes from AIDS and another one where a brain goes off, persons become mad at a very young age.

(Talk, evening before Diwali 1985)

MORGAN, A. (2000) Sahaja Yoga: an ancient path to modern mental health Transpersonal Psychology Review Dec 2000]

24. Multiple Scerosis

Multiple scerosis comes from Mooladhar and Nabhi. Left Nabhi and Mooladhar get affected more. It is more left sided. Therefore one should give the treatment of the left side. Saying the name of Ganesha and of Gauri will work out. Establish your innocence; work with flame on your left Mooladhar. Ask for Mooladhar cleansing techniques in your ashram. Massage your muscles with vibrated vitamin-oil. The same treatment goes also for MUSCULAR DISORDERS. (Rahuri Q&A 13/4/86)

25. Muscular Problems

See comments under Epilepsy: This treatment is also the same for cancer and other psychosomatic diseases. It includes Muscular skeletal disorders. In muscular problems, the trouble comes from your disturbed Sri Ganesha. (Shivaratri 1987)

When the vibrations flow, they relax the muscles. The muscles, in reality, have gone into spasms due to tensions, e.g. Left Vishuddhi. The vertebrae start to twist (physical). When you put your chakras in me (in my care) they will be relaxed and then you can adjust by giving vibrations. These vibrations can be given to others. You need not touch the other person, but give vibrations by using circular movement by hand using mantra. (Shivaratri 1987)

And so when the Mooladhar is gone off, the first thing that happens is that you get a disease which you know as AIDS, but also you get all the diseases which have to do with the muscles. The muscles start becoming weak. Advice on the treatment of virus infections, Pune, 1/12/87)

26. Neurosis

Is a left sided disease, see DEPRESSION.

27. Osteomylitis

It is due to lethargic left side.

28. Paralysis

It affects the Left side as well as the right side. Depends where Paralyses is active, this side you should give treatment. Ask: "Mother, I humbly ask you to forgive me".

29. Parkinsons Disease

It is a clear left side disease. Balance the left side.

30. Polieomylitis

[Discussing left-sided people and their problems] Cancer and muscular discrepancies and weaknesses in which the muscles become extremely weak gradually and Osteomyelitis, polio myeltis, - all these are due to lethargy

31. Psoriasis

Psoriasis is nothing but a left side problem; it is the lethargic liver and gives you allergies. For Psoriasis, put your left hand towards the photograph and right hand on the mother earth and observe the flow of energy. Putting hot water bottle on the stomach or even giving bandhan to your liver with the light is all right. Now people might think Psoriasis is active liver or inactive liver. You see it comes to that point.

We have only two types, active or inactive. Now whether psoriasis is inactive or active we will know from one point that when the liver is inactive, you get the allergies and when it is active, you get other problems like nausea and also get biliousness. You don't eat much; you thin down- all these problems are there.

32. Rheumatic pain

It is caused by left side. Person wishes to give. Treat the left side. Use vibrated kerosene-oil with some other oil to massage the paining joints. Ask a Sahaja Yogi to put his hand on the paining joints and the other hand on Mother Earth. This Mother Earth will suck in the pain.

33. Sciatica

It is caused due to the left sympathetic. Left Nabhi and left Swadishtan. Put right to left, give vibrations to affected chakras. Use kerosene with oil massage.

34. Schizophrenia

On the left side, one starts getting many diseases like schizophrenia, in the upper level of this 'group'. This side, these same seven centers act to give you very serious troubles. One of them is that people become schizophrenic. It can be cured; it can be cured, if you can move that person to the center and by Kundalini awakening you can do it."

(Navaratri Puja 2000)

"Now, you see the disease of schizophrenia also can come from Mooladhar problem."

(Shri Ganesha Puja 26/8/90)

"All your incurable diseases, right from all muscular troubles like Mellitus and all that, all your incurable diseases right from Cancer onwards, all your psychosomatic problems right from Schizophrenia and everything come because of the disturbance in Mooladhar. When the roots are not all right, how can you cure the tree? If the roots are all right then any medicine can reach any center, any area, any place, and any fruit. But if the roots are not all right, how can you work it out"

(Establishing Shri Ganesh principle, San Diego, USA, 7/9/86)

"Apart from that [i.e. diseases of the physical side] we have the mental troubles with people. Like a left sided person will have a mental problem, like he will be a sly person, he will be a frightened person, he would not be talking to others, he would be nervous, he would not have self-confidence, and he will be running away from public. And also then, he becomes schizophrenic that he hibernates sort of thing in the house, becomes like a cabbage. He becomes that kind of a lunatic."

(Sickness and its cure, New Delhi, 9/2/83, Nirmala Yoga no.25)

35. Slip Disc
It is a left sided disease, see LUMBAGO.

36. Spondylysis
It is left or right depending on overwork or over activeness of persons due to one's responsibility. Correct the imbalance. Affected parts have to be treated by using vibrated kerosene-oil and any other oil. Foot-soak in luke-warm saltwater.

37. Stress Disorders
The common problem is the stress. Now why do we have stress? Ida and Pingala are two channels and they cross each other at optic chiasm. Pingala Nadi (Right sympathetic) creates ego balloon, Ida Nadi (Left sympathetic) creates super ego balloon (due to conditionings).

When you are too right sided then ego moves and covers the left side, so there is a block; whatever problem you have it cannot pass out of your body. Then you become weaker and weaker. That is how you have stress (New Delhi talk to doctors 6/4/97. Transcript in New Delhi Medicos 13(4-5):32-34)

[see also Chug, D., et al. (1989) New insights into the aetiopathogenesis of essential hypertension and role of Sahaja Yoga in its treatment and prevention Proceedings of the XIIth International Union of Physiological Sciences Conference, Kupio, Finland, 3rd March 1989 Rai, U.C., et al (1988) Some effects of Sahaja Yoga and its role in the prevention of stress disorders Journal of the International Medical Sciences Academy 2(1):19-23. Reprinted in Stress management through Sahaja Yoga. 2nd edition (1995):23-30; also in New Delhi Medicos (1997) 13(4-5):35-38

38. Swellings

Another problem those in the central channel may develop is that if they have taken too much vibration, they may develop a swelling their body. Under these circumstances, first of all they should find out if they are in the neighborhood of somebody who is anti- God because such swellings are developed when the vibrations are fighting anti-God activities of the person who is with you. Say your wife is negative. Then such a person might develop a swelling because his vibrations are fighting the woman. He should not mind the fighting. But he must know how to correct the woman. He must know how to put her right. Or the man who is like that, the woman might develop an anti-devil force within her which gives her that swelling. Different types of swellings might appear, with the vibrations jetting out with a great speed. (Sickness and its cure, New Delhi, 9/2/83, Nirmala Yoga no.25)

The whole forehead, if it is full of lot of bumps, then we must know that the Kalki Chakra is out of order. If it is out of order then the person is about to go into some sort of very bad calamity, it is a sign on a person when he is going to get it. When the Kalki Chakra is caught up, all your fingers start burning, on the hands, on the palms and the same time in the body you get terrible burning. A persons Kalki Chakra catching means that he will be down with a horrible disease like Cancer, may be leprosy or may be that he is about to collapse into some sort of calamity. (Talk on Shri Kalki, Nirmala Yoga no.12, 1982)

When you have a very inflated ego, then you'll find a big blob-like ego coming out on left side, a very big one. Or you have a super- ego you can see another big thing jutting out of the brain on the right side. So, on both sides you might get swellings if both the sympathetic are over-active. If you are not a very collective person you might get a blob here. So you might get the entire thing filled up with your ego, superego, and this Virat centre again blown up in a way that a person develops a face like a monster sometimes! (Ekadashi Rudra Puja, 17/9/83, Nirmala Yoga no.21)

The Ekadashi Rudra shows on your forehead, and you get a swelling over here. Most of the cancer patients, if you see them, they have, from left to the right side quite a lot, of bumps there, on the right hand side.

{Ekadashi Rudra Puja, Austria, 8/6/88}

When a chakra is caught up you find it coming out as a big lump in the right side, so you have to take the name of Mahavir to remove that pressure from the left side. (Mahavir Puja, Perth, Australia, 28/3/91)

39. Tintinitis[ringing in the ears]

Put your alternative hand over opposite ear, with the other hand towards the outside, changing after a period. (reply to Melbourne yogi, 1995]

40. Tonsils

For tonsils we put the thumb, very clean thumb, in an antiseptic way, and press the tonsils on both sides and also on top. So tonsils cannot grow after that; just tonsils cannot grow and this upper portion called uvula also doesn't grow. It is a very simple thing that can be done to children. (Talk to Mothers and Babies, 1983)

41. Tuberculosis

It is caused by malnutrition, lack of protein and left side imbalance in the Left Nabhi/Swadishtan and Heart. You should raise the vibrations from right to the left. Foot-soak with right hand palm facing downwards to the floor. Give vibrations to affected chakras.

42. Tumor

Left side is affected. Give vibrations to the affected chakras. Use full left side treatment.

43. Varicose Veins

Varicose veins come from standing too long or standing all the time and they work very hard. As soon as it starts it is better to cure that. You have to lie down every day, those who stand every day for more than say three or four hours should lie down on bed and do cycling every day. That will help. Reduce the weight maybe. Due to weight also, some people might get that. But I have seen those who stand for a long time without the heels, if you use the heels you might be better off. With the heels, the pressure is not so much; it is distributed more to the lower, those five chakras down below. That might help.

But best is to do exercise after you have stood for a long time. Just lie in the bed and do cycling. Slow massaging downwards also helps. It can work out with the ice cubes as well. You can put some ice before massaging, you can put the ice then and use very cold oil and rub it. It will work out. (Rahuri Q&A 13/4/86)

44. Viral diseases and viruses

"Viruses come from the left side imbalance. They are dead entities that settle into the collective subconscious." Shri Mataji revealed while addressing the Medical Conference at Moscow in June 1990 to an august assembly of scientists, researchers and scholars. On another occasion speaking at the Ekadashi Rudra Puja at Austria on 8th June

1988, Shri Mataji had explained that in the process of evolution there were many plants, animals that were destroyed because they were not in the centre. So they went into the collective subconscious and came as subtler entities to harm the people who were ascending. We see these viruses that attack us. These are the plants which had gone out of circulation.

"If somebody has viral attack, you may give him all kinds of antibiotics, it won't help. Only Sahaja Yoga can drive it out, because Sahaja Yoga can act on the left side problem."

In left sided diseases, you get into the collective subconscious, from where you collect Protein 52, viruses. These make you helpless sometimes."

45. Venerial diseases

This is caused due to an imbalanced Left sympathetic and a disturbed Shri Ganesha. Establish your innocence. Correct the imbalance of the left side.

Chapter 21

Healing the Right Side

Diseases of the right side are caused due to over-activity. Fever, heart problems, heart attack, palpitation, asthma, constipation, liver problems (hot liver), problems with the lungs, unhealthy skin, tension, cirrhosis of the liver, headache, diabetes, leukemia, kidney, high blood pressure, childlessness (flirting type and thinking that one is too much beautiful), insomnia, lack of memory, spondilytis, jaundice, malaria, hysterectomy, heavy periods, dyhoeria, excessive urination, lumbago, muscular lumbago, etc. are all diseases caused due to over activity of the right side. Over activity and the resultant problems of the right side are caused due to over development of ego, quarrelsome and aggressive nature, PSI, psychosis, telepathy, drug addictions (like LSD, cocaine, mushroom), Hitler-like ideas, over natural powers, sadism, over ascetic life, forced sex abstinence, all extremes sports, work-holism, materialism, fashion fads, greed for power, anthroposophy, Steiner, TM, shamanism, fanaticism, scientology, etc., mental disturbances, Idiotic ideas survive, hot temper, obnoxious, cruelty, troublesome nature (may not look mentally upset), old age defects like being very talkative, accusing nature, dominating, asceticism, martyrdom.

Hot Right Side

Put the right hand towards the photograph and raise left hand towards the ether. Ether takes away the heat, but what actually happens is that your right side gets the vibrations and the heat is pushed towards the left and passes into the ether. Now this heat has to go away.

Right sided peopleshould not use any light at all, should not sit in the sun, but should sit in Moonlight. They should read poetry and they should not tie up watches, they should not look at the time permanently and they should become very emotional people. They should sing songs of Bhakti. They should not do Hatha Yoga.

Right Side Problems

If you are feeling less, or no vibrations, or even heat in your right hand, then there is an imbalance in the right side.

There are several ways of correcting this imbalance.

1. Raising the left side and lowering the right side; in this way you take from the strong left and give it to the exhausted right side.
2. Right hand towards the photograph and left hand pointing towards the sky. In this way "Akash" (Ether) absorbs all the heat and all the fumes of the right side.
3. Right hand towards the photograph, left hand in cold or even ice water.
4. Use carbohydrate diet and lots of sugar to cool down your right side (Liver diet).
5. Use icepacks on liver and right side.
6. Stop futuristic attitude and over planning, stay in the centre.
7. Have rest during the day time.

8.   Ask in the centre for the right mantras. When there is a problem in the right side, it means that it is heated up; it has to be cooled down and soothed.

Some right side diseases and their treatments-

1.   Cancer

For cancer best treatment is of water, i.e. putting feet in the river, sea or in the water at home with the photograph. Water has the dharma of cleansing and hence Shri Vishnu and Dattatreya responsible for the dharma of human beings are to be worshipped.

They help you to cure also the local deity of the chakra that is attacked. Seating the patient before the photograph with the candle and his feet in the water, bring down your hands across the sympathetic nervous system towards the water. The patient will cool down gradually. If he gets realization, then he is cured.

{undated letter [1970s] to Dr.Rahul in Nirmala Yoga no.8}

You will be surprised, all those patients of deadly diseases, like cancer, etc, whom I have cured, all of them without exception were the victims of fake gurus and Tantric. I have not seen any cancer patient who was not connected with a false guru which is why it is said that doctors cannot cure cancer.

(lecture in Hindi, Delhi, 18/8/79, English translation in Nirmala Yoga no.17)

A persons Kalki Chakra catching means that he will be down with a horrible disease like Cancer, may be leprosy or may be that he is about to collapse into some sort of calamity. (Talk on Shri Kalki, Nirmala Yoga no.12, 1982)

So when a person is on his destruction, say for example a cancer has set in, you might feel a throb, here at the apex of your Void. It doesn't logically mean that if there is a throb there is cancer, but if there is cancer there will be a throb. That means the force of life is trying to push it. {Ekadashi Rudra Puja, 17/9/83, Nirmala Yoga no 21}

The Ekadashi Rudra shows on your forehead, and you get a swelling over here. Most of the cancer patients, if you see them, from left it rises to the right side quite a lot, or have bumps there on the right hand side.

{Ekadashi Rudra Puja, Austria, 8/6/88}

There are two sides of life, left side and right side, when they meet (when one side is overactive), you get the psychosomatic diseases. If the Kundalini rises what happens is that it nourishes those centers. But suppose you are using right side too much, left side breaks up. Then what happens is that your connection with the mains is lost. You are on your own and Cancer starts. Cancer can be cured not at a galloping stage but at an early stage. We have also tried some galloping stage patients. (New Delhi talks to doctors 6/4/97. Transcript in New Delhi Medicos 13(4-5)32-34)

2. **Blood cancer**

Blood cancer is the result of speediness. So, one has to be very careful that the spleen is alright. (2nd Sydney Talk, 27/3/81)

In the left Nabhi area is the spleen. The spleen is a speedometer and also an adjuster. When it adjusts and it is not properly done due to sudden change, it causes problem. So it has to suddenly provide its energies to either increase or decrease the flow of the red blood corpuscles. That is how the spleen goes crazy. This is also the root cause of Blood Cancer for people who are hectic. (Shivaratri 1987)

The spleen produces red blood corpuscles for all emergencies. Modern life is always an emergency. Constant shocks to the spleen make it crazy and vulnerable to cancer. At such a moment of vulnerability if something triggers from the left side then blood cancer accrues. (Address to Medical Conference, Moscow, June 1990)

3. **Breast cancer**

    the sense of chastity in the Indian women is so great that nothing can deter them as long as they are chaste. But if they are not chaste, then fear settles in them 'very' fast. Chastity is the strength of women. And that is why, those women who have fear, mostly, have a problem of their chastity being challenged. A woman, who is frightened that her chastity may be disturbed, also can develop a problem with the heart chakra. Such women can develop breast cancer, breathing troubles, and other kind of frightening diseases on the emotional level also. (Talk on the Heart Chakra, Delhi, 1/2/83)

4. **Throat cancer**

    If you smoke too much then this Vishnumaya gets very angry. She, she is the one who then causes cancer. She can spoil your throat. I mean all kinds of ear, nose, and throat problems can come in with the smoking because she doesn't like that smoke. ... With that if you smoke, smoking, you can become also very much vulnerable to cancer of the throat. (Shri Vishnumaya Puja, New York, 19/7/92)

    Another thing which people do not know is the mantras. Now Shri Vishnumaya is the Mantrika; she is the one who gives the power to the mantra. Now if you are not connected to this divine power then there is a short circuit, and if you go on saying this mantra you develop all the troubles of the throat, throat cancer. You can develop also stomach problems, because Krishna and Vishnu are the same in the Virat, so, you might develop also the problem of Virat. (Shri Vishnumaya Puja, New York, 19/7/92)

    See also comments under epilepsy: This treatment is also the same for cancer and other psychosomatic diseases (Shivaratri 1987)

    [See also: Rai, U.C. (1993) Sahaja Yoga for the treatment and prevention of Cancer. In his: Medical science enlightened pp166-174]

5. **Constipation**

All such people i.e. right-sided people have over-active organs. Due to overactive organs, they develop a very bad heart, which is overactive. Palpitations take place in the heart that pumps fast. He develops asthma in the lungs. In his intestines, he develops constipation; he develops a very-very bad liver and a very unhealthy skin. The skin is extremely sallow. And such a person is very-very quarrelsome and aggressive (Sickness and its cure, New Delhi, 9/2/83, Nirmala Yoga no.25)

The heat from the liver after some time collapses the lungs leading to asthma. When the liver does not get enough nourishment then it becomes overactive. The intestines dry up causing constipation. (Address to Medical Conference, Moscow, June 1990)

The best thing if you are constipated is to read the newspaper. It's a simple thing. And read horrid news. That's how I see some people, I have treated. They say: We are constipated, I say: Read a newspaper in the morning. (Talk to Mothers and Babies, 1983).

We have so many ways of removing constipation in India. Like, we take Ajwain ka churan with black grapes, dried ones, raisins, black raisins. Prunes with orange juice are good; or also milk, boiled milk in the night. (Talk to Mothers and Babies, 1983)

It is caused by dry right side. Use carbohydrate diet (not macrobiotic, it makes it worse). Put dry figs in hot water, leave it over night, and drink the juice.

6. **Diabetes**

Is the action by the right side, affected by the left side? Right side is vulnerable. Firstly when you think too much (uncontrolled thinking), pay no attention and remain to your habits, then a fear element adds to your vulnerability. All the fat cells are used for the brain. The right Swadishtan goes into action and neglects its left counterpart. The left side gets drained.

At this stage, if some fear comes in and you also start feeling guilty, diabetes develops. Correction is to use Hazrat Ali's name as mantra. Source is Swadishtan and Nabhi on the left. Nabhi gets first affected, by having fear of wife, or worries of any of the family members. Clear it by clearing your Agnya Chakra. Forgive with your whole heart, do not think too much. Go in thoughtless awareness. Put left to right.

Take more salt so that it neutralizes the action of the sugar excerption, because it has got water of crystallization. Use ice on right Swadishtan and Nabhi. Avoid sugar, take proper tests if necessary.

{Shivaratri 1987}

There is one more thing that happens to our eyes. When the Swadishtan Chakra goes out of order, it is represented here at the back [of the head], which is around this back Agnya. So when you have diabetes or anything like that, people start becoming blind. You have seen many diabetic people get this blindness. So first of all cure your diabetes through curing your Swadishtan. And also you can use an ice around your Swadishtan at the back. If it is Swadishtan you have to use the water [ice] but if it is just the possession, then you have to just use the light. That is how we cure our Agnya Chakra.

{Talk on the Agnya Chakra, Delhi 3/2/83, Nirmala Yoga no.18}

If a pregnant woman is over thinking then the child may have diabetes. (Address to Medical Conference, Moscow, June 1990)

7. **Diarrohea**

Too much stimulation of the parasympathetic in the sacral region causes Diarrhea. Use Gayatri Mantra initially. The treatment must also be backed by medicines. Give Ajwain dhuni (even for surgery patients).

8. **Headache**

Headache is mostly caused due to the right over activity, too much ego. Also caused through Vishuddhi problem, or also when right Swadishtan gives you pain on its region on the head. Balance yourself and try to be thoughtlessly aware. Ask: "Mother, please come in my head" and "Mother, please I humbly request you to forgive me."

9. **Heart Attacks**

Cause: Over-active, inactive or lethargic heart.

Overactive heart is of right sided people. In such cases, the heart can collapse. Especially it can happen at very young age. This is because their attention is too much on the outside. Due to this, their Atma departs. The Atma gets no attention, due to their extreme materialistic nature. Over activity can also come from too much worry about the family, and thinking too much of the future. The heart starts to pump more blood, and over works itself. It gets tired. In addition, the attention is not on the spirit.

For lethargic hearts, these people take all kinds of mantras and first spoil their Left Vishuddhi. They take tobacco and cigarette, creating a problem on their Left Vishuddhi. This makes the pumping of the heart difficult, and so it becomes tired, because it cannot pump. Due to extreme Left Vishuddhi, the lethargic heart gives you Angina.

Those are the two types of heart attacks.

The first type can be cured by putting ice on the stomach and on the heart on the right side. Also move from left to right. Sit in water. Do not use light at all. Sleep in darkness, stay more indoors. Take full rest. And repeat that I am the spirit. O Lord, please forgive me.

The second type can be cured by asking him to say "Mother you are my beej mantra. You are the Mantrika. Also I am not guilty, and say I forgive everybody Lord" - so that, all the hurts disappear. Use light and fire to clear the left side. (Shivaratri 1987)

Now according to Sahaja Yoga we have two types of heart attacks, one is massive heart attack; the other is lethargic like Angina.

So the first one, which is massive one, is where that heat from the liver reaches the heart. Say there is a boy who is playing tennis at the age of 21 or 22 and drinking also and competing with his father. If you continue this kind of things may be you might get one day a massive heart attack, specially the industrialist. Industrialists are so futuristic, so much calculative that they don't calculate that this will entail their heart problems. So this heart suddenly collapses and they die.

Another one is lethargic heart attack like angina, and happens if you feel guilty. Some people are very sensitive and very formal type and you know they feel guilty, I should have done this. For anything they start feeling guilty. Not only you develop spondilytis, you develop a situation where your heart cannot pump properly. That is the angina. (New Delhi talks to doctors 6/4/97. Transcript in New Delhi Medicos 13(4-5):32-34)

[See also: Rai, U.C. (1993) Role of Sahaja Yoga in the treatment and prevention of some heart diseases. In his: Medical science enlightened pp175-180]

10. Heart Collapse

Results from over activity on the right side, too much ego, domination and "I"-ness. Then the attention is not on the Spirit, the Spirit is neglected. This and the pressure of the ego on left heart will lead to heart infarct. The heart can collapse when the attention is too much outside. Then the Atma departs. The Atma gets no attention due to over materialistic nature. It can also come from too much worries for family members and thinking too much of the future. Then the heart overworks itself, it gets tired.

Cure: Put ice on the stomach and heart on the right side. Move left towards the right. Sit in water. Use no light at all. Use affirmation of left heart.

11. High Blood Pressure

High blood pressure is a right sided problem and caused due to over activity of the right side. Treatment is very easy, raise left and lower the right and it will work out very quickly.

12. HIV/AIDS

(Sydney Press Interview 1985)

When the Mooladhar is gone off, the first thing that happens is that you get a disease which you know as AIDS, but also you get all the diseases which have to do with the muscles. (Advice on the treatment of virus infections, Pune, 1/12/87)

[See also: Rai, U.C. (1993) Behavioral modification through Sahaja Yoga a strategy for the prevention of AIDS. In his: Medical science enlightened pp181-186. Also in New Delhi Medicos (1997) 13(4-5):48-50]

13. Hot Liver

Hot liver is caused due to much thinking and planning, living in the future, overwork the liver, then it becomes hot. As the liver represents the attention, our attention becomes weak, we cannot keep it within. The symptoms are like JAUNDICE, we have to cool down the liver by using liver diet (see LIVERDIET). Put the vibrations from left to right 108times, with left hand on the liver and say the mantra: "Mother, please purify my attention" and "Shri Chandrama". Give icepack to the Swadishtan and also massage the liver with ice. With your left hand on the liver use the affirmation: "Mother, verily you are my guru".

14. Hypoglycemia

Hypoglycemia or low blood sugar comes from over activity. You should not think so much. Agnya chakra gets affected. One should surrender yourself to Christ, it will work out. (Rahuri Q&A 13/4/86)

15. Hysteroctomy

In Hysterectomy cases, where the uterus is removed, the problem is of Sri Ganesha and fear element. (Shivaratri 1987)

16. Infertility

Such people who are right-sided can become barren women, they may not have children at all. Especially women who are very-very flirtatious type and who think they are very beautiful, and also they are having a very active life, can become completely barren. (Sickness and its cure, New Delhi, 9/2/83, Nirmala Yoga no.25)

If somebody is not having a child, then she has a left Swadishtan problem. (Shivaratri 1987)

17. Insomnia

This is the result of an overactive right side. Put left to right.

Mantra: "Ya Devi Sarva bhuteshu, Nidra rupena samstitha, namastasyai, namastasyai, namastasyai, namo Namah".

18. Jaundice

Right Nabhi and right Swadishtan are affected. Put left to right 108 times. Do Foot-soak in lukewarm water.

Use affirmation: "Mother, verily you are my guru." Follow a strict liver diet for 2 weeks. Make tea from fresh radish leaves, sweeten with candy sugar and take instead of water for three days. Drink also much glucose water.

19. Kidney Problems

Right Swadishtan is affected. Take cool foot-soak. Use icepack on right Swadishtan. Put right hand on right Swadishtan at the back, taking the mantra: "Shri Brahmadeva Saraswati". After the mantra has finished, brush down three times. Repeat it six times. Diet without salt, drink much vibrated water, no meat.

20. Lack of Memory

This is caused by overactive right side. Put the left to right 108 times and take the mantra: "Ya Devi sarvabhuteshu, Smruti rupena samstitha, namastasyai, namastasyai, namastasyai, Namo Namah".

21. **Leucamia**

See BLOODCANCER.

22. **Malaria**

Comes from the right side, cool down the right side in every.

23. **Palpitation**

It is caused due to right side. Put left to right 108 times. Balance the right side.

24. **Paralysis**

At the level of the brain the right sided people become ego- oriented. The ego can go to that level, that they can develop paralysis. Paralysis is possible in both the cases. Even the left side person can get it or the right side person can get it. But mainly people get the paralysis on the right side. It comes from left side but affects the right side of the body. (Sickness and its cure, New Delhi, 9/2/83, Nirmala Yoga no.25)

Third disease that I told them will be coming very soon, where people who suffer from ego will be captured by ego. In that case the conscious mind will be taken over by ego. That means unconsciously you can walk, you can move about, but consciously you won't be able to even move your finger. That means you will be completely immobilized. The West is in great danger. Because, in the West only, you find this horrible disease called racialism. All the racists would be first, completely paralyzed. (Talk, evening before Diwali 1985)

Left side affects also the right side. Depends where Paralyses is active, this side you should give treatment.

Ask: "Mother, I humbly ask you to forgive me".

25. **Period Heavy**

This is also due to an over active right side. There is too much stimulation in the sacrum region.

26. Skin Diseases

All such people [i.e. right-sided] have over-active organs. Due to overactive organs, they develop a very bad heart, which is overactive. Palpitations take place in a heart that pumps fast. In lungs he develops asthma. In his intestines he develops constipation; he develops a very-very bad liver and a very unhealthy skin. The skin is extremely sallow. And such a person is very-very quarrelsome and aggressive. (Sickness and its cure, New Delhi, 9/2/83, Nirmala Yoga no.25)

27. Tension

Right sided problem. Use treatment of the right side.

Chapter 22

Chakra Cleansing and Achieving a Balanced State

In this chapter we shall see the qualities of each chakra, how they get affected and how each of them can be cleansed so that their bloom forth their splendor in the light of the spirit.

1. Mooladhar chakra

Mooladhar means the centre which is the support of the root of creation. The Mooladhar chakra is placed in the lowest region of the trunk of human beings about one inch above the centre of the seat. This most vital and important centre is in a subtle form. The gross expression of this centre is the pelvic plexus which surrounds the subtle centre.

The chakra has four petals, which appear as ripples in arrow like lines. The petal that points downwards has three further arrows, representing harmony, sense of balance and the sensitivity of the subject to innocence. All three threaded together, when developed fully through dedication, innocence and chastity gives the person a joy as identified with the joy of creation.

Qualities:
Eternal childhood, wisdom, purity, Holiness of Mother.

Causes of catches:

Unauthorized person tries to raise the Kundalini. Sin against the Mother, her holiness, her innocence and purity has been under the attack all the time. The causes include misuse of sex, sex outside marriage, sex for indulgent enjoyment, perversion of sex. Some false gurus know that and attack the chakras, and slow down or even ruin the seeker. It is also caused by misused tantrism, free sex and initiations by false gurus.

Treatment:

Central Mooladhar

1. Give vibrations to the chakra, left hand toward the photo, and right hand on the sacrum bone and between the legs.
2. Use the mantra of Shri Ganesha and Shri Gaurimata.
3. Use affirmation: "**Shri Mataji**, kindly make me innocent."
4. Sit on mother earth while taking vibrations (Mooladhar is made of the earth element) and mother earth will powerfully absorb the negativity in the chakra.
5. Take foot-soak treatment and allow all the negativity to go into the salt water.
6. Maintain purity of eyes and thoughts.
7. Take Ajwain smoke treatment.
8. Shoe beat the problem.
9. Watch Mother Earth.
10. be honest with yourself. No impurity in thoughts and words.

Left Mooladhar

As the above for the centre

1. Use the mantra of Shri Ganesha and Shri Gaurimata.

2. Use affirmation: "**Shri Mataji**, by your grace I am the pure innocence of a child."
3. IMPORTANT! Make Puja to Shri Ganesha in **Shri Mataji**.
4. Stop all tantric and occult practices.

Right Mooladhar

1. Dissolve all puritan ideas of sex; all austere attitudes and rigidity of any kind must be neutralized.
2. For constipation use carbohydrate diet for some time (Not macrobiotic).
3. Perform Puja to Shri Kartikeya in **Shri Mataji** praying that he destroys all the demonic forces and casts them to hell.
4. Use the mantra of Shri Kartikeya.
5. Use affirmation: "**Shri Mataji**, verily you are the killer of demons."

2. **Swadishtan Chakra**

Qualities:
Creativity, aesthetic

Center and Right Swadhishtan
Centre and right are one and the same.

Qualities:
Essence of creativity, external aspects, pure source of thinking, energy of the liver.

Causes of catches:
Thinking, planning and organizing make you lose your spontaneity, also extreme book learning and courses.

Treatment:

1. Left hand toward Photo, right hand on the chakra, give vibrations.
2. Left hand on the right Swadishtan, use affirmation: "Mother, please take away all my thoughts and doubts and give me inner peace". Or: "Mother, truly YOU are the creator and I do nothing at all".
3. Left hand on right Swadishtan, use the Shri Himalaya mantra (cooling).
4. Use cold or even ice water with salt for foot soak.
5. Icepack on right Swadishtan and liver.
6. Stop over planning and thinking and being futuristic.
7. Dissolve and shoe beat the tendency of anger.
8. Surrender your creativity to God, try to be spontaneous.
9. Use liver diet, lots of sugar, and brush down the right side.
10. Awaken the left side with Shri Shiva-, Chandradev- or Mahakali- Puja, which is the cooling aspect within you.

Left Swadhishtan

Qualities:
The knowledge of the divine techniques, truth and arts. Pure knowledge of truth, of how the divine works.

causes of catches:
Something unauthorized has entered in you; you have to be yourself.

Treatment:

1. Warm saltwater foot-soak, with a candle in the back of Swadishtan.
2. Bandhan with candle around your front Swadishtan.
3. Take Shri Ganesha mantra as quickly as you can 4 times.

4. Make from cotton wool a string, make 6 knots taking the mantras of the left side. Soak thread in mustard oil, light it and while looking at the flame, take Shri Shuddha Ichha mantra till the thread is burnt fully.

5. Use Shri Nirmal Vidya mantra (Pure knowledge) and Shri Shuddha Ichha mantra (Pure desire of God).

6. Use affirmation: "Mother, by your grace I am the pure knowledge of truth."

7. Stop indulging in impure knowledge, like teachings of false gurus.

8. Give vibrations to chakra by right hand on left side.

9. IMPORTANT: If there is a spirit possession, use Matka treatment and with the words: "In the name of **Shri Mataji Nirmala Devi,** the incarnation of the Holy Spirit, all the negativity which is possessing me – go to hell". Have a candle near the left Swadishtan and the right hand pressed on the left Swadishtan.

10. Write poetry, sing Bhajans, awaken the expressive side of your nature.

Other Affirmations:

"Mother, please give me the divine techniques and exclude all other techniques."

"Mother, by your grace I am the powerful knowledge of the divine and the truth."

Stop all involvement in past techniques of meditation. Stop all involvement in medium ship, clairvoyance, trance, clairaudience and other psychic practices.

Stop all psychiatric and psychotherapy treatments for mental disorders, and slowly reduce the intake of drugs given for the disturbance. Dispose off books, tapes etc. which are found to be giving bad vibrations (Pure knowledge comes from sources giving cool vibrations).

Note: A catch in left Swadishtan means, that there is some sort of spirit possession working. It manifests in your thoughts or in any chakra as a disturbance to the purity of YOUR subtle body. It has to be cleared out by:

1. Matka treatment
2. Shoe beating
3. String knotting
4. Paper burning
5. Candle treatment
6. Suitable treatment for chakra

Take food which helps to warm up. Improve the intake of salt. Combinations:

Right Swadishtan / right Nabhi - hot liver. Impatience, nausea, craving for salty food. Special liver diet.

Right Swadishtan / right Heart: possession by father.

Note: With all right side problems, one should sleep a lot, also in daytime.

3. Nabhi Chakra

Qualities:
Evolution, morality, nourishment, ethic, dharma (righteousness) ten commandments, honesty, welfare and well-being, maintenance.

Laxmi principle: Seeking God

Causes of catches:
Family and household worries, over-interest in food and money, suppress wife or husband, extreme use of pharmaceutical drugs, alcohol, immoral behavior, fanaticism, excessive fasting in the name of God. Unhealthy nourishment.

Treatment:

Center Nabhi Chakra

1. Use the mantra of Shri Laxmi Vishnu.
2. Use the affirmation: "Mother, please make me satisfied."

3. Give vibrations to the Nabhi.
4. Foot soaking in salt water. Water element is the most important in this chakra. It should be used in every way, like drinking vibrated water, foot soak, bathing etc.
5. In addition, there is some fire element in the Nabhi also.
6. Vibrate food and drinks which are not prepared by Sahaja Yogis.
7. Massage the mid back and stomach areas.
8. Massage your knees and elbows.
9. Eat enough food to keep your body covered with flesh, eat only until you are satisfied.
10. Be honest towards others and especially towards yourself.
11. Be satisfied with everything that happens to you; whether it seems nice or bad, it always is the right thing for you, and you should try to make happily the best out of it.

Left Nabhi Chakra

1. Use the mantra of Shri Gruhalakshmi.
2. Use Affirmations: "Mother, by your grace I am satisfied." "Mother, by your grace I am a generous person."
3. Give vibrations to the left side of the chakra.
4. Develop the habit of being satisfied with every aspect of life. Do not complain; be able to bear the problems. (This is a special quality of Gruhalakshmi.)
5. Develop the quality of auspiciousness and generosity. Remember the only value contained in matter, is the satisfaction it gives to others. Avoid miserliness.
6. When the role of husband and wife is reversed, correct it. Husband should be active, slightly stronger, and a little dominating, whilst the wife should be passive, and a little receding. She should draw her strength from her silent power as the Gruhalakshmi. (Men and women are equal but not similar.)
7. Abandon all tendencies to be "frantic" person, i.e. rushing meals, always doing things in a jerky manner and unable to

relax. This affects the spleen, our speedometer very badly, it loses control and diseases result.

8. Avoid precooked food. Chew your food well.
9. Increase the salt intake, especially if your problems are generally on the left side.
10. Foot-soak in warm water.
11. For overweight problems, take juice of three limes in hot water, 3 times a day.
12. For cold liver problems (causing allergies, hypersensitivity, rashes and dry skin problems) take 1/4teaspoon of gheru, 1 teaspoon of honey and warm water, 3 times a day.
13. Give bandhan with candle, clockwise around the left Nabhi. Left Nabhi also is to be cleared through the Agnya by forgiving.

Right Nabhi Chakra

1. Use the mantra of Shri Rajalakshmi.
2. Use the Affirmations: "**Shri Mataji**, verily you are the Royal Dignity in me." "**Shri Mataji**, verily you solve all my family / money worries and take care of my well-being."
3. Give vibrations to the right side of the chakra and to the liver. Massage with ice bag.

    (N.B. This catch will always be associated with right Swadishtan catch, when the liver is hot.)
4. Foot soak in cold or ice water.
5. Take to liver diet.
6. Stop worrying about money, work, family, material problems. All cheating and corrupt tendencies must be given up. Trust that GOD the Father will take care of you.
7. Where attention goes to these "outside" things, the Atma becomes covered or recedes and the joy is lost.

    By bringing the attention back to the Atma, attention is purified, problems get solved, liver cools down and joy returns.

Remember: liver problems are attention problems.

4. Void or Bhavsagar

Guru Principle Treatments:

1. Use the mantra of Shri Adi Guru Dattatreya and when appropriate, his 10 Incarnations. (Left: Janaka, Abraham, Lao-tse, Zoroaster, Sai Nath, Right: Moses, Nanak, Socrates, Confucius, Mohammed).
2. Use the Affirmation: "**Shri Mataji**, make me my own Guru / Master."
3. Give vibrations to the Void.
4. Where there has been adherence to a false guru, forget about it.
5. Throw away all Prasad, pendants, books, photographs, ashes, dresses and other objects given by the false guru.
6. Stop all techniques like chanting, fasting and special meditative techniques taught by the false guru.
7. Shoe beat the guru and the various forms of negativity you are suffering from him, e.g. recluse state, disturbed attention, anti social habits, etc.

Right Side

Incarnations:
Moses, Nanak, Socrates, Confucius, Mohammed

1. Understand that **Shri Mataji** gives you the knowledge, so SHE is YOUR teacher, guru or master.
2. Use Affirmation: "Mother, verily YOU are my master."
3. Use the mantras of the right side incarnations.

Left Side

Incarnations:

Janaka, Abraham, Laotse, Zoroaster, Sai Nath

1. Here, through the teachings and the grace of **Shri Mataji**, you are to become your own master.
2. Use Affirmation: "Mother, by your grace I AM my own master."
3. Use the mantras of the left side incarnations.

Severe Problems:

1. Take Matka treatment for weeks. Also use string knotting and paper burning techniques.
2. With stomach problems drink vibrated salt water.
3. Perform HAVAN to remove badhas of the false gurus.
4. There may be strong Agnya catch along with the void catch. In this case eyes may be unsteady, eyelids may flicker when closed. Keep the eyes open and simply watch **Shri Mataji's** Agnya chakra while foot soaking.
5. Foot-soak in warm salt water when left, and cold when right.

    A special case :When there is a strong devotion to one of the past incarnations of the Adi Guru, e.g. Shirdi Sai Nath, Confucius, etc., these devotees will often feel that by accepting **Shri Mataji** they are deserting the guru whom they loved and worshipped until Self Realization. This often causes a big obstacle for Kundalini's ascent and gives a serious left Vishuddhi catch. It has been explained that ALL the Incarnations of the Adi Guru have taken their place in **Shri Mataji** and they can be worshipped in HER. The Shakti is the same, and by worshipping them in HER, THEY are pleased. By not accepting that these Satgurus are now part of **Shri Mataji**, you are angering the Satgurus and they will harm you.

5. Anahat chakra

Center Heart

Qualities:
Holy Mother of the universe, physical mother, self confidence, fearlessness, sense of security, development of antibodies.

causes of catches:
Insecurity, fear, problems with the mother, childhood in unhappy families.

Treatment:

1. Use the mantra of Shri Jagadamba or Shri Durga Mata.
2. Use Affirmation: "**Shri Mataji**, make me a fearless person".
3. Give vibrations to the front and back heart.
4. Deep and relaxed slowly breathe in and out for a while.
5. Breathe in, keep the breath, in your mind say 12 times Jagadambe, breathe out; repeat 3 times.
6. Right hand on centre heart, 12 times take the name of Shri Jagadambe.
7. Candle treatment, if left Swadishtan is catching as well as centre heart.
8. Perform Puja with 108 names of the Devi.
9. Read Devi Mahatmyam.
10. Recite the 23 Psalm of the Bible.
11. If one has fear, write it on a piece of paper, put bandhan around it and burn or bury it.
12. Take the prayer: "Mother you are the most powerful Mother of the universe, and you are my Mother, You love me and protect me and nothing, and absolutely nothing can happen to me."

Left Heart

Qualities:
The Self, Atma, Spirit, to be (existence), Love, Joy (Ananda).

Cause of catches:
Disturbed relation with the mother, bad heartfelt relations, excessive physical and mental exercise, Mahayoga, blind faith, no confidence in God, anti God activities, outside attention, no seeking, and no interest in self.

Treatment:

1. Use the mantra of Shri Shiva Parvati.
2. Use Affirmation: "Mother, I AM the Spirit."
3. Give vibrations to left heart
4. Put **Shri Mataji** in your heart, and feel the JOY of HER presence and her love.
5. Keep the attention on the Atma.
6. Where left heart catches due to over activity of the right side, raise the left side and lower to the right side 108 times, and also ventilate the catch by putting right hand to the photograph and left hand upwards, pointing to the sky. Ether will dissolve the heat.
7. Ask for forgiveness for any mistake done against the Spirit without feeling guilty.
8. Use the practices listed under VOID, where the heart has been affected by false gurus.
9. Use candle and camphor as bandhan.
10. Use also the mantra Nirmala Atma Shiva.
11. Affirmation: "I AM the Spirit, only the Spirit, not this ego, not this emotion, not pain, only Spirit IAM, only Spirit." Do it several times with the whole heart.

Right Heart Qualities:
Dutiful happy blissful life as father, husband and king who gives us auspicious boundaries, responsibility.

Cause of catches:

Emotional aggression, father's problems, arrogant and reckless behavior, unauthorized dominion, economical and political suppression.

Treatment:

1. Use the mantra of Shri Sita Ram.
2. Use Affirmation: "**Shri Mataji**, verily you are the responsibility in me." & "**Shri Mataji**, You are the boundaries of good conduct and the benevolence of a good father."
3. Give vibrations to the right heart chakra, and also icepack.
4. Don't take too much responsibility, also don't be under responsible.
5. Develop the qualities of strength and protection of a father and husband. Correct any wrong relationship, which is coming from you as a father, husband, a son or a brother. Wives should not give reason for their husband's protective qualities to withdraw.
6. Take proper care and responsibility of your family and develop a benevolent attitude in Sahaja Yoga and in the community.
7. Develop the boundaries of good conduct in family life and in society (Maryadas).
8. Where the right heart catches due to an overemotional nature, raise the right side and lower the left 108 times and clear out the right heart catch by putting the left hand to the photo and the right hand on Mother Earth, so as to release the left side problem which caused the right heart to catch.
9. Read the "RAMAKAVACHA".
10. If there is a spirit possession, tell the relative that "I am a realized soul now, you do not have to take care of me, and I am perfectly alright. Please take a new birth, **Shri Mataji** is alive now and you will also have your Self Realization."

6. Vishuddhi chakra

Center Vishuddhi

Qualities:
Divine diplomacy, playful witness, omnipresence, collective consciousness, (Thyroid gland).

Cause of catches: Aggression, arrogance, lack of collectivity, lack of witness power.

Treatment:

1. Use the mantra of Shri Radha Krishna.
2. Use Affirmation: "Mother, make me a detached witness", "**Shri Mataji,** make me part and parcel of the whole", "**Shri Mataji,** make me a discriminating and self-correcting person."
3. Give vibrations to the Vishuddhi Chakra.
4. Put your index fingers in your ears, extend neck backwards, looking towards the sky, say Allah hu Akbar16 times.
5. Develop quality of detachment and witness state.
6. Massage the Vishuddhi area with oil, ghee or butter, and take butter in your throat.
7. Take saltwater gargle night and morning. Use Tulsi tea, and burn camphor.
8. Ajwain dhuni to clear nasal passages, sinuses and bronchites.
9. Press your chin to the chest bone, roll the tongue back, like swallowing it, do not touch the gum, and breathe relaxed and slowly in and out for 1 minute.
10. Breathe in with your nose, keep the breath for a while and breathe out and keep a while. With every inbreathing you should take a little less air, till you reach zero. Repeat 3 times.
11. Sip a little vibrated salt water through the nose.

Left Vishuddhi

Qualities:
Brother-sister relationship, self respect.

Cause of catches:
Feeling guilty, immorality, insidious way of speaking, sarcasm, lack of self respect, being poor in words.

Treatment:

1. Use the mantra of Shri Vishnumaya (sister of Shri Krishna).
2. Use Affirmation: "Mother, I am not guilty at all, as I am the Spirit by Thy grace; how can I be guilty."
3. Give vibrations to the Vishuddhi Chakra.
4. Avoid excusing and feeling guilty after doing something wrong or indulging your ego.
5. Develop the quality of purity in brother and sister relation.
6. Face any immorality or other sins of the past and know that Mother forgives you and that you should not feel guilty.
7. Evaluate yourself as an expression of the love of GOD; don't feel "useless" or inadequate. Don't be dominated by others.
8. Talk about Sahaja Yoga to others with confidence.
9. Sing Bhajans with your whole heart. Use your voice for worshipping
10. **Shri Mataji**.
11. Be not sarcastical or cynical.
12. If you have been using a mantra of a false guru, it has to be neutralized by affirming "**Shri Mataji**, You are the Source of all the great Mantras" or "Sarva Mantra Siddhi".

Right Vishuddhi

Qualities:
Witness of self, sweetness in sound, words, thoughts and behavior.

Cause of catches:

Cold, excessive responsibility, smoking, swearing, harsh talking, sinuses, too much singing and talking.

Treatment:

1. Use the mantra of Shri Yeshoda of Shri Vithala Rukmini.
2. Use Affirmation: "**Shri Mataji**, verily you are the sweet countenance of my words and deeds." "**Shri Mataji**, please take away all my aggression and dominance, give me a sweet voice, and make me a sweet and collective person."
3. Give vibrations to the right Vishuddhi.
4. Speak less, and if you do, try to avoid any tendency to dominate others by your voice.
5. Develop the quality of speaking sweetly to others.
6. Pay less attention to the taste of food.
7. Forgive everyone and dissolve your anger.
8. Don't argue with people or spend a lot of time convincing people of your point of view.

Medical Treatments of Vishuddhi

The best for Vishuddhi treatment is: Ghee-Butter-Oil and Salt. Oil is for the Krishna-principle very important, salt for the Master-principle. Both principles are mixed in the collectivity. When every single one is taking responsibility then the collectivity starts.

Eyes

1. When the eyes become weak due to much reading, learning or watching inauspicious things, use Netranjan or Kajal on your lower eyelids before sleeping.
2. Special for the lower chakras we recommend the following method:
   a) Rub a little Tiger balm under your nose.
   b) Rub a little honey on your lower eyelid.

c) In general looking in the sky, the green grass or earth.

Ears

1. Drop oil of primula.
2. Some garlic in olive oil, warm it up a little, soak cotton wool and before sleeping put in your ears.

Nose

1. Drop Ghee mixed with a little camphor in your nose, or use "Cold stop". Use it daily for your Hamsa.
2. Put Tiger balm in front of your nose.
3. Smell fragrant flowers, it clears your Agnya.

Mouth

1. Watch your teeth, brush them at least twice a day. Use a soft brush and dental floss is important.
2. Massage gums with finger using oil and salt. Very hard food is not good for the teeth; do not allow anything to stick between your teeth.
3. Clean the surface of your tongue.

Neck and Shoulder External

1. Massage daily with oil (any oil which contains vitamins). After cover yourself with shawl, oil dissolves the tensions and also affects the skin.
2. Massage your neck, chest and shoulder with Tiger-or Essential balm or Vick Vapo Rub. Afterwards cover yourself always, don't go into the cold.

Internal

1. Gargle with warm salt water or sage tea twice a day.

2. Eat honey, helps with severe problems.
3. Chew raw licorice.
4. Melt some butter or ghee in hot water and take it.
5. Mix Haldi with black pepper and ghee and take it.
6. Melt a little bit of butter on your tongue.
7. Roast some onions and inhale the steam.
8. Roast onion skin and put on your sinuses for 15 minutes.
9. Put Tiger- or Essential balm in hot water and inhale it.
10. Ajwain dhuni: Burn Ajwain on charcoal and inhale the fume.

Face and head

1. Massage with olive oil the sinuses, neck and shoulder, especially where you feel pain.
2. Massage your head with fingers, so that the scalp is moving. Once a week massage your head with oil (coconut or almond) sleep with the oil and wash next day.
3. Pull the hair in the region of the Nabhi. Above Back Agnya on the culmination.

All the above should be carried out religiously for a period of - say - 10 days, or a month in severe cases, and repeated after a while.

7. Agnya Chakra

Qualities:
Thoughtless awareness, forgiveness, compassion, resurrection.

Cause of catches:
Uncontrolled thinking, too much reading or looking at TV, Jewish or Christian "Fanaticism", worries, psychopharmaca, sexual fantasies, flirting, pornographic, unforgiving nature.

Treatment:

1. Use the mantra of Shri Jesus Mary or Shri Mahavishnu or Shri Mahalaxmi.
2. Use Affirmation: "Mother, make me a forgiving and sacrificing person."
3. Give vibrations by directing the vibration to the centre Agnya chakra, located inside the head at the point of crossing of the chiasm optical is at the pituitary gland.
4. Know, that when the Kundalini rises to your Agnya chakra, all your past sins are forgiven and your karmas are dissolved. Forget the past. The future doesn't exist, just be in the present.
5. Develop the state of thoughtless awareness: alert but not thinking. Nirvichar Samadhi. Use this state to dissolve your tendency to think too much.
6. Pray the "Lord's Prayer" with the whole heart.
7. Watch in a relaxed way, the Agnya of Mother's photograph.
8. Apply vibrated kumkum or sandalwood oil or balm on the forehead to protect the Agnya Chakra.
9. Let the down flow of the "Brahmashakti" remove all the angularities in your thinking, so that your thoughts and attention gets purified.
10. Use the light element, the subtle aspect of fire element, to enlighten this chakra.
11. Where there has been any "initiation" by a false guru, longer treatment may be required to remove the "badhas" put into the Agnya by the false guru. (Clear your Void also.)
12. Look through a flame at the photograph of Mother.
13. Smell scented flowers.

Right Agnya Qualities:
Ego, "I-ness"

Cause of catches:

Wrong ideas about GOD, doubt, worries, violence against others, aggressive attitude, egoism

Treatment:

1. Use the mantra of Shri Maha Kartikeya - Maha Hanuman - Maha Buddha - and Maha Saraswati. Forego use these mantras and in addition use Mahat Ahamkara.
2. Use Affirmation: "**Shri Mataji**, I forgive everybody, including myself" and "**Shri Mataji**, by your grace, keep me in your divine attention."
3. Give vibrations to the forehead, whole right side and also left top of head.
4. Reduce the pressure of the ego by stroking from the left temple over the forehead towards the right side, keep stroking downwards on the right side towards the right Swadishtan Chakra (Maha Saraswati Shakti).
5. Where there is an excessive over bloating of the ego, the Super ego becomes squeezed and "memory problem" shows up. Treatment as above.
6. Forgive everyone. Do not hold grudges or unforgiving attitudes, as others can manipulate your thoughts. To forgive is the simplest thing when seen in this light and it is also a great power of protection from malevolent thoughts. The power of forgiveness makes you very strong, and beautifully opens the way of Kundalini to the Sahasrar
7. Try to see that Lord Jesus Christ was opening the way to the spiritual rebirth. When this Agnya Chakra clears, our awareness fills with the light of HIS being, now in **Shri Mataji**.
8. Allow no unrealized person to touch your Agnya between the eyebrows or your eyelids.
9. Where there is excessive heat in the front and left side, or top, put ice bag.

10. Do not be "futuristic". The future does not exist in the present. If right Swadishtan is caught, very often Agnya also is caught. This gives serious problems and should be corrected by the treatments given above.

11. Forget the many wrong "conditionings". See the essence that was Christ.

12. Stop all meditative practices which involve the Agnya. Do not use concentration or visualization techniques and abandon "mind control" methods, clairvoyance, hypnosis and other "Siddhis" of the right Agnya Chakra. They are possessions and must be removed.

Left Agnya Qualities:
Constitution, remembrance, capacity of seeing (eyesight).

Cause of catches:
Harm yourself, self pity, conditionings, if you cannot forgive yourself.

Treatment:

1. Use the mantra of Shri Maha Ganesha - Maha Bhairava - Shri Mahavir - and Shri Mahakali and in addition Shri Manas Ahamkara.

2. Use Affirmation: "**Shri Mataji**, by your grace, please forgive me."

3. Give vibrations to the back of the head, and for superego to the whole of the head.

4. Without feeling guilty ask for forgiveness.

5. Avoid all impure use of the eyes. (This is also connected with the left Mooladhar).

6. Use candle treatment on the back head.

7. Tapping on the back of your head with right palm, left hand towards Mother's photo.

8. Reduce the pressure of the superego by stroking your left temple across the back head, downwards until the Swadishtan Chakra. (Mahakali Shakti).

9. Where there is excessive heat in the back or on the right side of your head, use ice-packs instead of candle treatment.

10. Sometimes superego becomes over bloated that it squeezes the ego and presses down the Vishuddhi at the base of the skull and neck. (This is sometimes wrongly treated as a Vishuddhi problem; it can be cured as above).

11. Do not live in the past. Reflecting on past events and relationship and nostalgic attitudes feed the superego. Break any useless conditionings and habits.

12. Surrender to the Super Ego of **Shri Mataji**.

13. in severe cases use burning camphor bandhan on the back head.

8. Sahasrar chakra

Qualities:
Integration, collective consciousness, silence.

Cause of catches:
Atheism, doubt in GOD and **Shri Mataji**, anti-God activities, anti-Sahaja activities.

Treatment:

1. Use Mahamantra.

2. Use Affirmations: "Mother, please give me Self Realization." "Mother, please be in my head."

   "Mother, please establish my Self Realization."

   "Mother, please accept my complete surrender and my sincerest thanks for making me a Sahaja Yogi /Yogini."

3. Give vibrations to the crown of your head, by massaging your scalp clockwise, using any of the affirmations, given above.

4. Develop the dedication to **Shri Mataji** through your meditation. (Not just recognition, but dedication).Know that She is in every molecule of creation and that She has created the creation.

5. Know that she alone has given Self Realization. (None of the other incarnations gave you realization but now they can be worshipped in **Shri Mataji**).

6. Know that through her only, the collectivity of all realized souls is being achieved. Know that she is the fulfillment of the prophecy of Lord Jesus Christ, when he said: "I will send you a Comforter, a Counselor, a Redeemer, the Holy Spirit, who will teach you all the truth".

7. Know that all the power which destroys all the negativity is working through HER Collective Being, first as the Ekadashi Rudra and ultimately as Shri Kalki.

8. Strengthen your connection to the divine, by stabilizing your Kundalini at the Sahasrar Chakra. Then only will the Brahma Shakti increasingly purify your being and give you the joy of Self Realization.

9. For your left Sahasrar problems, use the Affirmation: "**Shri Mataji**, verily YOU are the Victory overall the challenges to ascent" (Shri Kalki's Shakti).

10. For right Sahasrar problems, which indicate a left side problem, use the Affirmation: "**Shri Mataji**, by your grace, I am protected from the challenges and I will be victorious over all the challenges to ascent."

"Shri **Mataji**, by your grace, I am fortunate to be in the Attention of the Holy Spirit" (**Shri Mataji's** Shakti).

11. Finally, know that **Shri Mataji** has fulfilled all our desires as seekers. Now we have to fully establish our place, as realized Souls in the Kingdom of GOD.

Recognitions from the world

- Shri Mataji was invited by the United Nations for four consecutive years to speak on ways to achieve world peace between 1989 - 94
- Shri Mataji was an official guest speaker at the Women's Conference in Beijing and was official guest of the Chinese Government to speak to the people of China in 1995
- Shri Mataji was nominated twice for the Nobel Peace Prize
- St.Petersburg, Russia (1993) [Appointed as Honorary Member of the Presidium of the Petrovska Academy of Art and Science. In the history of the Academy only 12 people have ever been granted this honor, Einstein being one of them]
- Romania(1995)
- [Awarded Honorary Doctorate in Cognitive Science]
- St Petersburg, Russia (1998)[Inaugurated the International conference of Medicine and self-Knowledge]
- Doctorate in Cognitive Sciences from The Ecological University Romania (1995)
- Moscow(1989)
- [Shri Mataji had a meeting with the head of the Ministry of Health in USSR, following which Sahaja Yoga was granted full Government Sponsorship including funding for promotion of Scientific Research]
- Brazil(1994) [The Mayor welcomed Shri Mataji at the airport and presented her with the key to the city, and sponsored all of her programs]
- Italy(1996)
- [Declared "Personality of the Year" by Italian Government]
- London(1997)
- [Separate personal tributes paid to Shri Mataji from Claes Nobel (Grandnephew of Alfred Nobel) and Ayatollah Rouhani (leader of the Shia Moslems in Europe) at the Royal Albert Hall]
- India2001 [Manav Ratna Award in Pune]

Chapter 23

A Vision for the Future

It is a very privileged place for you to enter, into the Sahasrar of the Virat (The Cosmic Whole), to reside in the brain as cells of Sahasrar. These are specially created cells through the working of the Swadishtan. Passing through all the chakras, when they arrive at Sahasrar they are equipped to handle the brain's activity without getting involved with other elements in the body. The first thing that happens to a Sahaja Yogi at the Sahasrar level is that he becomes 'Beyond', (Atita). He transcends so many things; he goes beyond time, (Kalatita). Time is his slave. If you have to go somewhere then suddenly you discover that everything is working at the same time when you are able to do it. Like you are, say, to catch a train and you arrive late at the station, you find the train is late for you. Things work out in such a way that you feel they are all active for your complete convenient to go beyond time that is Kalatita.

Then you go beyond dharma (Dharmatita). That means dharma becomes part and parcel of your being. Nobody has to tell you, "You do this" or "you do that" - you just do it. Whatever you have to do, you do it.

When you go beyond all these dharmas, that are the human dharmas - human dharma is that one's attention gets attracted either with lust, greed to something, and then one cannot draw one's attention away. Then the attention becomes 'Dharmatita'. That means the attention loses its dharma.

The dharma of the attention is such that we have to use the dharmas taught by the prophets to control it because, we are coming (in evolution) from the lowest level. So these (lower) dharmas exist in our being and start showing, and when they attack us, then we have to have some measures with which to control them. So we build up our dharmas, OUR OWN SELF-REGULATION, and control those dharmas which have come to us from lower conditioning. This is the greatness of human beings, that they have made their own dharmas, established on top of the lower dharmas.

But with the Sahasrar ascent the attention loses that quality, which means you do not need to put dharmas, restrictions upon yourself. You do not have to discipline yourself, but you get disciplined automatically. The attention does not get attached to, or attacked by, anything whatsoever, it is so pure. Like water does not stay on the Lotus leaf, so you become 'Kalatita', you become 'Dharmatita'. You become 'Gunanita'. Means, you go beyond the three 'moods' (Gunas) with which you are born, left, right and centre.

The left one in the one by which you have emotional attachments of your attention. The second one (right) is the physical and the mental attachments. And the third one (centre), is the attachment to the dharma, attachment to be righteous and to make other righteous, of disciplining others and disciplining yourself... Where a person tries to control all his enemies of lust, anger, pride, vanity, attachments and greed.

All these restrictions on the attention get lost and you become a free person of complete wisdom. Your attention itself becomes dharmic. So you lose all your gunas and you become 'Satgunis', means virtuous, not by discipline, but spontaneously. You become righteous spontaneously.

So you reach a state which can be described with the word 'a' that means 'without'. So such a person is without thought; he does not think. Such person is without greed; such a person is without lust, devoid of it. Such a person is said to be 'ascesa': 'Out of which nothing is left out'. Like when you want to make a vacuum, you go on creating the vacuum. Reach any point and the vacuum cannot be completed because it reaches a point all the time where you find some part of it remains. You cannot have a complete vacuum. But such a person has a complete vacuum - a vacuum of all the negative, aggressive qualities - complete, they do not exist.

Such a person is an eternal being nobody can kill, nobody can harm, and nobody can hurt. The anger of anyone or respect of anyone does not touch such a person. He is not disturbed by insults or non-insults. He is not elated by prayers, because he is devoid of the capacity to enjoy the boons of the ego.

So at the third state he reaches he gets the blessing of the word 'Nih'. Nih is the first word of my name, but in Sanskrit, when you combine it with 'Mala', then it becomes 'Nirmala' (Pure). But the word is Nih...

...But this word nira or nih is used in two forms... One for say: 'Without' or 'Devoid of '. Then another form is: 'The only', 'The absolute joy, nothing but joy. It is complete freedom. So you have all kinds of joys, as I told you before. You have Svananda - the joy of the spirit, and then you have got Brahmanand - the joy of well-being. You have got Leelananda and Krishnananda - where you have the joy of the play. But when you reach the state of Sahasrar it is NIRANANDA - means, sheer absolute joy.

Although the name 'Nira' is my name, it means 'Absolute'. So when you put such an adjective before anything else it becomes absolute. Thus YOU become absolute. And when you are at that state of absolute then there is no place for anything. Let us see what 'Absolute' is? That means it is not relative, it has no relative qualities. Absolute cannot be compared (Atuliya) it cannot be compared. It cannot relate to anything, it is absolute. It cannot be comprehended because it cannot be related to anything else through which we can comprehend. It is absolute. Whatever way you try to know it, you go away from the absolute. Wherever you try to analyze the absolute, you are away from it. So this is what at Sahasrar you get - 'Niranand' (Sheer joy).

In different stages of Sahaja Yoga we had to start from 'Sarirananda', means the Ananda (Joy) of the body; 'Manasananda', the joy of the 'Manas', the psyche. Then you can say 'Ahamkarananda', where you have to have the satisfaction of the ego. But the state that now has to be established within us is of 'Niranand'. Then what is the question of fear? What is the question of talking about it? You cannot talk about it, because how will you relate it? I cannot say "It is like this, it is like that". There are no words to describe the Absolute.

Only by negation: 'not this, not this' and what remains is absolute. So you reach the state of absolute and that is the state where a complete communication is established and in that communication you have nobody else but the absolute within you. That is the level to which you should aspire. That should be the ascent. We should be established within ourselves. We do not have to go to the Himalayas; we do not have to do anything drastic. Remaining in this world, we have to become the Absolute, the 'Only' (Kevalam). There is nothing like "How?" for it. You just become. You just become, like a flower becomes the fruit. It is all built in. Allow it to work out.

Just by surrendering you become. Surrender it and you will be surprised; you will be at the state where you will enjoy your absoluteness. It is absolute love, it is absolute compassion, and it is absolute power. The words stops, the description stops. You just become the absolute and feel your absoluteness through it with the oneness. If somebody is not with you, you do not worry. There is no company needed. You are alone enjoying the Absolute. Only there can you also enjoy the Absolute in others, in the best form, without seeing anything else but the Absolute.

May God Bless You!"
Sahasrar Puja -1985.
Our Humble Pranams at Your Holy Feet Param Pujya Shree Mataji

PART II

The Mystery of Music

Foreword

It is with a profound and deep sense of understanding of the Divine Grace's blessing of this work that I am today penning these words as a foreword to this book written by Saraswati Raman. I remember my husband, Dr Arun Apte's first introduction of Saraswati to me when he showed me the e-mail she had written, describing beautifully the sublime effect his music had on her and how it had cured her of the unique problem she had of waking up at one-thirty every night for sixteen years.

It was so touching that my eyes swelled with tears. She was one of his students at the music class that he conducted at Parag Raje's house in Thane, when he used to drive all the way from Pune every weekend, and on some occasions, I too, had the privilege of being present with all those devoted students. I was so surprised that Music Therapy could do such magic on people, that in spite of my initial apprehensions, I began to be convinced of its efficacy.

Although he had a background in music, having come from a family of musicians; where his mother was a student of Pundit Paluskar and he himself having been trained under Pundit Jitendra Abhisheki, his obsession for doing research in music and the relation of music and the *Kundalini Chakra* began after a performance in 1993 as a guest artist at Cabella on the occasion of *puja* of Shri Mataji Nirmala Devi. We had been invited to perform before Her Holiness, and the vibrations during the performance were tremendous. After the program, many Sahaja Yogis who were listening to him came back to him and said that their Kundalini was dancing as he sang. That performance was the turning point when Arun just plunged into the world of music and never looked back after that.

His approach to application of music centered around observing and contemplation on the effect of *Swaras* on each chakra. We used to have several Sahaja yogis coming to our house and experimenting and discussing on the effects of notes on the Chakras.

After realization from Her Holiness, Shri Mataji Nirmala Devi, his depth in music intensified and his creative energies manifested in the form of music *Bandishs* (Compositions), all of which started coming to him naturally and automatically. Even though he was involved with all of us externally, like driving his scooter or watching movies on the TV with us, his attention was on the movement of Kundalini within him and the effect of external sounds on his Kundalini energy as She meandered within his subtle system.

My musical journey attained some stature under his nurturing care and tutelage. Although I was already a radio artist in Goa; after marriage, it was under Arun's training in *riaz* of the *sur*, pronunciations, *taranas,* etc that it grew. He was my husband, guru, and best friend, all rolled in one. My whole world was centered on him, but his journey in this life with me was shortened and perhaps that was divinely ordained.

In the last couple of years, somehow, he seemed to have fast tracked his work on this Earth, and he did several CDs consisting of *Bija* mantras, *Bija Aksharas*, Om therapy, chanting of *Slokas* on the deities of each chakra, and Music Therapy.

Saraswati has captured here some of the subtle discoveries that he had made in the use of swara phrases composed by him which had links with the glands and energy centers in the body. By making proper use of these combinations, one can cure most psychosomatic diseases, stress, and depression and bring a healthy balance of energies in one's life.

I hope that lovers of music will find their seeking in this book.
Jai Shri Mataji! Surekha Apte
14th January 2012.

Introduction

It was around 12-30 in the afternoon of Friday the 15th May 2010 when I received an SMS that Dr. Arun Apte is in the ICU of Poona Hospital. During lunch break, I freed myself around 2-20 and reached there. I was told he was on bed 34 Medical ICU. Some nurses were arranging tubes around him. There was nobody else there. Nobody asked me anything. They just allowed me in. I asked the nurse in Malayalam, how bad was he. They said that he was in very bad shape. I asked what happened. Some gastro problem they said. I asked, when he was admitted. They said around 12 that day. I saw the breathing was very slow, around 4 in half a minute. I asked, whether I could stay there for some time. They said fine.

Dr. Arun Apte, had brought out a CD on Music Therapy, that had ragas for every energy center, beginning from Mooladhar, and I had it on my mobile. I used to play it often when I was on official visits and had to stay alone in hotels. I asked the nurses whether I could play music. They said okay but in low volume. I started playing. It started from the first energy center in Dr. Arun Apte's voice. As it started, his breathing became faster. I began to cry uncontrollably. He started to slowly open his eyes. The nurses were surprised. They asked me who he was. I told them that he was my music teacher. As it went on I noticed him shake his head as if singing along with it.

After some time they told me to go on the other side as they wanted to adjust the tubes. I went on the other side, and saw him looking at me blankly as if trying to figure out who I was. I noticed tears at the edge of his eyes. I told him you'll be fine. He then flashed his eyelids as if in recognition. I continued playing- tears running down my cheeks.

Then the nurses told me to go on to the other side as they adjusted some tubes into his mouth this side. He slowly opened this eye. I had my hands holding his all the time. They were cold. When the music came to the portion of " Allah ke samne jab jaoge, poochenge, baat, baat, vegun gun gyan... I noticed him visible shaken up within. Then suddenly his face flinched in pain, and his grip tightened in my hand. I looked around in hopelessness and helplessness.

Then his hands relaxed as he settled back into the overwhelming unconsciousness. I could take it no more.

Such souls come rarely in one's life. I was fortunate to have known him and shared those last moments. I had lost yet another wonderful soul to that inevitable leveler of all. He was my music guru, who had transformed a nightmare that was my life into something worth living, and left a treasure of research in music.

It was around that time that I decided to write this book, as a tribute to one great son of Holy Mother, Shri Mataji Nirmala Devi, who had made music his life and explored music to his heart's content. I felt that the various insights that he discussed and shared with us, when he used to sing his heart out, and describe the subtle knowledge that he had acquired due to Shri Mataji's Grace and blessings, should be brought home to every lover of music so that they can delve into those very depths and drown in the ocean of love, pure awareness and absolute bliss.

I dedicate this book, to this great music teacher who walked with me a few steps in the journey of my life, and showed that life is indeed, worth living.

Nada Brahma Resonates from Dr Arun Apte - A Devotee's Tribute

It was the 6th of November 2004 when I first met Dr. Arun Apte personally. That day what he said made a lot of sense to me. Sahaja yoga was not merely a waving of hands or fingers and generating motions of unseen things in ether but direct awareness of that unseen force working within as an expression of one's activities or thoughts in one's own work area or field. Chakras are active in each one in a more or less degree depending on each one's constitution – in tune with the blue print with which one is born. One could exercise his will in directing this flow of physical bio- energy through long per- sistent efforts.

Years of relentless search within, into the secrets of the work- ing of the human mechanism of mind and energy, through observa- tion and attention, through concentration and single pointedness, has culminated in connecting individual awareness with cosmic awareness - the all pervading stillness through which all things and in which all things are existing, growing and perishing all activated by that vibrant, powerful and ever existing Kundalini or Adi Shakti.

I saw a *jhalak* of this when Arun Apte began giving voice to the accompaniment of his harmonium. I felt myself dissolving in the notes of his voice and merging with the 'm' sound of "OM". As I shut myself from the group amongst whom I sat, I felt it so easy to be one with the sound that was emanating from somewhere in the depths, which was so gentle and yet so rich in vibrations. I could have lifted off to anywhere in space had I persisted for long in that degree of concentration and minuteness that Dr. Arun seems to be evoking so easily and so effortlessly.

I started practice in right earnest with harmonium and notes the next morning but found the sounds different. I felt my harmonium may be defective - the case of bad workman blaming the tools – I tried for some 20 minutes but didn't find it convincing - so I put it away. I then put on some Bhajans on my walkman, closed my eyes and slowly drifted into it. It was Sunday.

I had decided to catch up with some important assignment in office – I worked all day with little success. I had taken out all the records. It was 7.15 p.m. I was almost giving it up. I tried humming to myself recollecting the morning Bhajans. All of a sudden I could hear Arun Apte's voice in my ears – the notes that he sang came from nowhere. A silent pleasure seemed to rise in me. I kept repeating it to myself. I felt relaxed. My eyes and mind continued the work in front of me. My voice started picking up bits and pieces of Bhajans and songs I loved. The tunes also seemed very accurate.

And all of a sudden I located the Rs. 6/- difference I had been searching for the past 2 days and 10 hours. My joy knew no bounds. I said a silent thanks to Dr. Arun - reflecting on it I realized it was precisely 7.15 – 7.30 p.m. the time I was with him the previous day.

Isn't it a scientific fact that the body has a rhythm and anything that goes into the deepest part will work with clockwise precision? I remembered my "out of the body" experience that I had when I was at the Ashram precisely in July 1986. I had been meditating deeply after the evening's prayer, aarti and Bhajans at the temple and had gone to sleep. I found myself drifting in space and I had gone very far away. Suddenly when my physical body's eyes opened it could feel emptiness.

There seemed no sensation in the hands or body. The eyes looked all around. It seemed to try to connect to something. But could not do so. The time was 1.30 a.m. - After a long time the link returned. The heart pounding could be felt. The numbness gave place to feeling and the face smiled. But it was a strangely disjointed experience. There was no ecstasy. There was no joy. But there was freshness. It was a fully wakeful experience. It was like I had been asleep for so long – that I had woken.

But that experience was the beginning of a nightmare for 18 long years. I had, since then woken up every night at precisely 1.30 am and could not sleep until I had worked myself up till I got tired. I would do anything from doing my office files, correspondence, or washing clothes or cleaning up my closet, shelves or room, reading books, or simply crying until I had drained myself.

My subtle body's rhythm had been affected by that nocturnal journey beyond the peripherals of the physical body. My awakening with shock and full consciousness every night at 1.30 even after 18 years of that experience goes to show how when we go deep within the deepest part of our internal system during our wakeful state it can stir up your subtle system .

It was Monday. My head had been aching and I struggled to fight my sanity and calmness. I couldn't stand the pain. I felt I would never be able to cope up. Tears welled in my eyes as I tried to focus on my work. I looked at Shri Mataji's photo – those eyes spoke. Those very eyes had pushed me from my seat on Saturday to keep my appointment with Dr. Arun Apte. I had felt the same sense of exasperation and she had come to my rescue - gently persuading me to leave everything and go.

Now at 12.30 at night as I write this listening to the cassette of Dr.Arun Apte as he sings – the music floating all over me- the vara-dadevi – premadayini following Uma Uma Shiva Shankar that melts my heart every time I listen -. every Twamewa Sakshat can direct your attention to the goddess of the center embracing the consort of her own center whether it is Uma with Shiva Shankar, Saraswati with Brahma or Radha with Krishna - the dance of Shiva and Shakti, the blending of music to rhythm, of voice to beat, of harmonium to tabla.

I felt I needed his voice within me to guide me more closely. With a slight hesitation I asked Parag Raje whether I could tape his class. He said that I should ask the Master himself for permission. With a lot of fear I rang up Dr. Arun Apte and told him I wanted to catch on tape his spontaneous and subtle nuances of tone and voice - to which he immediately replied I could tape his music not his words. I was more than thrilled.

I had taped the notes that he taught that Saturday. I played it every day morning for three days. But I woke regularly at night at 1.30. But there was a difference. I was able to sleep at around 3.00. But this was not so satisfying. I was tired the next two days and had skipped listening to the tape. But on Friday night I remembered one point he had made - I should listen and sing with the tape for about 20 minutes after 10 O'clock – the time I usually went to bed.

Very religiously I put on my walkman and sang with the tape. I sang slowly and feelingly. Soon I was so absorbed that I realized it only when the tape was over. I slept off peacefully, and when I woke up - and as was my usual practice to see the time in the watch - I couldn't believe myself. It was 6.30 a.m. in the morning. I had not woken up at 1.30 at night for the first time in 18 years. And I felt fresh and light that Saturday morning. From the depth of my heart I felt a strange sense of reverence and gratitude to Dr. Arun Apte and tears rose to my eyes. I cried profusely.

That evening when I told Dr. Arun Apte about it, he just said it was the working of the raga. If he had realized what a sea-changing exploration he had made in music he didn't say it but seemed only to rejoice in more heartfelt music which he simply showered that evening. I just felt myself dissolve and melt in his soul stirring voice. As I closed my eyes I found an expression rising from the emptiness of silence. At last I had found someone who had delved into what he had loved most and made it speak to him - music - he asked her his queries and she answered him with her subtle meanderings. He had found his answer to life as it were. Music was his life.

As I type this out it is 10 days that I have not got up at 1.30 at night. And I now realize that my subtle system had changed her course due to the grace and music of Dr. Arun Apte. In his own humble way he says that he has not performed any miracle but it is only a scientific working of music. Yet had he not discovered that subtle way in which music works? To this he again humbly says it is Shri Adi Shakti Nirmala Devi's discovery. He is only a disciple. That speaks of his greatness and his contribution to music as a therapy where medicine had failed.

The power of music and the right intonation can alter the course of working of the subtle system. But it cannot be overnight as he rightly says. His own effort had been over a considerable period of time and sustained continuously due to sheer will power and love of music. He has tapped the spirit of music and has brought the nectar for the benefit of music lovers.

I feel it the great divine destiny had her role to play in bringing a non entity like me in the shadows of a beautiful soul like that of Dr. Arun Apte.

Chapter 1

Sound of Cosmos

The origin of music dates as far back as the origin of sound itself. When the Divine mother or the Feminine power of God Almighty manifested herself, the first sound was created. This sound is called "OM" or Omkar. The Divine and Primordial Mother created the entire universe with the power of this sound; the OM.

OM is the manifestation of the three powers of the Divine mother:

"A" – The power of pure Desire
"U" – The power of Action "M"
– The power of evolution
a combination of the three syllables A-U-M forms "AUM," or the sound "OM."

OM or Omkar is the beginning of music.

The entire universe was created by the energy of the Primordial Divine Mother through the Primordial Sound "Omkar." From the Omkar, five elements were formed: first, space and ether; second, air; third, fire; fourth, water; and last, Earth.

These five elements combined to form the Galaxies, stars and planets, as well as the human body. Each element contributed to the evolution of the entire human body, right through the stages of amoeba to the present human form.

Thus, the human body is a miniature form of the Cosmos, since the Cosmos and humans are composed of the same five elements. Our bones are composed of the Earth element; our blood and other fluids of the Water element; vital energy of the fire element; and our movements employ the Air element. And, our bodily form is shaped by the space element.

The initial creative impulses arose in the Cosmos as a thought vibration or spandan in the Absolute being. The sound that emanated from the vibration was AUM. AUM is the synthesis of all the sounds of the highly vibrating life forces. This cosmic sound continuously flows in the ether.

The cosmic sound of AUM is the combined vibration three phases of Nature the "A" of the "AUM" means the Mahakali energy having the power of desire and existence. The "U" is the Maha Saraswati Energy having the power of action and creation. The "M" is the Mahalaxmi Energy having the power of evolution and awareness. "A" is the Tamoguna; "U" is the Rajoguna and "M" is the Sattwa guna.

The Aum of the Vedas became the sacred word Hum of the Tibetans, Amin of the Moslems, and Amen of the Egyptians, Greeks, Romans, Jews, and Christians. Amen in Hebrew means "sure, faithful". Aum is the all pervading sound emanating from the Holy Ghost as it performs its work of creating and maintaining the Universal structure.

Aum is the voice of creation, testifying to the Divine presence in every atom. In the yoga sutra of Patanjali Aum or Om is spoken of as the symbol of Isvara or God. Patanjali refers to Aum as a cosmic sound continuously flowing in the ether. The Cosmic sound is spoken of in the Christian Bible as follows: "In the beginning was the Word, and the Word was with God, and the word was God." The Bible also refers to the word as the Holy Ghost or Intelligence- the ghostlike unseen vibration that is the creation of all forms of nature.

Om kar is the beginning of music and for this very reason music has become the universal language. This Omkar is also the Adi Sangeet which Adi Shakti gave to Lord Brahma. The four Vedas are nothing but the continued manifestation of this Adi Sangeet, Lord

Brahma gave this music to Devi Saraswati. From Devi Saraswati music went to Maharishi Narad, Guru Narad taught music to the Gandharvas, Apsaras and Kinnaras. Music was destined to come to man for his physical, mental, emotional and spiritual ascent.

In its transcendental aspect it is difficult to establish contact with the Supreme Being. The nearest approach is Sound. Super charged with transcendental soul force, sound is in all creation, the one powerful principle that widely influences and controls all other manifestations. Self realized beings, the Siddhas, discovered a definite relationship between sound and mind. The mind, in the process of being attracted towards sound, loses awareness of the external world altogether.

Through meditation, seekers following the path of Siddha yoga endeavor to establish contact with the divine sound, the Anahat Naad that helps in subduing the turbulent mind- that keeps roving in the pleasure garden of sensual objects – and giving it a new, inward direction. As the seeker delves deep within, he realizes that his physical and astral bodies, his senses and the mind- all have sound as their basis.

Anahat Naad also forms the basis in all the six chakras or plexus located within the Sushumna that extends from the base of the spine to the crown of the head – the Brahmarandra or the tenth door. Since the lower three chakras- the Mooladhar, the Swadhishthan and the Manipur are dominated by the earth, water and fire elements or tatwas, the Naad is not clearly heard in these chakras.

Anahat chakra, or the heart chakra which corresponds to the cardiac plexus in the physical body, is the centre of Vayu tatwa or the air element. The Anahat Naad, the sound of the Shabda Brahman, emanates from here. The Anahat Naad is the unstruck, mystic sound that occurs spontaneously and is not the result of striking or beating of things. Depending on the intensity of concentration and the level of the mental purity of the seeker, the Anahat Naad can be distinctly heard in deep meditation, paving the way for the seeker's evolution to the highest level of consciousness.

Anahat Naad manifests itself in different ways ranging from the sound of the lashing waves of the sea, the deafening peals of huge bells, the holy sounds of the conch or the whistling swish of winds.

When the seeker hears the flute, his entire being is permeated with Divine bliss and he loses his body consciousness the sound of the kettledrum bestows the seeker with powers of clairvoyance and the ability to see distant objects. But the Naad that leads the seeker to the ultimate goal of yoga, the Nirvikalpa Samadhi, is the megha Naad, the sound of thunder.

It is said by the Siddha yoga masters that constant hearing of the meghanaad for some days in deep meditation enables the seeker to enter the abode of chitta, pure consciousness, where one experiences the tranquility of the supra-causal state of consciousness. We come to know that there are two dimensions to the chitta; one that is supremely pure transcendental which transcends the world, and the other, which we hear as sound, in which by free will, there is differentiation, attribution and the projection of the wondrous universe on the canvas of the Supreme Being. Despite appearing as the universe with its innumerable dimensions, chitta still retains her immaculate purity and remains absolutely untainted.

The immense potential of the power of Shabda (cosmic flow of sound) hidden in music was well recognized by the ancient Indian sages and they had devised several musical patterns emanating from the "Omkar" for chanting of the Vedic hymns and for distinct spiritual effects. The Shastric schools of music discovered musical octave (sa, re, ga, ma, pa, dha, ni, sa) indwelling in the subtle sounds of Nature and invented the basic classical ragas for activating specific streams of natural powers and effects; a wide variety of musical compositions were generated consequently.

Thus, music originated in the heavens and has its origins in spirituality. The Gods brought it to earth by giving it to saints and scholars who were gifted with the ability to detect and understand it. They then created the notes and various forms of music with appropriate, rules, structures and methods. There is no doubt that musical sounds are divine and have a strong correlation with spirituality and divinity.

Interpretation of the Vedic scriptures or Nada Vidya implies that Classical Music helps synergetic augmentation of the panch pranas or the five vital energies in the human body. Research in energy medicine and pranic healing through classical music shows those specific shastric ragas enhance the level of vital energy. It has been found that it is the deficiencies and disorders in the vital energy distribution in the mind body system, which is the root cause of its ailing state.

The smooth and increased flow of vital energy rejuvenates the mind and empowers the immune system as well as the auto-regulatory healing mechanism of the body. This is how classical music generates new hope, joy and enthusiasm in the otherwise dull or depressed mind and removes the disorders and relieves one of the unnecessary pressures, anxieties negative emotions of inferiority complex, despair, fear, anger, and conditionings.

Music therapy based on classical ragas is being used or advised these days for the treatment of insomnia, migraine, hypertension, chronic headache, anxiety, and stress relief. It empowers the immune system as well as the auto-regulatory healing mechanism of the body. It has been also found effective in the cure of psychosomatic disorders.

There are several historical examples of the immense remedial power of music. In 1933, when the Italian dictator Mussolini was terribly suffering from insomnia, no medicine or therapeutic mode could help him get sleep. Pt. Omkarnath Thakur, a great shastric musician was visiting Europe around that time.

When he heard of Mussolini's affliction, he agreed to perform remedial musical programme to allay the latter's sufferings. His performance of the raga Puriya indeed worked magically and Mussolini went into deep sleep within half-an-hour. This and similar incidents attracted the attention of many contemporary musicians, scientists and physicians and triggered research in music therapy.

Because of its impact on the chakras which are the energy vortices Classical music not only vibrates and soothes the mental strings, but also energizes and balances the organs of the body. According to Dr. W. H. J. Wales, the Indian classical music can cure the problems of the digestive system, liver including the diseases like jaundice. Dr. Jane remarks that this music rhythmically vibrates the tissue-membranes of the ear and, relaxes the nerves and muscles beneath the temple and in the brain; as a result of which the sensory and motor systems are energized and activated.

Chapter 2

The Subtle Energy System -The Kundalini Energy System

Kundalini is the reflection of the primordial energy within us.

What are the mechanics behind how the two powers - the Spirit within and the Kundalini energy unite in human beings? Nature intended this union to be scientific and logical. The spirit and the inner energy or reflection of the two powers within us is part of a larger package known as the Subtle Energy system. To understand how this union takes place, we must first understand how the energies themselves are formed inside human beings.

When the child is in the mother's womb, the all-pervading power or the Primordial Energy enters the child's brain. The human brain evolves into the shape of a prism with three sides and a base. When the energy enters, it passes through the surfaces of the brain at the fontanel bone area into the medulla oblongata which is the lower brain structure that is continuous with the spinal cord and controls functions such as respiration, circulation, etc, it splits into two forming the two subtle energy channels – the Ida Nadi and the Pingala Nadi.

Our nervous systems at the gross level consist of the central nervous system and the autonomic nervous system, including the parasympathetic and sympathetic nervous systems on both sides of the body.

The residual energy from these processes settles into the triangular-shaped sacrum bone at the base of the spine as the reflection of the Primordial feminine energy. This is the Kundalini energy. These energy channels are subtle and invisible, just as the energy itself is subtle and invisible.

Before the residual energy settles down as the "Kundalini," the energy flow forms specific energy centers at specific points along the three energy channels. Again, these energy centers are subtle, but they're expressed at a gross physiological level as the plexuses that are easily discernible to the medical world. We can see the medulla oblongata and plexuses, but cannot see the subtle energy channels or energy centers within which are called chakras.

Each of these energy centers is associated with specific functions and qualities. These energy centers are subtle and so are the qualities attributed to them. The stronger these energy centers are, the stronger the qualities within us that each of the energy centers represent. Conversely, the more we develop and strengthen those qualities within us, the stronger our energy centers become. These can be strengthened through enlightenment which is brought about by awakening the Kundalini energy within us and allowing it to work out within our nervous system.

Self- Realization or the Actualization of Enlightenment

This powerful Kundalini energy is dormant in us unless it's awakened through specific spiritual techniques or under the guidance of expert spiritual gurus. Once awakened, this energy, which is placed in the triangular sacrum bone, rises and passes through the six energy centers that are distributed along the central nervous system.

This energy establishes a connection with the cosmic energy or the all-pervading divine energy once it reaches the fontanel bone area. And once this connection is established, the energy centers vibrate in resonance with the Kundalini and cosmic energy, and one can actually experience the vibrations of the energy centers through the nerve endings on the fingers and toes. This energy awakening and sensation of the vibration of the chakras is the actualization of spiritual awakening in human beings.

This awakening provides several benefits, including the ability to understand your energy centers and remove imbalances and obstacles that are the root cause of all our physical, mental and emotional problems in life. After spiritual awakening, you become relaxed. You gain tremendous inner powers and energy that will empower you to solve all problems and lead a healthy, happy and peaceful life.

The seven basic Swaras or musical notes of an octave have a one-to-one correspondence with these chakras. The lower most chakra, the Mooladhar Chakra is associated with the swara "sa"; that means, the practice of chanting this particular musical note will have impact on awakening or activation of this particular chakra. Similarly, the chakras successively moving upwards in this direction namely, the Swadishtan, Manipuri, Anahat, Vishuddhi, Agnya and the top-most Sahasrar Chakra… have correspondence respectively with the Swaras "re", "ga" "ma", "pa", "dha" and "ni".

Energy Centers, Qualities, Musical notes and Ragas

Note	Frequency	Energy Center	Quality	Musical Instrument	Ragas
Sa	240 Hz	Mooladhar	Innocence, Wisdom	Shehnai	Hindol, Shyam Kalyan
Komal RE	254 2/17 Hz	Left Swadhishthan	Pure knowledge.	Veena	Gunari Todi, Yaman,
Normal Re	270 Hz	Center & right Swadhishthan	Creativity	Veena	Hansadhwani
Komal Ga	288 Hz	Left Nabhi	Satisfaction	Santoor	Malkauns, Abhogi
Normal Ga	301 Hz	Center & Right Nabhi	Contentment, attention	Santoor	Bhim Palas, Hindolam
Normal Ma	320 Hz	Center & Left Heart	Sense of Security	Tabla	Bhairav, Ahir Bhairav
Teevra Ma	338 14/17 Hz	Right Heart	Fearlessness	Tabla	Mayamalava Gowla, Durga
Pa	360 Hz	Left, right & center Vishuddhi	Diplomacy, speech, respect	Flute	Jayjaywanti, Desh
Komal Dha	381 3/17 Hz	Right Agnya	Forgiveness	Sarod	Bhup, Mohanam
Normal Dha	405 Hz	Center & Right Agnya	Discrimination	Sarod	Bhageshri
Komal Ni	432 Hz	Sahasrar	Collective Consciousness	Sitar	Darbari, Kanada
Normal Ni	452 4/43 Hz	Sahasrar	Integration of energies	Sitar	Sindhu Bhairavi

NOTES COMMENTS

Indian classical music has twelve notes. These twelve notes are used for absorption and energizing of the subtle system. These notes were the result of contemplation by the Rishis and Munis in the ancient times. Sa is from peacock, re is from bull, ga is from sheep, ma is from cuckoo, dha is from horse and ni is from elephant. In Indian classical music they are known as normal notes.

Besides this there are five other notes, flat re which is between normal sa and re, flat ga between normal re and ga, sharp ma between normal ma and pa, flat dha between pa and dha and flat ni between normal Dha and ni Sa and pa are static. Thus in all there are twelve notes in Indian classical music.

The normal notes Sa is for Mooladhar, Re is for Swadishtan, ga is for Nabhi, Ma is for Anahat, Pa is for Vishuddhi, Dha is for Agnya, and Ni stands for Sahasrar chakra. Sa is for left, right and central Mooladhar. Flat re is for left Swadishtan, and normal re is for central and right Swadishtan, Flat ga is for left Nabhi while normal ga is for central and right Nabhi, Ma is for central and left heart, sharp ma represents right heart, Pa is static and common for left Vishuddhi central and right Vishuddhi, flat Dha is for right Agnya and normal Dha for central and left Agnya because at Agnya the left channel and right channels cross each other. Ni is for Sahasrar.

Each musical note carries a particular frequency. The frequency of Shadja or Sa is 240 and the related musical instrument is Shehanai; that of komal Rishabh Re is 254 2/17 while that of Shuddha Rishabh Re is 270 and the related musical instrument is Veena; komal Gandhar or Ga is 288 that of Shuddha Gandhar Ga is 301 17/43 and the related musical instrument is Santur; the frequency of Shuddha Madhyama is 320 and Teevra Madhyama is 338 14/17 and the related musical instrument is the tabla; the frequency of Pancham or Pa is 360 and the instrument is Flute; the frequency of Komal Dhaivat or Dha is 381 3/17 and Shuddha Dhaivat Dha is 405 and the musical instrument is Sarod and lastly Komal Nishad Ni the frequency is 432, Shuddha Nishad Ni is 452 4/43 and the related musical instrument is Sitar.

When a person listens to music after his Kundalini has been awakened and the chakras have been enlightened, he listens to music not through his ears but though the chakras. Chakras become the ears and Kundalini ascends followed by spiritual emancipation. This is Sahaja yoga, the yoga for the whole world discovered by Her Holiness Shri Mataji Nirmala Devi.

Chapter 3

Chakras and Bija Mantras

As a tree is contained in the seed, so also the power of a Mantra lies potentially in a Bija mantra. Just as the tree grows out of a seed, so also a mantra evolves from Bija mantra. Hence Bija mantras are the source of creation. The Saints, Sages, Rishis and Munis, realized that the Bija mantras had potencies. When properly intoned the mantras have the power to activate the creative forces and produce the desired results.

Divine protection and guidance are the general characteristics of all seed mantras. Each of them has its own specific transformative power. Bija mantras contain the potential of the Divine to manifest into a grand tree of spiritual illumination. They are like the engines pulling a train, and therefore they are often called as Shakti mantras. Om is the Bija mantras of universal consciousness.

Vaikhari or the power of speaking was made to have the transformative potential by the realized people, by framing mantras containing the Bija mantras that are related to each chakra or energy centre. Every letter of the Sanskrit language is a mantra, that emanated from the meditative contemplations of the yogis and they have all come from the sound that emanates when the Kundalini energy moves within a human being.

When Kundalini energy moves it emanates a sound like sha. sh...sh...at the Mooladhar chakra. At every chakra it emits different sounds. To awaken the Kundalini energy, the Bija mantra is Reem.

Shri Mataji once said in her talk in 1988 at Pune, India, that "Ra" is the energy Radha. One who sustains the energy is Radha. She is Mahalaxmi that is why she sustains the Kundalini. "Eee" is the Primordial Mother, and "Ra" is the energy that is Kundalini. So "Reem" means that you have the energy passing through the body towards the Primordial Being.

All the petals of the seven chakras have a particular letter which was seen and heard by the great Rishis during meditation. These letters are charged with the specific power of that particular petal and when chanted give the desired result.

The Mooladhar chakra or the Pelvic Plexus is placed below the sacrum bone and controls the excretory functions, as well as sexual activity, and exerts a general control on the left sympathetic nervous system. The Bija mantra of this chakra is "Lam". It has four petals which carry the sound of four Bija aksharas namely, Wam, Sham, Sham, Sam. Influence of these sounds affect the prostate gland, vas deferens, Cervix of the uterus, and fallopian tubes.

Sounds affecting this chakra or can be altered or positively induced to promote its inherent qualities of innocence, wisdom, chastity, sense of direction, balance, auspiciousness, simplicity, joy and purity. This is related to the Earth element and connected to the nose or sense of smell.

The Swadishtan chakra or the Aortic Plexus is placed above the sacrum bone and plays an important role in controlling the abdominal organs such as the liver, kidneys and the large intestines. The Bija mantra of this chakra is "Wam". It has six petals which correspond to the six Bija aksharas of Bam, Bham, Mam, Vam, Sham, Lam. This chakra has the power of sustenance or the Dharana Shakti.

The reproductive organs of a woman are also partly controlled by this center. Being governed by the water element it is related to the tongue. Music related to this center can influence, kidneys, liver, pancreas, spleen and the lower abdomen.

This center caters to the creative instincts of a person and this is the center that is focused for inducing qualities of creativity, pure attention, pure knowledge, inspiration, and observation, power of concentration, Aesthetics and arts.

The third Chakra is the Nabhi Chakra or the Colic plexus which controls the stomach, the pancreas and many other organs around the solar plexus. The Bija mantra is "Ram". It has ten petals which emit the sound of the Bija aksharas which are Dam, Dham, Nam, Tam, Tham, Dam, Dham, Nam, Pam, Fam. This chakra has the power of transformation promote qualities like, complete satisfaction, generosity, peace and contentment, righteousness or Dharma, inner sense of morality, evolution, sense of dignity, and that of a good host. The chakra carries the fire element and is connected to the eyes.

The Anahat chakra which is the fourth chakra is the Cardiac Plexus and supplies air, blood and vibrations. The Bija mantra is "Yam" and has twelve petals carrying the sounds of the Bija aksharas such as Kam, Kham, Gam, Gham, Gam, Cham, Cham, Jam, Zam, Nyam, Tam, Tham.

This chakra enhances the Divinity and Immunity power in children up to 12 years through the Thymus gland, which produces T-Lymphocytes and B-Lymphocytes. Music and ragas carrying the frequency of this chakra can promote compassion, pure love, and complete sense of security, confidence, and a joy of the spirit. It helps in nourishing the anti-bodies. Being connected to the air element this chakra is related to skin or a sense of touch.

The Vishuddhi chakra or the cervical plexus which is the fifth chakra is governed by the Bija mantra "Ham". It has sixteen petals which respond to the sounds of the Bija aksharas, Am, Aam, Im, Iim, Um, Uum, Rum, Ruum, Lrum, Lruum, Em, Aim, Aum, Oum, Am, Ah. Vishuddhi chakra is a Divine confluence of the five elements and controller of five sense organs.

That is, pancha Tanmatras and pancha jnyanendriyas – nose with the earth element carrying smell or gandha Tanmatras; the tongue works for the water element carrying the taste or rasa tanmatra; the eyes work for the fire element carrying vision or the teja tanmatra; ears work for the ether element carrying the Shabda tanmatra; and skin works for the air element carrying the sparsha tanmatra.

Vishuddhi chakra is the Divine door of vocal music. This centre is also important for its control over the hands. Its qualities are divine diplomacy, detachment, witness state, collective consciousness, self-esteem, pure relationships, connection with the whole and Madhurya. It is connected to the space element or Akasha and hence connected to the ears.

The Agnya chakra or the Optic Chiasm is located at the base of the brain, and sits behind the forehead. The Bija mantra is "Om" and has two petals carrying the sounds of Ham and ksham. When the Kundalini passes the Agnya chakra, our mental activity ceases, silence and enlightenment takes place. The Agnya chakra governs pineal and pituitary glands, Hypothalamus, Retina, Optic Chiasm and the optic lobes.

The cleansing of this chakra promotes vision and light into life which brings the qualities of humility, forgiveness, dissolution of the ego, conditionings and false ideas. This chakra controls the sense of sankalpa – vikalpa.

The Seventh chakra is the Sahasrar chakra in the limbic area which looks like a lotus of a thousand petals. Its Bija mantra is "Om" and it has no sound, but a pure Anahat Naad- the throbbing in a purest form and in the heart there is A La Ta La Ta A La. Its physical expression is the thousand nerves distributed under the surface of the skull.

It is the integration of all the lower chakras and their power. It integrates all the chakras, and there is an absolute perception of reality as it is, on our central nervous system, and brings about a state of thoughtless awareness.

Bija mantras contain the potential of the Divine to manifest into the grand tree of spiritual illumination.

Chapter 4

Energizing Chakras

Indian classical music has twelve notes. These twelve notes are used for absorption and energizing of the subtle system. Sa is for Mooladhar, Re is for Swadishtan, Ga is for Nabhi, Ma is for Anahat, Pa is for Vishuddhi, Dha is for Agnya, and Ni stands for Sahasrar chakra. Sa being static, it is the same for left, right and central Mooladhar. Flat Re is for left Swadishtan, and normal Re is for central and right Swadishtan.

Flat Ga is for left Nabhi while normal Ga is for central and right Nabhi, Normal Ma is for central and left heart, sharp Ma represents right heart, Pa is static and common for left Vishuddhi central and right Vishuddhi, flat Dha is for right Agnya and normal Dha for central and left Agnya because at Agnya the left channel and right channels cross each other. Ni is for Sahasrar.

In the morning when you wake up we should see whether we are left sided or right sided. Very few are in the center. The ideal would be to be in the center, but we are all striving to be in the center. We all have stress. Stress is a very important thing in our life. As it is stresses that make us do things in life. Stress makes us do action in life. We must have the ability to adapt to overcome the stress. You must increase your stress bearing capacity. This is possible only through Sahaja yoga meditation. When we sing, first thing that will happen is that your wandering mind will come to attention. Your wandering attention will come within.

You know what kind of personality you are. If you are a left sided personality, use all sharp notes. Such as Sa Re Ga sharp Ma Pa Ni Dha Sa.

This is see-saw theory. If you are left sided it will be balanced by the sharp notes of the right side. If you are on the right side, use flat notes. All flat notes are for the Ida Nadi while normal notes are for the central channel, while normal and sharp notes are for the Pingala Nadi. If you sing flat re and try to think about the future you cannot think. Thinking about the future is a right sided activity. If you sing Flat re, the frequency of the ray is matching with the frequency of the left Swadishtan hence you cannot go on the right side. Hence you cannot think about the future.

Sa gives you wisdom, Re prevents the thought, with Ga you get satisfaction and contentment, with Ma you will get compassion and fearlessness, with Pa you will develop your personality and Dha will remove your negativity, you will become positive, if someone will tell some work, he will always tell it is not possible. If you sing more and more of Dha that is your Agnya chakra you will develop positivity.

Mr. Apte narrated to us one incident in his life, when he used to work with TELCO his boss used to often tell him several things to do because he knew that he would do it. For each such instruction he used to always say yes. He used to say, "Yes, I will do in two minutes, I was not doing it always, but I would say yes." To develop positivity sing dha. He also narrated an incident that Shri Mataji had told him once. "Once, Sir C P wanted tea at midnight. Shri Mataji asked one devotee to go and bring tea. But he said no the shop would be closed as it is twelve in the night. Then Shri Mataji said that we all shall go. So they all went and that day the shop was open. It so happened that Sir C P was to inaugurate that tea shop and when they returned they were all given a huge present of tea."

There are several connections between chakras. Mooladhar is connected with Agnya chakra. You know a person is a flirt, by looking at his eyes, he will have roving eyes. Swadishtan is connected with Agnya chakra because thoughts are linked to the Agnya chakra. Source of thought is Swadishtan. If you sing Re, particularly komal

Re you will get attention, your attention will become very sharp. Attention is very important in meditation.

Re plays a very important role in improving your attention. Try to think, think, and think and then sing flat re, it will also help in cooling the system. Many times we use ice packs to cool the liver. But by singing flat Re, the ice pack will be within you. Sa is for Mooladhar. dha is Agnya chakra. Re is Swadishtan chakra, so Swadishtan is connected with Agnya chakra. Ga is for Nabhi. Nabhi is connected to Vishuddhi. Sound is from energy. Sound comes from Nabhi chakra. If you want to give vibrations to Vishuddhi chakra, you will have to clear the Nabhi, so we have to sing Ga and then Dha which is for Vishuddhi. Ma is heart and Ni is Sahasrar. When you are giving vibrations to one chakra you should give vibrations to other chakra also.

If you want to clear the Mooladhar, you have to give vibrations to Agnya chakra also. You have to sing Dha of the lower octave and Sa for Mooladhar. This is for left Mooladhar. Every time you have to clear the Mooladhar as Sa is the basic note.

Sa Dha
Dha Sa,
Dha Sa

For Swadishtan, Sa is for Mooladhar, every time you have to clear the Mooladhar.
Dha Sa Re Ga Re Sa

For Nabhi, Sa is compulsory. Nabhi is connected with Swadishtan, so Re should be there, Nabhi is Ga and Vishuddhi is Pa. So Sa Re Ga Pa for Nabhi clearance.
Sa Re Ga Pa
Pa Ga Re
Sa

For Anahat, Sa is compulsory; Anahat is connected with Swadishtan, Nabhi and Anahat. and it is connected with Ni

Ni Sa Re Ga Ma
Ma Ga Re Sa

For Agnya chakra, it is connected with Mooladhar and Swadishtan
Dha, Sa Re Sa.

Now we will activate the right channel. From Mooladhar to Agnya
chakra.

Sa Dha Sa
Dha Sa Ga Re Sa
Sa Re Ga Pa Ga Re Sa
Ni Sa Re Ga Ma Ga Re Sa
Ga Sa Pa Ga Re Sa
Dha Sa Re Sa

So you have to activate from these notes. When you sing all the
notes, there will be one note that will help you most and that is Sa
– It is your note, what note you are using to keep yourself balanced,
that note is your note.

You can keep balance through meditation and music is a powerful method of maintaining your balance. If you are in balance you
can immediately make use of the notes to balance yourself. If you
are left sided make use of sharp notes, if you are right sided uses flat
notes. If your Nabhi chakra is not in balance, use sa re ga pa ga re sa
with flat ga.

The three Mahamantra can help to increase your vibrations.
We have ragas in Indian classical music. The combinations of notes
which are sweet to hear are called ragas. Ragas consist of notes in
ascending order and descending order. There are certain rules for
these ragas. The three Mahamantra are in Rag Jayjaywanti. It is for
Vishuddhi chakra. In Indian classical music there is meend which is
the swing with which we come from one note to another.

Indian classical music, consists of several things like meend,
khatkas murkhi, taanas mantras, - all of which help in increasing the
vibrations. In Rag Jayjaywanti, there is a swing and a khatkas

First we will learn to sing Om. Om is a combination of A U and M. A kar U kar and Ma kar. While singing Ma kar if you keep your palm on the fontanel bone area, you will get vibrations. When you are in stressful situations if you practice Ma kar it will keep you in balance. Ma kar helps to activate the central channel. When the central channel is vibrating, the left and right channels are in balance. Sing Ma kar in stressful situations.

Like notes we have ragas. There are two types of ragas, one for left side and one for right side. Every note can be sa. Depending upon the sa the next note will be re and so on. Every body's Sa is different. How you sing Sa is important. It is like coming back home.

The Left channel can be activated or energized by Raga Miyanki Todi, the right channel by Maru Bihag and Central Channel by Raag Jog.

The different ragas for chakra exercitation and balancing are:

1. Left, Central and Right Mooladhar - Hindol, Shyam Kalyan, Hansadhwani
2. Left Swadishtan – Gujri Todi
3. Central and right Swadishtan – Yaman
4. Left Nabhi – Bhatiyaar, Bibhas, Lalit, Gunakali,
5. Central and right Nabhi – Abhogi, Bhimpalas,
6. Void- Malkauns, Bhimplas
7. Shri Lalita Chakra – Jogkauns
8. Shri Shri Chakra- Shree
9. Left Anahat- Bhairav, Ahir Bhairav
10. Central and Right Anahat – Durga
11. Left, Central and right Vishuddhi – Jayjaywanti, Des
12. Left Agnya- Bageshri
13. Central and Right Agnya- Bhup
14. Sahasrar- Darbari and Bhairavi.

Nourishing the chakras by the use of appropriate ragas and notes helps cleansing them which ultimately brings a soothing silence and internally blissful state.

Chapter 5

Sound of Silence

Creation is born out of the womb of meditative silence. Spiritual theory and practice have a deep legacy of silence. There is physiological silence and there is self-stilled silence. Physiological silence, a function of our body-mind complex is the one experienced by our auditory nerves when we place our palms over our ears and shut out sound. It is a silence many of us need desperately to be able to think clearly, or even to sleep.

Self-stilled silence is the silence of being as opposed to becoming. It is not a silence to be experienced but the silence of the experiencer, the witness. It is the silence of our unconditional self, a silence that exceeds the ego and reaches into the pure field of consciousness. It exists all the time within us, the answer of the Universe to all the sounds we generate. It is in this silence that the world recedes into the background or vanishes altogether and the Universe within us emerges.

Self-stilled silence is rooted in being in the present, in realizing the pure potential of the moment. This silence is the template of the interior, which the Bhagavat Gita says, "weapons cannot cut, fire cannot burn, water cannot wet, nor do winds wither ". It is the fount of deep detachment of the yogi, who regards joy and sorrow, success and failure, victory and defeat, all alike.

Self stilled silence is the language of communication with the Divine. In silence, we open to life and life opens to us and touches us in the centre of our heart. Our heart breaks open and another heart is revealed. This is the true heart, the one that knows how to meet life with open arms. Silence knows that thoughts about life are not life itself. Everything except wonderment falls away, the anger, the fear and the violence disappear as if they never existed.

Silence is beyond words. Silence knows only this moment, this incredible instant of pure life when time suddenly stops, when we breathe the air every moment, which winds around and binds together the strands of our DNA, the essence of who we really are. It is there like music between our thoughts, the light within our eyes, the rhythm of waves, the deep feelings within our heart that have no cause, knowing silence knows us. We only have to be still and allow that silence to engulf us and to enlighten us. This silence is the real teacher, the real teaching, and the real path. And in that silence, we shall discover our beauty, the eternal treasure of perfection itself.

Eckhart Tolle writes in his book "Stillness Speaks"- True intelligence operates silently. Stillness is where creativity and solutions to problems can be found. When you become aware of silence, immediately there is that state of inner still alertness. You are present. You have stepped out of thousands of years of collective human conditioning."

Chapter 6

Music induced Meditation

Meditation is a period of time set aside every day to quieten the mind. It is a way to slow down, chill out and get in touch with the eternal side of one's being. Initially in meditation, thoughts are slowed down, and eventually, thought stops completely. The height of meditation is a state called Samadhi where the mind is completely merged with worlds of perfect light. Meditation recharges you and helps you to get in touch with your inner self. It brings clarity of thought and insight into daily life- you can more easily determine what is really right for you.

Meditation makes you happy and bright. It also empowers you to accomplish things in the daily world by connecting you to the power of the universe. Eventually, dedicated meditation practice leads to enlightenment. Meditation helps to heal emotionally, has a calming effect on our nerves, balances blood pressure, has excellent stress reduction properties, and helps us to relax and to control pain. But whatever, the 'worldly' benefit of meditation, its most important application is spiritual growth, which is impossible without contemplative practice.

There are many methods of practicing meditation. They generally involve focusing on the energy centers in the body, concentrating on a picture, or image, chanting or breathing exercises. But Medicinal vocal music Therapy is the most powerful method for easy, quick, deep and effortless Meditation.

The term Indian vocal music therapy consists, of Indian music, vocal music and therapeutic value of music. Music consists of several aspects such as entertaining aspect, emotional aspect, devotional aspect, religious aspect and spiritual aspects of music. When we use all these aspects of music for therapeutic purposes it is called music therapy.

Music as a therapy has been recommended by several people for meditation. Through meditation, we can have other benefits such as stress management, depression management, blood pressure management, pain relief for pregnant women and ADHD (Attention deficit hyperactivity disorder). We have to train our attention through meditation.

But how does music help in meditation. When we are singing pure sounds we are connected with various sounds; the sounds are connected with sound, music and then silence. Everything goes to its origin. Silence is the source of sound and sound is the source of music. Therefore music leads to the state of silence which is meditation. Meditation means balance and when we are meditating nicely, the journey starts from disability to ability, illness to wellness, suppression to expression, and disease to ease.

As the sounds are heard the effects go to every cell and atom of our being. Sounds also affect the subtle Chakra centers. Sound is very powerful, sounds can create and destroy. It is all according to one's intention and the nature of the sounds themselves. Sounds are an ideal point of focus during meditation. The attention is naturally and effortlessly concentrated on sounds it perceives. Attention is the core of meditation, meditation is the core of yoga and yoga is the core of Spirituality. That is why Omkar, Bija mantra, Bija Akshar, Stotras, Slokas and particular melodious notes, are used repetitively in prayers and mantras which lead to the state of meditation.

"A" kar resonates in the center of the mouth and activates the left channel; the channel of pure desire "U" kar resonates at the back of the mouth and activates the right channel or the channel of pure action and "M" kar that is humming with the lips closed, resonates in the front of the mouth and buzzes through our head and activates the central channel which is the channel for achieving balance or a meditative state. It vibrates the central channel in the Sahasrar and as the sound moves through the nasal passage it produces a special effect. This is how Omkar is used for stress management.

"A" plus "U" is equal to "O" and "A" plus "U" plus "O" plus "M" is equal to "OM". There is a half moon on the picture of "OM" This half moon is represented by "AUM" which is pronounced nasally. This helps to clear the Agnya chakra. This is complete OM. OM is the engine of Mantra. OM kar is the sound of Kundalini. Your personality is connected with your name. Just as when someone calls you by your name, your attention goes there,because you are attracted by the sound of your name.

There is a connection between sound and attention. Sound attracts attention. Attention dissolves in sound. When you sing OM kar, which is the sound of Kundalini, it gets attracted and it rises. When Kundalini rises, you attain the state of meditation. Meditation is the breath of spirituality and yoga. When you are in meditation, you are in a state of thoughtless energy, which helps in saving the mental energy or the energy of the brain.

Even when we sleep, our brain is thinking. So all the time there is wastage of energy. When we meditate there is a gap between two thoughts, and this gap helps us in saving the brain energy. In this thoughtless energy state we can connect to the cosmic energy.

With the help of Kundalini we can connect to the cosmic energy which helps us receive several other kinds of energies from the cosmos which helps us in our ascent and spiritual growth. Music helps in easily achieving the state of thoughtless energy that we strive for through meditation. When we sing the OM kar we easily get to the state of thoughtlessness.

The aim of Meditational vocal music therapy is to purify and harmonize the gross and subtle bodies in alignment with their natural vibration, and to bring the individual to the highest state of awareness, the state of Yoga. The experience of this "unified state" is health and happiness and is our birthright. It is within our reach to enjoy a balanced life physically, emotionally and spiritually.

Sounds and rhythms have time and again contributed to that gentle sliding into meditation with effortless ease as it were. Several techniques have been adopted by the masters over time, some of which are discussed here.

Dr. Arun Apte taught us the woodpecker method. Just as the woodpecker, the bird which makes its nest in the form of a hole in a tree through small, regular beats. So also music can be used through the woodpecker method, by continuous repetition of notes for definite period of time, alternating aesthetically, to train our mind to gain more attention.

For e.g. Sa sa sa sa sa sa sa sa, re re re re re re re re, Sa sa sa sa sa sa sa sa. and so on with different combinations.

Like, ri, dha na na, ri dha na na, ri dha na na, ri dha na na, ri dha na na

This is sung at the note of Sa, re, Sa again and again. This trains our mind to focus its attention.

One of the most appealing examples of this transformation of life into art is that of the jhoomra tala, the most vilambit or slow tala in the Hindustani music, which consists of 56 beats, divided into frames of 12 and 16. The secret of the tala is that each frame of 12 must be played within the time period of 16, to get the rhythm going evenly. It is inspired by the gait of the elephant namely that of the constant sway or jhoomna in its walk.

When Ustad Amir Khan Saheb of the Indore gharana came to specialize his singing of the bada or slow khayal in the jhoomra tala, he found that it suited his deeply meditative temperament in the singing of the raga. And in this tala he took on the most serious of ragas from the classical repertoire to match.

When any student is struggling with the tala, Pundit Amarnath, who was also from the Indore gharana used to say that he must first come full circle within himself, withdrawn from external vrittis or tendencies before he attempts to meditate any raga using this tala. The student must first sway to the antar-laya or the inner cosmic rhythm within himself if he is to sing his raga using the jhoomra tala.

The sway of the tala lies in the interplay of the three beats with the four, expanded to a maximum of four times each to get the figure of 12 and 16. When these 12 beats are sung or playing into the time period of 16, to work out an even gait of the tala, it is done with a sway- like that of the elephant's sway within its heavy footed gait. It is this silence of the sway in the three beats along with the even four beat walk of the gait that brings with it the presence of the unheard in the heard tala. It is in these moments of joy that one is transported into states of non-materiality to the states of the abstract that become the window to meditation.

Initially this extra slow tempo of the khayal singing of the Indore gharana induces a deep sense of calm in the minds of the listener, but as the mind slowly begins to get absorbed in the gait, becoming one with it, it achieves absorption, or the antar-laya, which is the universal silence, which in turn lifts it to greater heights. This experience becomes liberating and deeply peaceful. Musicians who have absorbed ragas in this tala have been the most profoundly peaceful people, who reflected divine radiance which was almost God like.

Sound can be with support anchored to the vocal chords, i.e. it could be aadhaar or niraadhaar Naad, which fills the body like a fluid entity and can flow with the prana or vital breath. The navel, heart, throat, palate, lips, tongue, teeth, the head and the three energy channels – Ida, Pingala and Sushumna along the navel- head axis, construe the instrument – the gayatri veena, with which sound is produced. The singer, with his breath, plays this instrument created by the divine.

The most fundamental process of nada yoga is udatt, anudatt and swarit. These are processes of the prana, or the vital breath and can only be done by a singer who has mastery over niraadhaar Naad. These processes create different states of notes, and enable the singer to establish consonance or samvad between notes in a very subtle and complex ways. It is the consonance between notes that changes the character of the tonic or the sa, making it either tivrang or komalang that is higher or lower – and this changed music defines the character of the raga.

Raga Marwa for example is sung in the tivrang or with raised notes and the re is tejaswi or dazzling. The tivrang komal re of marwa paints a tonal picture of the appearance of the sun as a ball of fire on the horizon in the early evening, the notes change dramatically in Puria becoming lajjit or shy and komalang or lowered in pitch. For, puria pertains to the twilight hour, when the sun is below the horizon, and only a glimmer remains in the evening sky reminding us of its presence.

This is what the Dagars, who were masters of the marwa tradition, mean when they say that a raga is a personality or a living entity. It was more of a virtuosity of the inner world of the subtle shades of sound and microtones, and not an outwardly demonstrative virtuosity of executing complicated note permutations at high speed.

Chapter 7

Healing Power of Sound

Music is an important aspect of sound in our lives. Used properly it can be a powerful means to promote health, but used unwisely it can lead to dissipation of mind, unhinging of the passions and degeneration of the body. It can also kill if certain very low frequencies are utilized. To understand how the power of music can be utilized to enhance growth we can read in the ancient texts how Lord Krishna's flute playing promoted love and friendship in the forests and gardens of Vrindavan.

Mian Tan Sen, one of the nine sages in the court of the Moghul emperor Akbar, could make plants blossom as though spring had arrived, just by intoning devotional songs (ragas) to them. He could also make rain fall and light oil lamps in the same way. Tan Sen cured many diseases with his singing. He took the disease onto himself, and then another singer would take the disease from him, and so on, until it had been passed around, shared, and thereby dissipated of its negative, disharmonic force.

Many modern day researchers have shown that sound affects growth. P. Tomkins and G. Bird in their book The Secret Life of Plants report on experiments conducted by Mrs. Dorothy Rettalack of USA. She set up three sets of plants listening to 'rock and roll', classical western music and classical eastern music. Loud pop music caused the plants to lean away from the sound. Western classical, Bach organ preludes, caused the plants to lean 35 degrees towards the music. The sitar playing of Ravi Shankar, however, caused the plants to strain towards the sound at angles of more than 60 degrees, "the nearest one almost embracing the loudspeaker".

Music has a hypnotic effect, subduing not only man and plants, but also the most vicious and irrational brute in the animal kingdom as well. For example, snake charmers are famous for their flute-entranced cobras. The rhinoceros, camel, elephant and horse have also been tamed by instruments such as the stringed veena and the pungi (trumpet). Birds, of course, are music lovers and adept musicians in their own right.

KKT clinic in Mumbai recently made use of sound waves for treatment of spinal problems. The clinic says it is the first in India to treat spinal problems through non-invasive sound waves, sent from the start of the spinal cord in the neck down the whole length. The procedure has 20 sessions on an average and the patient is subjected to 10-15 minutes of sound wave vibrations in the spine.

The problem area is diagnosed with x-rays, 3D scans, and hip and shoulder calipers. Software is then fed the information, which decides the frequency and position for the patient. The patient lies on a side depending on the problem. A probe is settled over the neck which touches the skin and releases sound waves, which travel the length of the spine.

What do the sound waves do?

- The sound waves correct the bio-mechanical access to the spine
- improve micro-circulation within the blood vessels around the spine
- stimulate the nervous system and improve the reflexes of the person
- Help in regeneration of the tissues.
- it can help realign the distortions or dislocations in the spinal cord The treatment can be used for
- De-generation of the spine
- Spondylosis
- Accident or sport injuries

- Arthritis
- Alleviate Parkinson's symptoms

In a Cancer Centre in Pune, which works for the cancer patients in the advanced stages, frequently holds music programmes for their patients, for, as their director, Priyadarshini Kulkarni, feels that more than treatment for cure and recovery, what is important is to help them live their condition and music is a useful tool in that direction. As freelance counselor Neha Kulkarni, who was present on the occasion of the 900th program when Amol Dongre presented some soulful ragas for the patients, said, "Music can distract you from present worries, traumas. If the patients can forget their pain for even one hour, we have achieved our goal."

According to Dongre, playing for the patients, selection of the ragas should be done carefully, as it should not be something that will excite the patients. Again, it should not be something that brings back memories to them. Therefore, he says, "I focus mostly on peaceful ragas like Ahir- Bhairav, Madhuwanti, Bageshri, Pahadi-dhun and so on. Instead of playing traditional alap, jod and jhala, I perform only the alap and jod as the fast tempo of jhal may excite the patients.

To understand the value of Vibrational Therapy, one must first accept that our bodies vibrate and so does everything else on this planet including sickness and disease. The secret of staying healthy is to keep our body's vibrations higher than that of sickness and disease. If through stress or unhealthy lifestyle choices, we lower our vibration to match that of a certain sickness or disease, our body will indeed take on this imbalance.

If there is an imbalance in this netting because of an emotional or spiritual conflict, the shield will deteriorate and mirror this imbalance on the physical body and develop what we know as sickness or disease. The sickness or disease first occurs in our energy body and if the energy body lacks Vibrational nutrition, this sickness or disease will manifest itself in the physical body and we come to know it as heart disease, liver congestion, nervous disorders, allergies, etc.

It is therefore pertinent that we feed this shield and nourish it so it can support us. This leads us to focus the healing on the first line of defense, our first energy system being the auric field, then the chakras and finally meridians. Just as a balanced diet nourishes our physical body, Sound, Color, Gems and Crystals, Affirmations, Symbols, Aroma and Homeopathy nourish our energy systems: the auric field, chakras and meridians.

Evelyn Mulders, author of *"Western Herbs for Eastern Meridians and Five Element Theory"*, *"Full Spectrum Vibrational Healing for the meridians, chakras and auric field"* and *"Vibrational Healing with the Chakra Sound Essences"* and founder of the Sound Essence products believes in the healing effects of sound. Inspired to capture these healing vibrations and make them accessible and practical for all Sound Essence utilizes sound waves from various sound sources to structure the molecules of pristine Canadian spring water. Sound Essence products are meridian or chakra specific holding various other vibrations in support of the characteristics of the meridian or chakra.

Sound Essences has utilized sound waves to structure the molecules of pristine Canadian spring water through the use of Tibetan singing crystal bowls and meridian specific tuning forks. The sound wave vibration imprinted in the water assists in balancing the entire organism. Sound Essence products raise the vibration of the whole body to counteract these physical and emotional challenges and used as preventative therapy these essences help maintains your body's balance.

Everything in our world has its own unique essence, its own unique code. The air around us connects us all and we are affected by all that we come in contact with, whether positive or negative. Our bodies all have energetic fields within which our grosser physical lives take place. We are affected on the energetic level instantly.

The effects of our environment on the physical body may take minutes, hours, days, weeks, months and even years to show up in the physical. Once they do, the reversal of the process is slow and difficult to achieve. Surrounding ourselves with positive vibrations assists us in being balanced throughout every aspect of living.

We have all experienced the physical effects of sound on our bodies, whether at car racing, rock concerts or the symphony. The psychic responds to the sound waves at their energetic level. Each note has a different wave pattern and a different energetic code, which our subtle body not only recognizes but utilizes.

The fact that there is stress in the body indicates that the electrical circuitry has been overloaded. Any injury such as a bruise, sprain or swelling is an insult to the electrical circuitry of the body. Sound can be positively used to promote the recovery and recuperation of the electrical circuitry. Positive sound vibrations help to reconnect and stabilize the weakened electrical area while the body goes through the necessary healing process.

Sound produces vibratory feelings in the body depending on the frequency and amplitude of the sound used. They influence the geometric patterns and organization of cells and its connection to the various glands. The use of various patterns of sound to induce relaxing and meditative experiences has exploded over the last decade.

Various devices, apart from the bio- acoustic tapes and CDs, devices like the brain machines that use different auditory and visual stimuli causing the user to experience a kind of hallucinating virtual reality, have all tried to offer new ways to achieve meditative and creative states.

Binaural signal generators and personal computer software programs have been developed that utilize the binaural-beat technology of the hemi-synch tapes. By combining these methods with subliminal message imprinting, these systems allow a user to create custom sound tapes to achieve various states of consciousness, relaxation and creativity.

A wide variety of meditative and healing sound tapes have evolved that, when combined with brain machines, offer users a way to tap into some of the brains hidden abilities. Richard Gerber, in his well researched and documented book Vibrational medicine, writes about how the vibration technologies involving sound and healing are making their way into the everyday world.

However, research and experimentation with sound done by several people across the globe, like Sharry Edwards, creator of the Bio-Acoustics method, as well as my own music teacher, Dr. Arun Apte, have found, that sound can produce remarkable healing effects if the people themselves sing, or use their own unique note or sound frequencies.

I can recall, the first day, I met Dr. Arun Apte, before anything else, he told me to sing Sa, the first note of the middle octave. When I sang the note Sa, his immediate response was, "Your Sa is very nice." To a layman this might sound a very casual remark. But when we look at it deeply, one can realize that what he actually meant was, that the Mooladhar Chakra, to which that sound frequency is related to is strong and hence the base is very strong. He had the capacity of identifying which were the energy centers that were weak or were affected merely by listening to the sound and the tonic quality of the various notes that a person sang before him.

Sharry Edwards, on the other hand discovered through her experimentation on the recordings of various sound frequencies and the healing effects it had on listeners that different healing effects were noted when they heard their own personal sound or unique note frequency. She discovered that a person's key note frequency could also be deduced from computer analysis of his or her sonic voice patterns.

Another sound healing approach developed by Nicole LaVoie, utilizes a series of sound frequency tapes referred to as Sound Wave Energy tapes. The tapes are designed to harmonically stimulate and balance various energy levels in the human energy field. There are five series of tapes. The first series consists of seven tapes produced to harmonically balance the seven major chakras.

The spiritual series of tapes attempts to sonically assist with relaxation, love, and transition to inner harmony, and with opening the self to experiencing miracles. The emotional tape series works with releasing imbalances and blockages relating to fear and doubt; it also assists the individual in awakening to Christ Consciousness.

The physical series of SWE tapes was created to vibrationally assist with cell rejuvenation, circulation, bones and joints, and hearing. Nicole LaVoie, also utilizes computer analysis of speech patterns to arrive at the frequency of a person's Soul Note.

The Chinese medicine also makes use of music based on the five elements of creation, namely fire, earth, metal, water and wood, each of which is associated with a particular organ system. Melodies with emphasis on particular elemental notes have been developed in China to stimulate healing of the various organ systems of the body, for which analysis will be made on the basis of the Meridian system used in Chinese medicine. Intricate musical tone studies done by the Shanghai Chinese Traditional Orchestra resulted in a series of six tapes, collectively known as Yi Ching Music for health. Yi Ching music is actually a healing music based on the Five Element Theory of Chinese medicine.

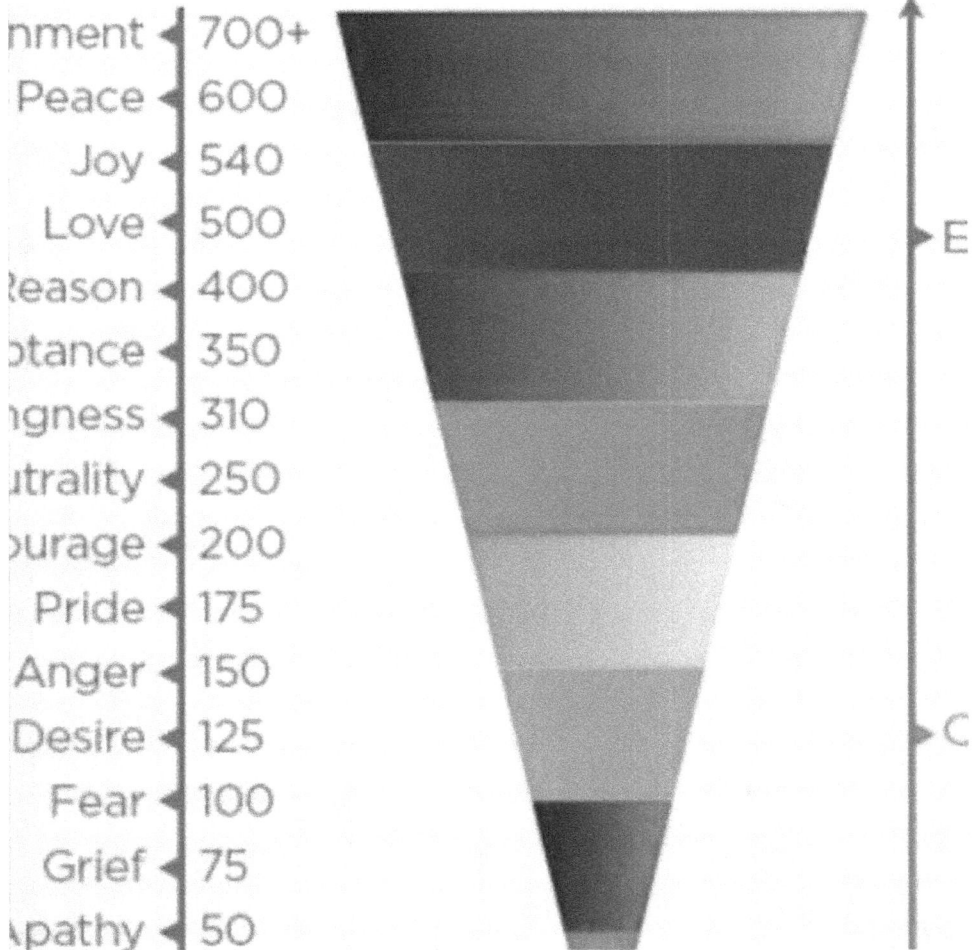

nment	700+
Peace	600
Joy	540
Love	500
Reason	400
ptance	350
ngness	310
utrality	250
ourage	200
Pride	175
Anger	150
Desire	125
Fear	100
Grief	75
Apathy	50

20:55 📞 📷 in ✂ •   📞² 📶 ◎ ᴵᴵᴵ ᴵᴵᴵ 🔋

Levels Of Consciousi

Level	Scale (Log of)	Emotion	Life View
ightenment	700-1000	Ineffable	Is
Peace	600	Bliss	Perfect
Joy	540	Serenity	Complete
Love	500	Reverence	Benign
Reason	400	Understanding	Meaningful
Acceptance	350	Forgiveness	Harmonious
Willingness	310	Optimism	Hopeful
Neutrality	250	Trust	Satisfactory
Courage	200	Affirmation	Feasible
Pride	175	Dignity (Scorn)	Demanding
Anger	150	Hate	Antagonistic
Desire	125	Craving	Disappointing
Fear	100	Anxiety	Frightening
Grief	75	Regret	Tragic
Apathy	50	Despire	Hopeless
Guilt	30	Blame	Condemnation (e
Shame	20	Humiliation	Miserable

When we look at the above two charts we find that if we vibrate at low levels like 20, 50, 75 etc we invoke qualities such as misery, anger, apathy, guilt etc. While if the vibration is above 500 we invoke, love, calm, peace and above 700 enlightenment. Here it must be remembered that these numbers are amplitude or attenuation and not sound frequencies. We can see that at high amplitudes the frequency will be very low.

It is just like deep breathing. When we breath deeply right up to the nabhi, and exhale slowly the number of breaths per minute will just be 4 or 5. This should be kept in mind while using sound frequencies for energy activation, enhancement and balance.

Chapter 8

Ragas of Indian Music

Ragas are pieces of Indian classical music. They are compositions of pleasing sounds or swara, conveying definite sentiments and possess the power to create pleasant impressions in the mind, calm the emotions, and thereby influence the condition of the body. Listening to the most beautiful, intricate and powerful pieces in specific ragas, has a great deal of practical application in the field of therapy.

Raga" is derived from the Sanskrit root "ranja", meaning to color the mind with the sounds emanating from the cosmic vibratory Nada called "AUM" transmitting pranic energy. Technically speaking a raga is a sequence of notes or Swaras which manifest from the universe -both internal and external. But there is a lot more to this, as there are many characteristics required to establish the many fine features of any particular raga. Raga describes a generalized form of melodic practice. It also prescribes a set of rules for building the melody, the tempo and coming back to its Sam.

Much information on Indian classical music is to be found in the ancient ayurvedic medical books such as Sushruta, Charaka, and so on, which date back to the second millennia BC, and beyond. Ragas were used to ease and erase conflicting mental disturbances. They were also used in physical disease in combination with other therapy. One great physician, Dhanvantari of Ujjaini, during the reign of King Vikramaditya said that musical sounds pleasing to the ear should be used as therapy for mental ailments.

Ayurvedic philosophy is based on the concept of the three doshas - vata, pitta, and kappa - which have been literally translated as wind, bile and phlegm respectively. These elements are found in every part of the body in the combination appropriate to that part. Imbalance in these combinations leads to disease, and the ragas act by altering and regulating the balance of these three elements. However, there is more to them than their literal meaning. For example, the Charaka Samhita states the following:

"Vata is the source of both structure and function. It is that which is represented by the five forms of body energy: prana, udana, samana, vyana, and apana... the controller and guiding force of consciousness; the stimulant of the senses; the companion of sensations; the organizer of the elements of the body; the principle of synthesis; the storage battery of speech; the cause of feelings and perceptions..." (1, 12: 8)

"Kapha is the nectar. It is the fertile water for the play of life; it is living fluid, the protoplasm which sustains all life processes." (1, 12: 12)

"The normal function of pitta causes: power of cognition, fire of digestion, fresh complexion, clarity of thought, body temperature, hunger and thirst, and nimbleness of mind." (1, 18: 50)

Any healing which can affect, and thereby regulate the balance of these three elements deserves investigation to establish its practical value in the healing sciences. For example, it is said that raga Bhairava controls ailments arising from dominance of kapha (phlegm) such as fever, constipation, etc. Malhar, Sorat, Jayajayavanti ragas are said to increase body energy, calm the mind and subdue anger. Asawari tranquillizes all afflictions arising from blood, semen, phlegm, and the iris. Bhairavi stimulates the mind and helps regeneration, especially in respiratory illness, colds, flu, bronchitis, pleurisy, TB, and so on. Gurjari, Vageeswari and Malkauns clear diseases of phlegm such as asthma. Saranga eliminates pitta disorders such as headaches, bilious fevers, etc. Palasi, Multani, Pata-deepak and Pata- manjari clear eye problems. Darbari alleviates heart pain and rheumatism. Hindola is for disorders of the spleen and Pancham is for gastric troubles.

The ragas are also associated with different times of day, different plants, animals, and the four elements of earth, water, fire and air. Thereby the elements themselves can be influenced when ragas are performed according to certain rules. Thus music can be used to establish harmony between the outer world and the cosmos.

When the heat energy (Fire element) in our stomach mixes with the Air element in our lungs and uses the Space and ether elements in the sound box or larynx in our throats, the Human Voice emerges. The Spirit wishing to express itself prompts the will; the will awakens the energy in the body, which in turn prompts the breath. The breath rises higher, step by step... through the chest, up through the throat

Ragas are designed to help activate specific chakras, which allow the Kundalini energy to rise easily and energize and nourish the chakra. The raga also influences the chakra to maintain its optimum spin and balance, ensuring a balanced energy supply to different organs that are connected to the specific chakra.

The raga Shyam Kalyan helps activate the Mooladhar chakra. It helps to allow the Kundalini to rise easily, naturally and gently. Chastity, innocence and wisdom are established in the process. This raga develops the quality of the Earth Element, i.e., gravity within, and our sense of smell and direction. This raga gives strength to Apana Vayu which is responsible for activities in the lower abdomen and excretion and sex sublimation. Para Vaani gets enlightened which further leads to Pashyanti vani and makes our personality fragrant.

The raga Gurjari Todi (close to Subhapantuvarali in Carnatic Music) has a capacity to cool down the Liver. This raga and the raga Yaman help activate the Swadishtan chakra that governs our attention. Both ragas help focus wandering or wavering attention, which is crucial for effective meditation. Diseases of psychosomatic nature are due to unsteady attention and imbalance in the sympathetic and parasympathetic nervous system.

Yoga has observed that the Swadishtan chakra governs this function an overworked brain needs constant supply of energy which is done through supply of fat particles from the Swadishtan chakra. As a result less energy becomes available to manufacture insulin thereby leading to diabetes, and other disorders of the liver, gynecological problems, and imbalance of the fluid contents of the body.

These ragas also develop the quality of the Fire Element and make our personality creative, balanced, closely attentive and spiritual. Raga Todi helps to cool the right Swadishtan, while Raga yaman helps to heat up the left Swadishtan.

The raga Abhogi helps activate the Nabhi chakra and stimulate the digestion process. When the Kundalini enters this Chakra, the Chakra is cleansed, bringing about a change of attitudes and inner transformation. This raga is also known to bring about de-addiction in human beings — it helps one give up vices, impulsive and compulsive habits. This raga helps develop the quality of the water element. This raga gives strength to Samaan Vayu which is responsible for assimilation, digestion and excretion.

Pashyanti Vaani gets enlightened which further leads to Madhyama Vaani. The Raga Abhogi makes our personality contented, righteous and generous.

The ragas Bhairav and Durga have a power of Divine bliss and protection. Both help activate the Anahat chakra. When the Kundalini touches the heart chakra, Raag Bhairav activates spirituality in the person. Raag Durga boosts self-confidence and helps develop the quality of the air element. These ragas also enhance the Divinity and Immunity in children, by stimulating the Thymus glands which produces the T-Lymphocytes and B-Lymphocytes up to the age of 12. It gives a rhythm for the whole life and strengthens the Vyaan Vayu which works at the subtle movements of the organs. Madhyama Vaani gets enlightened which further leads to Vaikhari Vaani.

The Raga Jayjaywanti helps activate the Vishuddhi chakra, the controller of the sensory organs and the essence of the five elements this raga also develops the quality of the ether element and the expression of voice, and helps make one's personality loving and sweet. This raga gives strength to Udaan Vayu which is responsible for energy and strength of speech. Vishuddhi chakra is considered to be the Divine door for vocal music. A person with an enlightened Vaikhari Vaani becomes sweet and melodious in his speech and music.

The Raga Bhup corresponding to Raga Mohanam in Carnatic music helps purify and open the Agnya chakra. It helps relieve tensions, anger and mental fatigue. The mood created by this Raga helps the Kundalini pass through the Agnya chakra and enter the Sahasrar in the limbic area of the brain. This causes the person to reach a state of thoughtless awareness and has a tremendous impact on our ability to forgive. This raga strengthens the Praana Vayu and is useful to release tension, stress and mental fatigue.

Ragas Darbari (Darbari Kaanada in Carnatic) and Bhairavi (Sindhu Bhairavi in Carnatic) are helpful in prolonging the state of meditation and thoughtless awareness. The notes of these ragas help relax and calm the emotionally-related limbic area. The Kundalini energy then soothes and nourishes the Sahasrar chakra and the brain. The result is that one feels, joyous, energetic, peaceful and relieved of tension and depression. The person also enjoys the sensation of a cool breeze on the finger tips and achieves the state of Self-Realization or enlightenment.

Regular meditation in this way can open a new dimension of self knowledge which objectively indicates the current condition of one's own chakras on the finger tips by means of warm, cool or tingling sensations, and that of the collective consciousness and also an objective indication of the state of other person's chakras on the finger tips. Mediation in this manner can effortlessly achieve a state of complete balance and well-being.

Chapter 9

Spiritual Sadhana – Nada Yoga

Good music is a kind of spiritual sadhana. Guru Nanak and other spiritual gurus and seekers have expressed their devotion to God through singing songs often to the accompaniment of musical instruments. It was not only Sufi dervishes who danced to the rhythm of music, but also saints like Chaitanya Mahaprabhu, Sur-Das and Mirabai who sang their hearts out to win the beloved's love. At Dargahs like Ajmer Sharif, devout qawwalls soulfully seek benediction of Gharib Nawaz.

It is often through music that a saint relates his mystical experience. It is difficult to imagine expression of devotion at hallowed places like the Golden Temple without the timeless aid of music, the universal language.

The musician Tansen, one of the navratnas or nine jewels in the mughal emperor Akbar's court, was so talented and popular that there are several legends and fables about his music. When he sang the raga malhar, it is said that clouds would get heavy with rain. When he sang the Deepak raga earthen lamps would begin to glow with light.

Akbar, one day expressed a desire to meet Tansen's guru and hear him sing. Tansen said to Akbar," My guru, Swami Haridas, will not come to your court. He is not employed by you like I am. He lives in a hut in the jungle. He sings only when he feels like; so no one can command him to sing." "If he will not come, we will go to meet him," said Akbar.

When Akbar and Tansen reached Swami Haridas's home, they found him sitting outside, silent, with his musical instruments beside him. Tansen requested Akbar to wait while he himself started singing. After a while, he deliberately made a mistake, at which Swami Haridas said benignly, "Don't sing like this, Tansen"

Then Swami Haridas began to sing, casting a magic spell all around. Akbar was in a trance, transported to a state of spiritual bliss, broken only by the cessation of the melody. The emperor left for his palace but the song haunted him throughout the journey.

Akbar asked Tansen, "Why don't you sing as well as Haridas does" Tansen folded his hands and said, "You're Lordship! Between Guru Haridas and me there is a vast difference. I sing for my king while he sings for the Lord of the Universe. He is a musician of a much higher court." On hearing this profound truth, Akbar fell silent.

According to eastern spiritual traditions, the soul separated from the supreme beloved pines for a reunion. The soul's agony has often been expressed in spontaneous poetry set to music. The original composers as well as devout seekers who sang these compositions lost themselves in the rhythmic expressions of love and devotion. Delving deep within, the evolved musician transports listeners to another realm, and the experience is like that of a transforming prayer. Music is then an offering, a thanksgiving. There is no difference between the inspiration and the music.

Music has been regarded as a sacred art. It is related to values which are sublime and permanent but intangible. In the Vedic age, religious songs were sung in India in simple chants. Later on, Gandharva music was seen by the Creator in His contemplation and later performed by seers and saints. It was considered as the surest means of attaining liberation.

Jaydev Goswami was one of the first mystical singers of Vaishnavite Bhakti. His Geet Govinda is regarded as a classic of devotional music. He sang of the love of Radha and Krishna with great emotion and sincerity. Chaitanya of Bengal too sang of the mystic love of Krishna and Radha. Swami Haridas, Tansen's teacher, was an expert in the Dhrupad style of devotional music.

The first five Sikh gurus were also great musicians. They regarded music as a means of spiritual sadhana. They affirmed that singing the praises of God stabilized the mind. In Bengal, Rabindranath Tagore evolved the Rabindra Sangeet style. He wrote:

"When Thou commandest me to sing,
it seems that my heart would break in pride,
And I look to Thy face and tears come to my eyes.
Drunk with the joy of singing,
I forget myself and call…
Thee friend who art my Lord."

Music is an integral part of Sufi devotion. They call it Samai Hakani or spiritual trance. The Chisti mystics of northern India encouraged the qawwals or musicians to sing the praise of God and then got into a situation of rapture when all danced together in a sort of mystic trance.

In India Bhakti movement gave an impetus to sacred music. There are nine traditional stages of Bhakti according to the scriptures:

1. Sunnan or hearing the holy word.
2. Kirtan or singing the praise of God
3. Simaran or remembrance of the Lord
4. Puja or love-worship of God
5. Pad-sevan or surrender of the self at the lord's feet
6. Vandana or supplication to the Lord
7. Dasa-bhava or service to the Lord.
8. Maitri Bhava or friendship with the Lord and total dependence on Him and
9. Atma-nivedan or surrendering oneself to the Lord as an act of total dedication and surrender.

Anhad Naad, the unstruck or Naad has been mentioned by saints like Kabir and Meera, as the music heard within the depths of one's being. Anhad Naad is a divine melody, a celestial music which is transcendent beyond the senses and intellect. It can neither be sung nor heard. It can be contacted by the soul alone. Anhad Naad and soul are in essence the same as God. There is therefore a natural spiritual magnetic attraction between them. So when a listener's soul is turned towards the anhad Naad within it is drawn like a needle to a magnet. In the niraakaar the unmanifest supreme God, like everything else in Creation, is in its potential state so also music too is in its potentiality only. But this potentiality is the thing that eventually takes form, the aakaar as music in the physical world when it is sung or played.

The pleasure or satisfaction experienced by the listener as rasa and rang is due to the union of the manifest music with the unmanifest anhad Naad deep within the listener. Everybody does not appreciate or enjoy music to the same extent or intensity. This is because the fine-tuning of the body and soul differs from person to person.

The relationship between the listener's soul and anhad Naad within the being is like that between the struck- baaj ke taar – strings of a sitar and its unstruck sympathetic strings or tarben which resonates only by the vibrations caused by the struck strings. The musicality of the sound produced by the struck strings is hollow and incomplete without the complementary sound lent by the sympathetic unstruck strings. That is why the sitar maestros give so much time and attention to the fine – tuning of the tarben.

Only a perfect maestro can join the disciple's soul with the anhad Naad within. We cannot achieve this by reading books or listening to the record of past maestros. Anhad Naad is a transcendent entity and therefore cannot be conveyed or given to others indirectly. Only a living person can open the current of the divine melody within us. If his own soul has awakened to this anhad Naad he can awaken other souls too. Every lover of classical music may not be aware of the anahad Naad within, like an accomplished singer.

According to the Vedic Philosophy, yoga and music both are part of Nada Vidya. Yoga deals with realization of Anahat nada the sublime sound of the eternal force of cosmic consciousness. Music pertains to the perception and expression of the infinite spectrum of the rhythmic flow of the Anahat nada pervading in Nature. Both have direct impact on the chakras hidden along the endocrine column and hence affect our physical as well as subtle bodies. Moreover, music also happens to be the best means for expressing the inner feelings. This is why good music is often described as the voice of the heart.

The original ragas of the Indian classical music or shastriya Sangeet are the fusion of Divine knowledge of Prana movement and sounds emanating from it. They are created according to the deep knowledge of harmonious consonance between the seven Swaras and chakras. This is why classical musical compositions are found to have significant positive effect on the mind-body system and also have the potential to awaken the otherwise dormant faculties.

Nada yoga involves long and rigorous practice. The method of training in the Dagar family for example, was long and rigorous involving the practice of the 12 fundamental alankars or grammatical elements for many years before going on to the study of alap and compositions. These elements are aakar, ghamak, lahak, dagar, dhuran, muran, kampit, andolit, sphurat, meend, hudak and soot. Practice is done with a long chain of beads, - the tezbi, with 1100 or 1500 beads strung on a chord, and the student sings each phrase or exercise and keeps count on the tezbi by sliding a bead forward. In addition to the 12 fundamental ornaments there are 40 elements and principles that have to be learnt later.

Voice should be able to enable us to establish a direct connection with the Divine. In Hindustani classical music this is called saakshatkaar. It is the development of a voice that sings using the halak or full breath rather than the vocal chords alone. Singing "aa"-wise, mouth opened in the aakaar, is to be replaced by singing haa-wise, mouth opened to the haakaar, so as to open the voice channel and make space for the breath to flow without constriction or congestion. For the sound must travel from the umbilicus and through the entire thoracic sound box, before the vocal chords and the mouth will articulate it. In gharana language, this is the cultivation of the halak awaaz, the voice of egolessness, or the true voice.

In the Indore gharana voice culture begins with a unique preliminary exercise. The student is asked to sing the Haa, not the Saa, after inserting between the front teeth, the bone between the two knuckles of any finger of the hand. This is done to measure how wide the mouth has to be opened throughout. Care is taken to make sure that the voice moves through the tract without hitting the sides of the thoracic cage, so as not to pick up any kind of materiality. With long hours of practice the voice unites with the naada, the sound of timelessness that lies at the innermost recesses of each being, and runs through all of God's creation.

This naada is similar to the sound you can hear if you put your ear to the heart of any large sea-shell- like the strong sound of the ocean running through it. In the earlier days, when there were no tanpuras, ustads would have four to six disciples sit around them singing the Haa - Saa to provide the pitch or drone for their singing, which later came to be developed into the four or the six stringed tanpura, which is now played as the shruti in the singing of classical music.

Indian voice culture includes vocalism known as the gamak, developed by using the breath rather than just the vocal chords, which is also developed through the halak. In Living Idioms in Hindustani Music, Pundit Amarnath says, gamak comes from the root gama, meaning to acquire peace. Gamak, which comes from the word garmana- which means to beat up, begins from the note preceding it, filling each note with a heavy, rich and rounded quality of tone. When the note gains momentum by the energy of the naada, the gamak comes to life as it were, and the Swaras or notes themselves are the strings of the naada. Gamak is introduced to the student only after he has perfected the Haa-Saa and established in it.

A great emphasis has been laid on the Kharj Saadhana by ancient and contemporary musicians. Kharj Sadhana is practicing the key note Sa as well as the other notes in the lower octave. This kind of practice develops the tonal quality of the voice and improves the stamina and capacity of the singer. The training of the voice pro-ceeds step by step.

To begin with one should sing the note Sa for sometime in a clear open voice, in one breath, as long as the sound can continue without tremors. After this the second step is to sing the other notes of the lower octave in the same manner. The notes should be sung followed by Aakaar. When the normal notes have improved, the sharp and flat notes are to be practiced. This is called Kharj sadhana.

Bharat Muni in his Natya Shastra has described nine moods of dramatic art called the Nava rasa. Ragas express various moods. A voice that is made flexible through proper training can express various emotions by modulating it into soft, loud, tender, forceful, serene or melancholic. Notes, intervals, techniques, styles of rendering the ragas can culture the voice according to needs. Ancient musicians expressed certain emotions through specific notes, like Sa and Re for love and laughter, Ni and Ga for heroism, wrath and wonder, Ma for compassion, Pa for peace and so on.

Celebrated veteran vocalist late Pundit Omkar Nath Thakur had cultured his voice in such a way that each and every emotion would speak for itself. Voice culture in Indian music apart from its technical development is also an intellectual development and refinement of the voice for expression of the sentiments of music.

When naada speaks through the voice, it endows it with a spiritual character. Ordinarily the speaking voice is both congested and constricted, but even so, all voices have it in them. Some realize it, some don't. The voice that does realize the naada, acquires an eternal beauty, a honey like intonation, a deep layer of peace, and the hush of eternal silence. This is the saintly voice, the deeply consoling voice, the voice of a realized soul.

Chapter 10

Spiritual Harmony

Music can bring about a spiritual experience to both the listener and the performer. But, how do we arrive at what a spiritual experience is? A spiritual experience is similar to an experience when we forget one's self, where time stood still and we get carried away by the moment, only that it is more intense, and powerful enough to have the potential to transform one permanently over time – and there is no going back. Music has the potential to bring about such a permanent change in the listener, but the intensity of the spiritual experience is completely determined by the quality of the musician.

The musician develops this proficiency towards manifesting the spiritual energy through the medium of music by sustained practice. This kind of music may not necessarily be soothing or even nice-sounding in the beginning, in the way we have come to believe as soothing or nice-sounding. Different music forms have different shades of aesthetics or beauty within the particular music form. A musician accomplished in a particular music form has internalized all relevant aspects of that music form including the aesthetic aspect.

However this particular spiritual energy can occur in any music from across the world, anytime and anywhere not necessarily in a temple, church, or a dargah, but even in a coffee shop or a concert hall or even in the living room. And when it occurs, transformation will occur, when we open ourselves up to it, without being judgmental or rationalizing it with the mind.

Everything in our world has its own unique essence, its own unique code. The air around us connects us all and we are affected by all that we come in contact with, whether positive or negative. Our bodies all have energetic fields within which our grosser physical lives take place. We are affected on the energetic level instantly. The effects of our environment on the physical body may take minutes, hours, days, weeks, months and even years to show up in the physical. Once they do, the reversal of the process is slow and difficult to achieve. Surrounding ourselves with positive vibrations assists us in being balanced throughout every aspect of living.

Contrary to popular belief that spirituality is based solely on faith and has no scientific or logical proof. Spirituality or the presence of the Spirit within is actually based on a logically arranged system of subtle energy — energy channels and energy centers. The inner subtle energy system is the energy channels.

The energy centers may be thought of as electric switches or ports which are simply points of concentration for electricity or outlets for tapping the inner energy. The energy channels may also be explained as the manifestation of the power of our inner energy in complete form for full-body functioning. Each energy center has a purpose in our evolution that's related to specific bodily functions. The inner energy itself is called Kundalini. It resides in the sacrum bone, which is found at the base of the spine.

After its formation, the Kundalini energy is dormant in all human beings due to the closing of the limbic area of the brain. Your limbic system (emotional and motivational system) is the conduit that connects your inner energy to the main power supply. You can think of the limbic area and the crown of the head as analogous to the main switchboard that regulates the flow of electricity from the external power supply or circuit into the home.

So, spiritual enlightenment is the lighting up of "the house" within us. The main power supplies are switched on, as are all the switches, and the electricity or energy starts flowing through all circuits. The house that was in darkness is now fully illuminated, and we are able to see things clearly. Not only that, we're now able to apply this electricity or energy to multiple uses — lighting, appliances and other devices that exist for our comfort and allow us to fully control our lives.

Likewise, the Kundalini energy is awakened during spiritual enlightenment. It then passes through six energy centers placed along the central nervous system, fills the limbic area, penetrates the crown of the head, and connects or unites itself with the all-pervading power or the energy that is omnipresent in the universe.

This cosmic energy is the energy that drives the whole universe and everything in it, including human beings. Sure, each human is given additional special powers of control, such as an individual brain that can think, rationalize and control movements and behaviors. But the power of our brains is miniscule compared to the overall cosmic, all-pervading power.

Once enlightenment occurs, one can see oneself clearly- problems, limitations, emotions, ego, habits, behavior — everything. In other words, it is as if there is a core entity within that is separate from all these human aspects that is witnessing these aspects. This core entity is simply the Spirit or the soul. Thus, spiritual enlightenment leads to the discovery of one's soul or the Spirit within.

The result of our seeking ends with the finding of the Spirit, the ultimate truth and the core of our existence. This spirit is a reflection of the all-pervading cosmic power. Spiritual enlightenment thus causes us to find and realize that cosmic power within ourselves. This cosmic power which is in the nature of intelligent existence itself is the supreme power which manifests within us in the form of this entire subtle energy system.

The Spirit is a reflection of this cosmic intelligence that is physically located in the heart, the 7 principal energy centers (within our plexuses), the three primary energy channels and the Kundalini energy, or the desire power within us. The desire power within us grows stronger and stronger as we seek the ultimate truth. Ultimately, with the reflection of the desire power within us, the Kundalini, awakens, and connects with the all- pervading power, becoming one with it. Thus, the fully combined power is now flowing through our energy centers and energy channels.

What is the verifiable proof of enlightenment?

Once the subtle energy system is fully active and energized, one can experience a physical sensation in the form of a tingling in the fingers and a cool breeze at the crown of the head. This is real and verifiable. There's other evidence, as well; such as, a feeling of inner peace, emotional stability and an overall feeling of greater vigor.

Chapter 11

The Power of Music From teachings of Swami Svananda Saraswati

Music is the most ancient of arts. It is the medium for expressing emotion. Music kindles love and infuses hope. It has countless voices and instruments. Music is in the hearts of all men and women. Music is on their tongues. Music is in the wind and the waves. Music is in the nightingale. It is in cinema stars and musicians. It is in the concert, orchestra and theatres. There is music in the running brooks. There is music in the crying of children. There is music in all things if you have ears.

Sound is the first manifestation of the absolute. Super charged with transcendent soul force, sound is the one powerful principle in all creation that widely influences and effectively brings under control all other manifestations. Many examples can be quoted to bear testimony to this claim of sound regarding both the individual and the cosmos.

We have heard how Tansen was able to make it rain through the Megha Raga, how he lit the lamp through singing in Dipaka Raga. There are accounts of how the Tibetan lamas drove away and dispersed rain-bearing clouds, or gathered the clouds and made them rain by blowing horns and trumpets and beating drums.

We have also heard how the deer is entrapped by sweet sound, how the cobra is enchanted by sweet music. Nada entraps the mind.

The mind dissolves in sweet nada. Mark the power of the gentle, sweet sounds: Sa, Re, Ga, Ma, Pa, Dha, Ni, Sa. Music has charms to soothe a ferocious tiger. It melts rocks and bends the banyan tree. It enraptures lulls and energizes. It elevates, inspires, strengthens and invigorates. It vibrates in the memory.

Music fills the mind with Sattwa. Music generates harmony in the heart. Music melts the hardest heart. It softens the brutal nature. Music comforts, soothes and cheers the afflicted. It comforts the lonely and the distressed. Music removes worries, cares and anxieties. It makes you forget the world. Music relaxes and elevates.

Music is not an instrument for titillation of the nerves or satisfaction of the senses. It is a yoga sadhana which enables you to attain Self-realization. Music should be treated as yoga. True music can be tasted only by one who has freed himself from all taints of worldliness, and who practices music as a sadhana for Self-realization.

Tyagaraja was a devotee of Lord Rama. Most of his devotional songs are in praise of Lord Rama. He had direct darshan of Lord Rama on several occasions. Mira came face to face with Krishna. She talked with her beloved. She drank the Krishnaprema-rasa. She has sung from the core of her heart the; music of her soul, the music of her beloved, her unique spiritual experiences.

Music is nada yoga. The various musical notes have their own corresponding nadis or subtle channels in the Kundalini chakras. Music vibrates these nadis, purifies them and awakens the psychic and spiritual power dormant in them. Purification of the nadis not only ensures peace and happiness of mind, but goes a long way in yoga sadhana and helps the aspirant to reach the goal of life very easily.

Sweet melody exercises a powerful influence on the mind and physical nature of every living being. Trapped in music, the mysterious mind with its thousand hoods of vasanas and vrittis lies quiescently in the lap of the Sadhak; and he can make it dance to his tune, control it according to his will, and mould it as he pleases. The mind, the magic wand of Maya, the terror of all spiritual aspirants, is under perfect control in the hands of the music yogi.

The wonder of wonders is that not only is the mind of the musician thus controlled, but also the minds of all those who listen to the music. They become calm and blissful. That is why great saints like Mira Bai, Tukaram, Kabir Das, Tyagaraja, Purandara Das and others wove their experiences into sweet music. With the sweet music these sublime thoughts would easily get into the heart of the listener, which at other times is zealously guarded by the cobra of worldliness.

The Rishis of yore have invariably written their inspiring works either in the form of poetry or in the form of songs. The Vedas, smritis, puranas etc. are all set to music, and are metrical compositions. There is rhythm, meter and melody in them. The Sama Veda, especially, is unrivalled in its music. Music is an aid in the treatment of diseases. The sages affirm that many diseases can be cured by the melodious sound of a flute or violin, a veena or a sarangi. Harmonious rhythm caused by sweet music draws out disease. The disease comes out to encounter the music wave. The two blend together and vanish in space.

Music relaxes nervous tension and makes the parts of the body affected by tension resume their normal functions. When all other medicine has failed to cure a disease, Kirtan will work wonders. Try this unique medicine and realize its marvelous benefits. If you do Kirtan near the bed of someone suffering from a disease, they will soon be cured.

Music melts the heart of even a stone-hearted person. If there is anything at all this can change the heart in a very quick time, that is music and dance. This very method is made use of in Kirtan Bhakti; but it is directed towards God instead of towards sensual enjoyments. The emotions are directed towards divinity. The heart is easily purified.

Chapter 12

Music as Therapy

Medicinal Indian vocal music therapy is being evolved not only with music as a base, but by a unique combination and study of other sciences as well. These are science of the primordial sound and its energies, the science of the human body and its connection with the five elements, science of human voice, science of Music and science of spirituality. It is a complementary therapy that promotes the inbuilt natural healing process. It can be effective by itself and can also be used along with other therapies to provide comfort from the side effects. It has curative as well as preventive effects.

Music produces different effects such as heating, cooling and soothing the body and the psyche of the singer and listener. We rejuvenate our four bodies by matching individual sound frequency with the frequency of the cosmic sound through the singing of Omkar or the primordial sound, Bija mantras, Bija Akshar, different mantras, Stotras from Upanishads in different notes and specific Indian classical ragas. When we start singing in this manner, our individual frequencies start matching with the cosmic frequencies and there is an internal balancing and harmonizing taking balance. The central channel gets opened and the kundalini's ascent will be triggered off in an easier and faster way, and the Kundalini rises automatically. When the Kundalini ascends and emerges from the Brahmarandra or the fontanel bone area, the rest of the nourishment is done automatically and we reach the meditative state or Samadhi effortlessly.

When the person becomes enlightened in this manner, which is manifested by an inner blissful silence, he gets physical, mental, emotional and spiritual balance and the journey from disease to ease begins.

Music is a combination of three arts, vocal, instrumental and dance. In music there are three things, they are notes, rhythm and words. As the elements of rhythm, melody and harmony are carried out over a period of time, the change process is initiated and the creative process of moving toward wholeness in the physical, emotional, mental and spiritual self starts manifesting, in ways such as independence, freedom to change, adaptability, balance and integration.

Every energy center has its own frequency. We are all the time thinking about the past or the future. Only when we are in a thoughtless state we are in a state of meditation. We try to balance the frequency of the chakras through musical notes. Every energy center has frequencies that match the seven notes of a musical octave namely Sa Re Ga Ma Pa Dha Ni. When each chakra works at its ideal frequency we are in balance. Just as the frequency of the raga matches with the frequency of the energy center then it is in a state of balance.

Every raga has a mantra and represents deities of each particular chakra. When it is sung in this manner, the energy center gets activated and energized. Melodies induce a feeling of well-being which translates into regularized cardiac functions, lowered blood pressure, and appearance of alpha and theta wave frequencies in the EEG.

Music is perceived in the sub-cortical level, in the Thalamus which is the seat of emotions, feeling and sensations and this is automatic and unconscious. But what is essential is that the listener should be emotionally receptive which requires his involvement and knowledge. It is as much dependent on the quality of the performer. It is a creative therapy, in as much as emotions, aesthetics, and creativity are used predominantly to establish a rapport with the patients.

The Musical Life Panorama project as a facilitating method in the field of clinical and socio-cultural music therapy was introduced by the Nordic Journal of Music Therapy, in psychotherapeutic and socio-therapeutic issues. It works with the emotional meanings of experiences, events and memories that are connected with music in one's life's experiences, and this is talked and discussed so that an individual can be assisted to cope up with problems in his life style.

The effect of music is always dependent upon the context and mood linked with emotionally significant events and periods in our development, and releases the memory and feelings that were linked to the specific situations and events in life at that time.

Music is a visionary artistic creation not merely psychological. Strange visions emerge from the abyss of our memory; primordial experiences that passeth human understanding, sublime, pregnant with meanings arising from the timeless depths, a revelation whose heights and depths are beyond fathoming.

Each of us has two minds: conscious mind and subconscious mind. Sub conscious mind is more powerful than the conscious mind. Sub conscious mind influences many of our actions and reactions. Music, which uses to influence the subconscious mind, tries to put hidden messages into it. The brain has its own opium like chemical called endorphins which reduce pain and give a feeling of happiness. Listening to mind power music releases these endorphins in your brain and prepares you for change, quickly and easily.

Mind power music puts a person in a meditative state which induces all the resultant effects on the body, like that of reducing the blood pressure, reducing the oxygen consumption of the body, relaxation, reducing stress, and releasing endorphins. It also releases the alpha and theta waves, thereby making the mind into relaxed states which facilitate learning. It also makes a person use both sides of the brain thereby promoting a holistic growth of the individual.

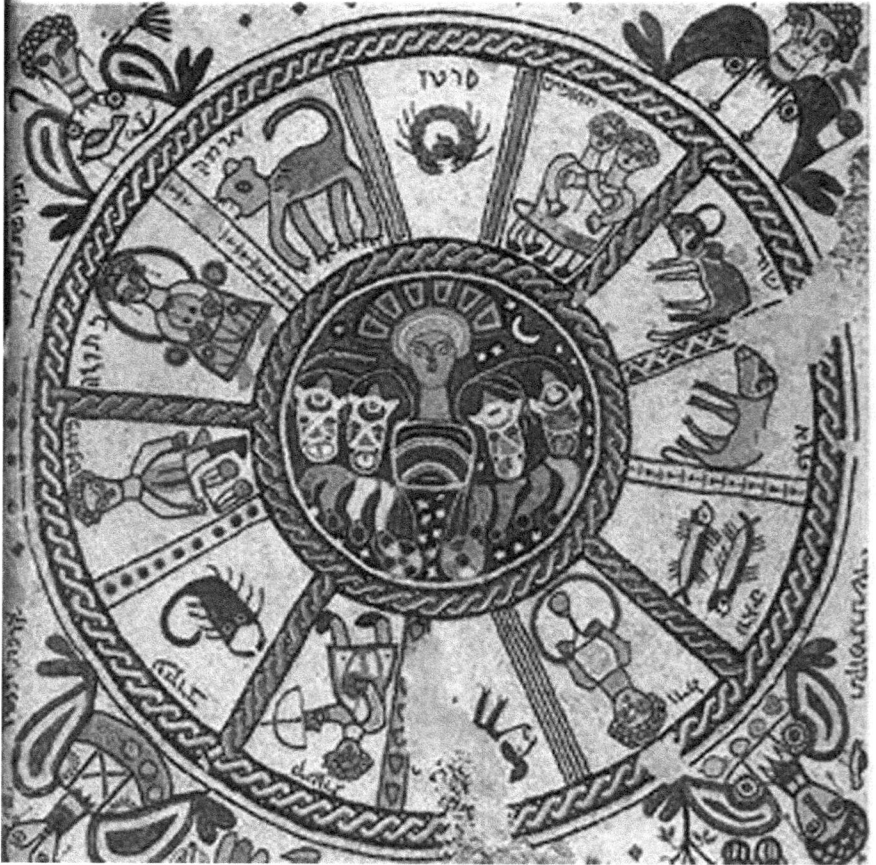

PART III

Incarnations – Steps to Momentum in Human Evolution

Preface

The inspiration for the study of Avataras was none other than Dr. Annie Besant, the greater revolutionary leader whose role in the Indian Freedom Movement is well known and who played a pivotal role in putting the Indian culture, the Indian heritage and eternal wisdom of the ancient sages and saints of India on the International arena.

On the occasion of the twenty fourth annual meeting of the Theosophical society at Adyar, Madras in the year 1899, Dr. Annie Besant had delivered a four-lecture series on the role of Avatars. This book is an adaptation of some of the contents of those lectures delivered together with the information and knowledge provided by Shri Mataji Nirmala Devi, who incarnated from 1923 to 2011.

Speaking on several occasions particularly during the major pujas across the world, Shri Mataji has thrown light about the timing and purpose of incarnations over the ages and how they were instrumental in bringing about that much needed push for human beings to go to the next step in their evolution which is reflected in the activation of the energy vortices at the Virat or Cosmic level which later on percolates in the microcosmic forms.

Avatars and Incarnations has been a subject that has fascinated men of all generations when they ventured out to study the great mysteries of life.

Even the great visionary like Dr. Annie Besant expressed how mighty the horizon opens before our thoughts and how narrow the words seem when we try to sketch such an exploration. Struck by the grandeur of the Eternal Self in the Universe, all that we know that is in this world, is like nothing beside Him when he incarnates as an Avatar, as man, as one among all His manifold manifestations.

Study of Avatars itself calls for a deep humility, patience, reverence and humbleness of heart. It is only with the deepest reverence and profoundest humility that we can study His works; more so when we try to understand what is meant by an Avatara, what is the meaning, what is the purpose of such a revelation?

In all the faiths of the world there is a belief in such manifestations, and that ancient maxim as to what Truth is - it is whatever has been believed everywhere, at all ages, and by all people that is true, that is Reality, just like the Hall Mark indicates the purity of gold and silver.

The age in which we are passing through from century to century, from millennium to millennium, knowledge seems to have become dimmer, spiritual insights rarer, and those who know about it, fewer and those who speak with clear vision of the spiritual Truths are lost amidst the crowds of orators who have honed their public speaking skills and chosen spirituality as their subject without actually living it.

This is not all; today the ones who wield power over traditions fail to understand the origins of those very traditions. The priest and the prophet have come into conflict with one another. The priest carries on the traditions of antiquity and too often he has lost the knowledge that made them real.

The prophet, on the other hand, coming forth from time to time with the Divine word, speaks out the ancient Truth and thereby illuminates tradition. But they who cling to the words of tradition are apt to be blinded by the light of the one who speaks the Truth that they have lost. Therefore, in religion after religion, when some great teacher has arisen, there has been opposition, and even rejection, because the Truth he spoke was too mighty to be confined within the limits of narrow thinking.

Therefore, many times when we are dealing with the subject of Avatars we may have to counter some of the beliefs that have been passed down over generations, repeated by memory rather than because it was either understood or the Truth beneath it fully grasped. But certain grooves or ruts have been formed in the human mind and therefore it may seem to be clashing with details of tradition. However, let us look at Truth as it illuminates the mind. Truth however true is not yet Truth for you, unless your heart opens out to receive it, as the flower opens out its heart to receive the rays of the morning Sun.

An Avatar has two great aspects to the world. First, He is a historical fact. When we are reading the story of the great Ones, we are reading history and not fable. But it is more than history; the Avataras act out on the stage of the world a mighty drama. He is, as it were, a player on the world's stage, and He plays a definite drama, and that drama is an exposition of spiritual Truth. And though the facts are facts of history, they are also an allegory under which great spiritual Truths are conveyed to the minds and to the hearts of men.

The history of an Avatar is an exposition of spiritual verities; but though the drama be a real one, it is a drama with an object, a drama with distinct outlines laid down by the author, and the Avatar plays His part on the stage at the same time as He is living out His life as man in the history of the world. That must be remembered; otherwise some of the great lessons of the Avatar will be misread.

Then He comes into the world surrounded by many who have been with Him in former births, surrounded by celestial beings born as men, and by a vast body of beings of the opposing side also born as men. They are not born into the world alone; they are born with a great circle round them of friends. It is as if there is a great host before them of apparent foes, incarnated as human beings, to work out the world-drama that is being played.

Chapter 1

Who is an Avatar?

Yada yadahidharmasya glanirbavati Bharata | Abhyutthanamadharmasya tadatmanam srujamyaham || Paritranaya sadhunam vinashayacadushkrutam || Dharmasamsthapanarthaya sambhavami yuge yuge |||

"When Dharma,—righteousness, law—decays, when Adharma— unrighteousness, lawlessness--is exalted, then I myself come forth: for the protection of the good, for the destruction of the evil, for the establishment firmly of Dharma, I am born from age to age."

That is what Krishna tells us in the Bhagawad Gita of the coming forth of the Avatar. That is, the needs of His world call upon Him to manifest Him in His Divine power.

When in the great wheel of evolution of this Universe another turn round has to be given, when some new form, new type of life is coming forth, then also the Supreme reveals Himself, embodying the type which He seeks to initiate in His Cosmos. He takes an Avatar to bring about that evolutionary change to turn around the wheel of Time.

An Avatar is a manifestation of the Supreme, the Holiest of the Holy, those manifestations of God in the world in which He shows Himself as Divine, coming to help the world that He has made, shining forth in His essential nature, the form which is just a thin film scarcely veiling the Divinity from our eyes.

Dr. Annie Besant explored the two words that marked a certain distinction in the nature of the manifestation, namely one, the word "Avatar," and the other, the word "Avesha." The literal meaning of the word points to the fundamental difference between the two. The word "Avatar," has as its root "tru," passing over, and with the prefix which is added, the "ava," you get the idea of descent, one who descends. That is the literal meaning of the word.

The other word has as its root "Vishwa," permeating, penetrating, pervading, and you have there the thought of something which is permeated or penetrated. While in the case of an Avatar there is the thought of a descent from above, from Isvara to man or animal; in the other, there is the idea of an entity already existing that is influenced, permeated, pervaded by the Divine power, and specially illuminated as it were.

And thus we have a kind of intermediate step, if one may say so, between the divine manifestation in the Avatar and in the Cosmos. The partial divine manifestation that is permeated by the influence of the Supreme, or of some other being that practically dominates or permeates the individual.

What really is an Avatar?

Fundamentally He is the result of evolution. Since the earliest times, going into the distant past, beyond the past Kalpas, in worlds other than this, into Universes earlier than our own, those who were to be Avataras climbed slowly, step by step, the vast ladder of evolution, climbing from mineral to plant, from plant to animal, from animal to man, from man to Jivanmukta, from Jivanmukta higher and higher yet, up the mighty hierarchy that stretches beyond.

Those who have liberated Themselves from the bonds of humanity; until at last, thus climbing, They cast off not only all the limits of the separated Ego, not only burst asunder the limitations of the separated Self, but entered Isvara Himself and expanded into the all-pervading consciousness of the Lord, becoming one in knowledge with that eternal Life from which originally they came forth, living in that life, centers without circumferences, living centers, one with the Supreme.

There stretches behind such a One the endless chain of birth after birth, of manifestation after manifestation.

During the stage in which He was human, during the long climbing up of the ladder of humanity, there were two special characteristics that marked out the future Avatar from the ranks of men. One is his absolute Bhakti, his devotion to the Supreme. For only those who are Bhaktas and who have wed jynana, or knowledge to their Bhakti, can reach this goal.

As Krishna says, "By devotion, can a man "enter into my being.". And the need of the devotion for the future Avatar is this: he must keep the centre that he has built even in the life of Isvara, so that he may be able to draw the circumference once again round that centre, in order that he may come forth as a manifestation of Isvara, one with Him in knowledge, one with Him in power, the very Supreme Himself in earthly life.

He must therefore have the power of limiting himself to form, for form can exist in the universe only if there is a centre within it around which that form is drawn. He must be so devoted as to be willing to remain for the service of the universe while Isvara Himself abides in it and to share the continual sacrifice made by Him whereby the Universe lives. But devotion alone does not mark this great One who is climbing his Divine path. He must also be, as Isvara is, a lover of humanity.

Unless there burns within him the flame of love for men and for everything that exists in this universe of God, moving and unmoving, he will not be able to come forth as the Supreme whose life and love are in everything that He has brought forth out of His eternal and inexhaustible life.

"There is nothing," says the Beloved, "moving or unmoving, that may exist bereft of me;" and unless man can work that into his nature, unless he can love everything that is, not only the beautiful but also the ugly, not only the good but also the evil, not only the attractive but also the repellent, unless in every form he sees the Self, he cannot climb the steep path the Avatar must tread.

These, then, are the two great characteristics of the man who is to become the special manifestation of God-Bhakti, love to the One in whom he is to merge, and love to those whose very life is the life of God. Only such entities come forth in the man and he is on the path that leads him to be--in future universes, in far, far future kalpas-an Avatar coming as God to man.

Why does the Divine Incarnate?

Divine manifestation of a special kind take place from time to time as the need arises for their appearance. These special manifestations are marked out from the universal manifestation of God in His Cosmos for we must never forget that the Divine Principle is present in the lowest creature that crawl the earth just as much the Ishwara is present in the highest Deva. But there are certain special manifestations marked out from this general self-revelation in the Cosmos, and it is these special manifestations which are called Avatars.

Now, what are the occasions which lead to these great manifestations?

None can speak with mightier authority on this point than He who came Himself as an Avatar just before the beginning of our own age, the Divine Lord Shri Krishna Himself. When we turn to that marvelous poem, the Bhagavad-Gita, to the fourth Adhyaya, Slokas 7 and 8; there He tells us what draws Him forth to birth into His world in the manifested form of the Supreme:

Shri Mataji has mentioned in her speeches during Pujas, that in addition to those which deal with the human needs, there are certain cosmic necessities which in the earlier ages, called forth special manifestations.

"How does this need for Avataras arise?"

"Surely the whole plan of the world is in the mind of the Divine from the beginning, and surely we cannot suppose that He is working like a human being, not thoroughly understanding that at which He aims. He must be the architect as well as the builder; He must make the plan as well as carry it out. He is not like the mason who puts a stone in the wall where he is told, and knows nothing of the architecture of the building to which he is contributing. He is the master-builder, the great architect of the universe, and everything in the plan of that universe must be in His mind ever since the universe began.

But if that be so, how is it that the need for special intervention arises? Does not the fact of special intervention imply that some unforeseen difficulty has arisen? If there must be a kind of interference with the working out of the plan, does that not look as if in the original plan some force was left out of account, some difficulty was unseen, something had arisen for which preparation had not been made? Therefore it looks as though incarnations were brought about to meet unforeseen events. This is quite a natural, reasonable, and perfectly fair deduction.

Now the answer comes along three different lines. They are the three great classes of facts, each of which contribute to the necessity for the Divine to take on a particular manifestation.

The first of these lines arises from what may perhaps be called as the Nature of things. Our universe, our system, is part of a greater whole, not separate, or independent. Our Sun is a planet in a vaster system. Now what does that imply? As regards matter, Prakriti, it implies that our system is built out of matter already existing and already gifted with certain properties that spreads through all space, and from which every Divine takes His materials, modifying it according to His own plan and according to His own will.

When we speak of Mulaprakriti, the root of matter, we do not mean that it exists as the matter we know. It is the root of matter that forms are merely modifications. What does that imply? It implies that our great Lord who brought our solar system into existence is taking matter which already has certain properties given to it by one yet mightier than Him. In that matter three gunas exist in equilibrium, and it is the breath of the Divine that throws them out of equilibrium, and causes the motion by which our system is brought into existence. There must be a throwing out of equilibrium, for equilibrium for Pralaya to take place. When life and form come forth, equilibrium must have been disturbed, and motion must be liberated by which the world shall be built.

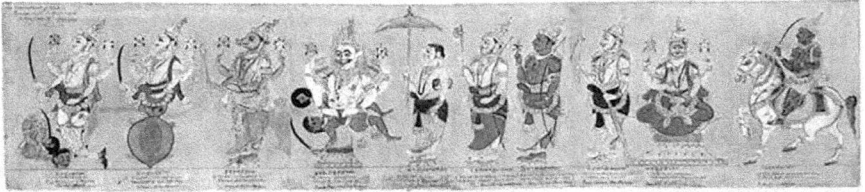

They mark stages in the evolution of the world. They mark new departures in the growth and development of life. Accounts of these Avataras are found in the Puranas. The Pauranic accounts describing the underlying truth of facts and events were given by Sages as they are seen on the higher planes.

A reading of the Puranas reveals that there are descriptions of strange forms and marvelous appearances that seem unlike anything that we have ever heard or dreamed of. The modern mind, with its somewhat narrow limitations, is apt to revolt against the accounts that are given.

Excavations and studies based on records in the small number of fossils collected may be within its limits. But these limits are exceedingly narrow, when measured by the sight that goes back kalpa after kalpa, where the Supreme is not limited to the manifestations of a few hundred thousands of years, but goes back million after million, hundreds of millions after hundreds of millions, and, the varieties of form, the enormous differences of types, the marvelous kinds of creatures which have come out of that creative imagination, and those which actually existed in the past kalpas through which the universe has gone, transcend in actuality all that man's mind can dream of.

What is a Purna Avatar?

A Purnavatara, is a full, complete, Avatar. What is the meaning of that word "full" as applied to the Avatar? We all know that Shri Krishna was a Purna Avatar. He is marked out especially by that name. Truly the word "Purna" cannot apply to the Illimitable, the Infinite; He may not be shown forth in any form; the eye may never behold Him; only the spirit that is Himself can know the One. What is meant by it is that, so far as is possible within the limits of form, the manifestation of the formless appears; as it came forth in that great One who came for helping the world.

Where the manifestation is that of a Purnavatara, then at any moment of time, at His own will, by Yoga or otherwise, He can transcend every limit of the form in which He finds Himself by His own will, and shine forth as the Lord of the Universe, within whom all the Universe is contained.

If for a moment we turn to that great epic "the Mahabharata" which is a storehouse of spiritual wisdom, to the Ashwamedha Parva which contains the Anugita, where, Arjuna after the great battle, forgetting the teaching that was given to him on Kurukshetra, asked his Teacher to repeat that teaching once again. And Shri Krishna, rebuking him for the fickleness of his mind and stating that He was much displeased, he uttered these remarkable words: "It is not possible for me to state it in full in that way. I discoursed to thee on the Supreme Brahman, having concentrated myself in Yoga." And then He goes on to give out the essence of that teaching, but not in the same sublime form as stated in the Bhagavad-Gita. That is what is meant by a Purnavatara; in a condition of Yoga, into which He throws Himself at will, He knows Himself as Lord of everything, as the Supreme on whom the Universe is built.

Again there is the occasion when, as Shri Krishna, He shows himself as Isvara, the Supreme. Once in the court of Dhritarashtra, the madly foolish Duryodhana talked about imprisoning the universal Lord within cell-walls. To show the wild folly of the arrogant prince in the court before every one's eye, He shone forth as Lord of all, filling earth and sky with His glory. All forms human and divine, superhuman and subhuman, were seen gathered round Him in the life from which they spring.

Then on Kurukshetra to Arjuna, His beloved disciple He gave the divine vision so that he might see Him in His Vaishnava form, the form of Vishnu, the Supreme Upholder of the Universe. And later on, on his way back to Dwarka, when he had a meeting with Sage Utanka, He and the sage came to a misunderstanding, and the sage was preparing to curse the Lord; to save him who was really His Bhakta, from the folly of uttering a curse against the Supreme, as a child might throw a tiny pebble against a rock of immemorial age, He showed him the great Vaishnava form of the Supreme.

What do those manifestations show? It shows that at will He can show himself forth as Lord of all, casting aside the limits of human form in which men live; casting aside the appearance so familiar to those around Him He could reveal himself as the mighty One, Isvara who is the life of all. This is the mark of a Purnavatara; always within His grasp, at will, the power to show Himself forth as Isvara.

But then why are not all Avataras of this kind, since all are verily of the Supreme Lord? The answer is that by His own will, by his own Maya, He veils Himself within the limits which serve the creatures that He has come to help.

Some of the Avataras came forth from Mahavishnu, who is concerned with our evolution and the evolution of the world. Mahavishnu, in His essential nature has no intermediary between Himself and the world that He comes to help. Vishnu as we know is a reflection of His glory, a reflection of His power, of His love, in more immediate connection with ourselves and our own world. He is His representative, as a viceroy may represent the king. But the Purnavatara comes forth directly from Mahavishnu.

Chapter 2

What is the source of an Avatar?

"What is the source of Avataras?" is a question that leads us deep into the mysteries of the Cosmos, the cosmic growth and its evolution.

It carries us to those far off times, almost incomprehensible to us, when our universe was coming into manifestation, when its very foundations, as it were, were being laid. It is recognized in all religions admitting Divine incarnations that the source of Avataras, the source of the Divine incarnations, is the second or middle manifestation of the sacred Triad. It does not matter whether with Hindus we speak of the Trimurti, or whether with Christians we speak of the Trinity, the fundamental idea is one and the same.

Taking the Christian symbology, the one Divine incarnation acknowledged in Christianity is that of the second person of the Trinity. No Christian will tell you that there has ever been an incarnation of God the Father, the primeval Source of life. They will never tell you that there has been an incarnation of the third Person of the Trinity, the Holy Spirit, the Spirit of Wisdom, or creative Intelligence, who built up the world-materials. But they will always say that it was the second Person, the Son, who took human form, who appeared under the likeness of humanity, who manifested as man for helping the salvation of the world.

If we analyze that phrase, we find that the sign of the second Person of the Trinity is duality. He is the underlying life of the world. It is by His power the worlds were made, and are being sustained, supported, and protected. While the Spirit of Wisdom is spoken of as bringing order out of disorder, Cosmos out of chaos, it is by the manifested Word of God, or the second Person of the Trinity. It is by Him that all forms are built up in this world, and man was made especially in His image.

So also when we turn to Hinduism, we find that all Avataras have their source in Vishnu, in Him who pervades the universe. As the very name Vishnu implies, He is the Supporter, the Protector, the pervading, all- permeating Life by which the universe is held together, and by which it is sustained. Taking the names of the Trimurti, the attributes of the Supreme Brahman, we have Mahadeva or Shiva, Vishnu, and Brahma: three names, just as in the other religion we have three names. But it is the middle or central one of the Three who is the source of Avataras.

There has never been a direct Avatar of Mahadeva, of Shiva Himself. He has come in form for special purposes served by that form but not as an incarnation or avatar going through the whole process from birth to death. If we look at the great epic the Mahabharata, we find Him appearing in the form of the hunter, the Kirata, testing the intuition of Arjuna, and struggling with him to test his strength, his courage, and finally his devotion to Himself. But that is a mere form taken for a purpose and cast aside the moment the purpose is served. Over and over again we find such appearances of Mahadeva.

In one most beautiful story, He appears in the form of a Chandal, veiling Himself in the form of an outcaste at the gateway of His own city of Kashi, when one who was especially overshadowed by a manifestation of Himself, Shri Shankaracharya, was coming with his disciples to the sacred city. For Him all forms are the same. The human differences are just like the grains of sand vanishing before the majesty of His greatness. He rolled Himself in the dust before the gateway, so that the great teacher could not walk across without touching Him, and he called to the Chandal to make way in order that the Brahmana might go on unpolluted by the touch of the outcaste.

The Lord then, speaking through the form He had chosen, rebuked the very one whom His power overshadowed, asking him questions which he could not answer and thus abasing his pride and teaching him humility. Such forms were truly taken by Shiva, but these are not what we can call Avataras. They are mere passing forms, not manifestations upon earth where a life is lived and a great drama is played out.

So with Brahma; He also has appeared from time to time. He has manifested Himself for some special purpose; but there is no Avatar of Brahma, which we can speak of by that very definite and well understood term.

Why is it that we do not find the source of Avataras alike in all these great divine manifestations? Why do they come from only one aspect, the aspect of Vishnu?

When we look at the Universe, or our solar system, which is one of the many solar systems in the Cosmos, each of which is complete in itself, in its turn is itself a part of a mightier system. Our Sun, the centre of our own system, is not the only Sun. If you look through the vast fields of space, myriads of suns are there, each one the centre of its own system, of its own universe; and our sun, supreme to us, is but, as it were, a planet in a bigger system, its orbit curved round a sun greater than itself. So in turn that Sun, round which our sun is circling, is planet to a yet mightier sun, and each set of systems in its turn circles round a more central sun, and so on.

It is impossible to know how far we may stretch the chain that to us is illimitable. Who is able to plumb the depths and heights of space, or to find a manifested circumference which takes in all universes! They are infinite in number, and there is no end to the manifestations of the one Life.

Now that is true physically. Look at the physical universe with the eye of spirit, and you see in it a picture of the spiritual universe. The story goes that, a Rishi speaking to one of His disciples, once said, "You always look at the things of the spirit with the eyes of the flesh. What you ought to do is to look at the things of the flesh with the eyes of the spirit." Now, what does that mean?

It means that instead of trying to degrade the spiritual and to limit it within the narrow bounds of the physical, because the human brain is unable clearly to grasp it, we ought to look at the physical universe with a deeper insight and see in it the reflection of the spiritual world, and learn the spiritual verities by studying the images that exist of them in the physical world around us. The physical world is easier to grasp.

Do not think the spiritual is modeled on the physical; the physical is fundamentally modeled on the spiritual, and if you look at the physical with the eye of spirit, then you find that it is the image of the higher, and then you will be able to grasp the higher truth by studying the faint reflections that you see in the world around you.

Just as there are many universes, each one part of a system mightier than itself, so in the spiritual universe there is hierarchy beyond hierarchy of spiritual intelligences who are as the suns of the spiritual world. Our physical system has at its centre the great spiritual Intelligence manifested as a Trinity, the Isvara of that system.

Then beyond Him there is a mightier Isvara, around whom those who are on the level of the Isvara of our system circle, looking to Him as Their central life. Just as the physical universes are beyond our thinking, the spiritual hierarchy also stretches beyond our thought. Dazzled and blinded by the splendor, we sink back to earth, as Arjuna was blinded when Krishna showed his Virat swarup.

We cry: "Oh! Show us again Thy more limited form that we may know it and live by it. We are not yet ready for the mightier manifestations. We are blinded, not helped, by such blaze of divine splendor."

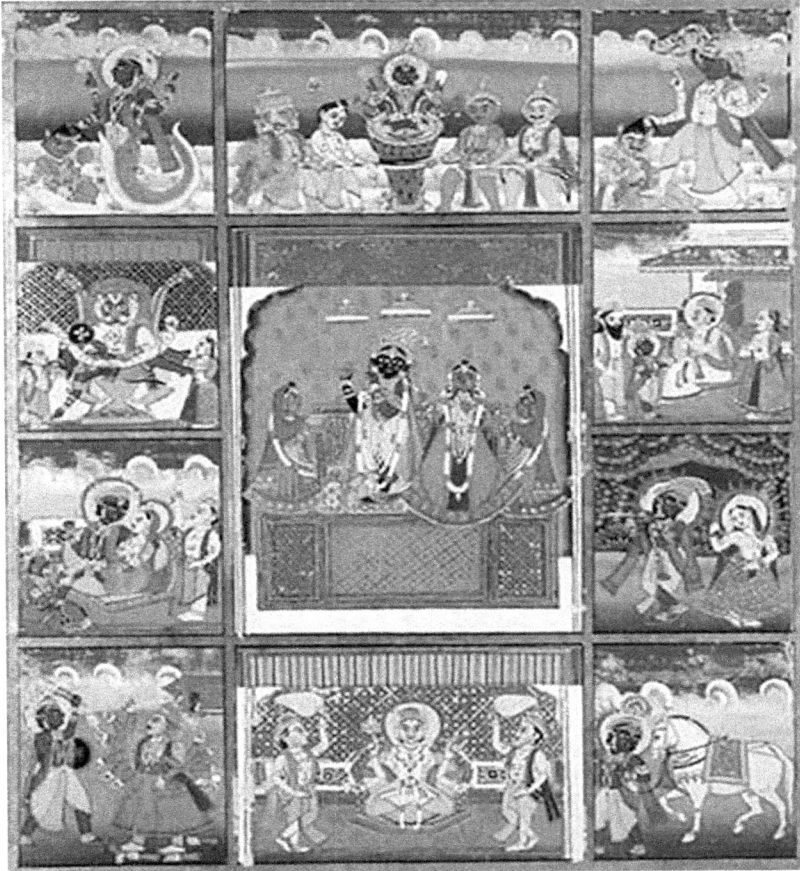

Picture of the Dashavataras as depicted in one of
the paintings from the epic Mahabharata

Chapter 3

The Twelve Ages of a Cycle
and the Avataras

The great cosmic cycles, or yugas as called in Sanskrit and their stages of evolution, covered very long periods of time which were beyond our comprehension and our range of observation, and hence the astronomers calculated the more tangible cycles congruous with our limited experience. The astronomers discovered (firstly in 128 BC by Hipparchus) a phenomenon called precession, which designates the slow rotation of the earth axis, and which describes a double cone having its vertex in the centre of our planet.

Every year, this movement causes the Sun to arrive at the equinoxes progressively sooner. This explains the name of precession of the equinoxes. The phenomenon can be noticed as a slow westward progression of equinoctial points due to the almost circular movement of the earthen axis around the poles of the ecliptic (the apparent way the Sun describes on the sky, under an angle of 23027' formed with terrestrial equatorial plane).

The progression on the ecliptic of the vernal equinox, and of its celestial co- ordinates, lasts 25,200 years. Starting from the vernal point, the astrologers divided the ecliptic in 12 equal sectors the zodiacs as we know them of 300 each bearing the
names of the respective constellations. The crossing of each sector requires 2100 (2000, roughly) years.

The North Pole of the terrestrial axis is now oriented towards Alpha of constellation Ursa Minor or Little Dipper (the present Polaris). Four thousand years ago it as directed towards another pole-star' namely Alpha Draconis, while in about 12000 years the axis of our planet will point at Vega. It is surprising to see that the measure for the divine Time in the Qur'an is "a day which is of the measure of fifty thousand years" (70.4) which equates two cycles of 25,000 years each, which means a deviation of only 0.8% from the precession of the equinoxes computed by the contemporary astronomers!

One cycle corresponds to the diurnal period when the Divinity is manifested in the Creation' and the other cycle covers the nocturnal period when Brahman remains unmanifest (deus otiosus). According to the ancient Persian belief, Zurvan akarana (Eternity) precedes and follows the 12,000 years of "limited time" [1]. In their turn' the Laws of Manu [2] and the Mahabharata [3] indicate for a maha Yuga a duration of 12,000 years (the sum total of the four yugas: 4800+3600+2400+1200 years). By adding an equal period of unmanifest (Zurvan akarana) one gets 24,000 years.

It is mentioned that at the end of the cycle, a Virgin, (representing Purity, Nirmala, in Sanskrit.) will enter the waters of a mystic lake. The Light of Glory (manifestation of the Kundalini) will be imminent in her body. She will bring up "one who will master all the evil deeds of demons and men". Considering the situation from this perspective, to each age, named after the respective constellation, it will correspond the manifestation of a different aeon, the revelation of a new divine attribute, at the same time with the incarnation of a new Avatar.

A Midrash written in the 3rd century AD admitted that the history of this world is divided in periods of 2000 years, and the last one will be that of Messiah's. The previous periods were supposed to be the time of the Law, and a void period (without the Law). According to this calculation, Jesus lived precisely at the end of the 4th millennium (computed from the origin of the biblical years)' after which ensued the 2000 years of the Messiah.

In his book on the Primitive Christian Symbols, Cardinal Jean Danni*Lou dedicated an entire chapter to "the twelve Apostles and the Zodiac" [6], where he quotes Hippolytus. In our opinion, that might throw a new light upon the connection of the zodiacal signs and the divine aspects governing each of them.

Eliade held that the Buddhism and the Jainism compare the cyclic time to a wheel with twelve spokes [7]' image used as early as the Vedic texts [8]. The twelve sectors composing the wheel of time depicted the revolution during the precession along the celestial circle divided into twelve zodiacal houses, signs or constellations corresponding to the twelve ages constituting the complete temporal cycle.

According to the Romans, the cycle duration was connected to number twelve revealed through the twelve eagles seen by Romulus [9]. During the time of Muhammad, according to Arabic tradition ghosts were allowed to ascend to the signs of the zodiac, could listen to the secrets of the heavens and afterwards they could impart them to the mortals. From Muhammad onwards, ghosts were driven away by blazing fire as soon as they attempted to go near the zodiac; the Quran students regarded them to be simple meteorites or falling stars. The Qur'anic text refers to "every accursed Satan... pursued by a manifest flame" (15.18)' and a hadith speaks of Abu Qatada who mentioned Allah's statement ("We adorned the lower heaven with lamps, and made things to stone Satans"; 67.5) and said: "the creation of these stars is for three purposes, i.e. as decoration of the lower heaven, as missiles to hit the devils, and as signs to guide travelers". Nevertheless, we think that the "stars" or the blazing fires were rather the luminous manifestation of the divine power intended to destroy negative tendencies.

Albertus Magnus, Thomas Aquinas, Roger Bacon, Dante Alighieri and many others also thought that the celestial bodies influence the cosmic cycles. According to the ratio of cosmic ages, the duration (4:3:2:1)' for a whole cycle turning round the twelve zodiacal houses, would require 4'8-3'6-2'4-1'2 eras for all the four yugas namely Kruta-Treta-Dwapara- Kali Yuga' respectively. As expected, the remotest periods of mankind existence left only vague and incomplete echoes. Hence, the far away ages of Capricorns (Goat)' Sagittarius (Archer) and Scorpio (Scorpion) left no traces in our memory but we can suppose that they corresponded to the golden age' the Kruta Yoga' together with the age of Libra (Balance) and that of Virgo (Virgin) amounting at about 4.8 eras.

The age of Leo (Lion) or royal fight against the evil together with that of Cancer (Crab, a well-known retrograde creature) and of Gemini (Twins) continuing the battle against the demons, were accompanied by the steady decay of the Dharma that started in the Treta Yuga. The age of Taurus (Bull) and of Aries (Ram) composed the Dwapara Yuga' while the age of Pisces (Fishes) corresponds to the Kali Yuga. At the end of the cycle, the Aquarian (Water-Bearer) age witnesses the opening of the Satya Yuga. Now we would analyze the nearest ages, named after the corresponding constellations in their sequence backwards in comparison with the apparent movement of the Sun.

The Age of Libra (c.14000 - c.12000 BC) named after the constellation sending to the perfect balance' the paradisiacal state, seems to have been included into the Golden Age of mankind-like the three preceding ages and the one that follows.

The Age of Virgo (c.12000 - c.10000 BC) is connected to the Great Goddess (Mahadevi) whose names designate her in many cases as a Virgin. This age refers, too, to a paradisiacal state since one of the most familiar names of the goddess is Gauri (Fair Virgin' Sanskrit.) who gave birth to Ganesha-Adam. Other eloquent appellations are Kanya (Virgin' Sanskrit.)' Kanya-Kumari (Virgin Girl' Sanskrit.) etc.

Remote echoes of those times can be found with the Gaura culture in Iran whose vestiges were unearthed from the prehistoric site Tepe-Gaura (tepe' hill' Iran.) north-east of Mosul' where a complex configured temple was found. Therefore, this age started through the manifestation of the Great Goddess who, according to tradition, incarnated 14,000 years ago to destroy the demons threatening the spiritual evolution of humanity.

Also Armstrong maintains the same situation "to the ancient world of the Middle East, where the idea of our God gradually emerged about 14,000 years ago". This qualification of Saviouress, or Redeemer, explains, too, other names given to her: Tara (Saviouress' Sanskrit.)' Jagaddhatri (Sustainer of the World' Sanskrit.) etc. When he spoke of the birth of civilization, the American archaeologist William Schiller estimated that this event occurred "about 13-15 thousand years ago".

Actually, that period was abundant in statuettes of the goddess, thus proving that she was then the dominant archetype and the society in those remote times was a Matriarchal one. Virgin archetype essence was preserved for a long period in all the spiritual cultures of mankind.

The Age of Leo (c.10000 - c.8000 BC) which belongs to the prehistory' too, also refers to the manifestation of the Great Goddess under the shape of Durga who is riding a lion (Sinha-rathi Sanskrit) in close relationship with the name of the age. Many goddesses had the lion (royal beast conferring the goddess the status of sovereignty) or other related felines as their vehicles.

The Age of Cancer (c.8000 - c.6000 BC). About this age there are not enough records to allow us the identification of the equivalent divine manifestation. However, because of the regressive character of the crab we can infer that humanity was faced with spiritual decline that will prepare the future rising of the patriarchal power. Indeed, the peaceful matriarchal tribal societies suffered afterwards a mutation into human communities dominated by aggressors, warriors (Kshatriyas Sanskrit.). The most famous Kshatriya was Parashuram who prepared the coming of the next Avatar, Rama.

The Age of Gemini (c.6000 - c.4000 BC) corresponded to the flourishing period of early Hinduism. It was under this sign that Rama, the seventh incarnation of Vishnu was manifested by the birth of two pairs of brothers regarded as twin souls: Rama and Lakshman on the one hand, Shatrughna and Bharata on the other. Rama himself had twin sons: Lav and Kush (in harmony with the name of the constellation where the Sun was at that epoch). Lav went to Russia (ego of the world), and from him we get the name of Slav.

The other son, Kush went to China (superego of the world); hence we get the name Kushan attributed in ancient times to the inhabitants of that great empire. These two divine principles were also incarnated as the Buddha Gautama and Mahavir, then as Shankaracharya and Dnyaneshwar.

In other eon, they were al-Hassan and al-Husain, the sons of Fatima and Hazrat 'Ali, the latter being the manifestation of Brahmadeva, the Principle of action ruling the right channel (channel of action). In fact, 'Ali was regarded as "the Prophet's right arm".

During the period of the Vedas people used to worship the twin gods Nastyas or Ashwins (horsemen; from ashram horse' Sanskrit.) echoed afterwards in Roman mythology through Castor and Pollex (dioskoœros Zeus' sons; from koœros' son' Gr.) riding winged horses. The Mazdaean tradition had the couple of goddesses with assonant names, Hauravat and Amaratat. According to the tradition, Rama incarnated during the Treta Yuga and lived 8000 years ago.

Then, the fourth chakra (Adi Anahat) was opened in the Virat. Anahat is an important centre of the human being. The central aspect is the seat of courage, fearlessness, confidence in God, in one's own Self, in the others and in the future; it is the subtle aspect that is mobilized for fighting the aggressions.

It secures the victory of the individual against all kinds of attacks as, for instance, the generating of antibodies to fight the pathogenic agents. This explains the relationship of the central aspect with the goddess Durga the destroyer of the enemies.

The right aspect manifests the qualities of Rama who was the perfect son, brother, husband, father and monarch, in complete observance of the existing rules (maryadas Sanskrit.). On the left side, on the level of the anatomic heart there is the seat of the Self (Atman' Sanskrit.)' the reflection of the divine Father (Shiva) as written in the Bhagavad-Gita: "The Lord abides in the hearts of all beings". "He is seated in the hearts of all".

Then, the Supreme Being says: "Abandoning all duties, come to me alone for shelter" thus rejecting all the cults known as religions (since they are external)' while the true and unique religion is the inner one because only it enables the integration with the Divine in Its inner manifestation. The Upanishads said: "In the heart resides the Atman, the Self. It is in the centre of a hundred and one little channels. It is in these moves... the life force, the breath".

The Zohar reads: "The Faithful Shepherd says: "... God leaves His throne... which is the Brain and sits on the throne of compassion that is the Heart, without which the world could not subsist". And indeed, the correspondent of the Anahat chakra on the head is the center of the opening of Brahman (Brahmarandra Sanskrit.). Besides, all the chakras have their specific projections on the head, this fact being well illustrated in the case of Samson through the seven locks of hair containing the power (shanty Sanskrit.) that was granted to him when the Spirit of God descended upon him (Judges 14:6'19; 16:17,19).

On the subtle field the Anahat controls the heart and lungs. This is confirmed by the Chinese, who believe that the heart organ follows the orders given by the central heart, while the lung is thought to exist only as a result of central heart commandment. Scarlet is the color of the Anahat chakra similar to the blood color. The graphic sign for Atman is a flame located in the heart. A biographer of the prominent Chinese alchemist Lie Ten (8th century AD) wrote: "the heart fire is red as the cinnabar. Or' the cinnabar (mercury sulphide) is scarlet and through the fire it releases mercury which in alchemy is characteristic for the left channel. We should add that mercury is also known as "quick silver" suggesting a living entity, i.e. Jivatman, while the silver designates the left channel. In Hindu symbolism, Atma is depicted as a flame above the Anahat heart chakra.

Likewise, in spite of the strong opposition of the Jesuits, the Roman Catholic Church introduced in the 17th century the image of the Sacred Heart of Jesus bearing a flame on its top, and Christ became "the King of the heart". The Self was described by Jesus as our treasure: when He said: "where your treasure is, there also will your heart be" (Luke 12:34; cf. Matthew 6:21). Consequently, in the spiritual doctrine of the old Church the heart is the dwelling of the "soul".

This subtle center is the seat of love in its purest form, i.e. divine love, a fact that, otherwise, is generally acknowledged. The epistles read about homo interior (Lat.)' "the inward man" (Romans 7:22)' about "inwardly... of the heart, in spirit" (2:29) and "the hidden man of the heart ' in the incorruptibility of a meek and quiet spirit, which in the sight of God is of great price" (1 Peter 3:4).

The end of the sentence points very clearly towards the pure relation between Atman and the meek, maternal, and most pure Kundalini, the Holy Spirit. Once more we are guided towards the deep significance of the ancient Greek urge expressed through the slogan: gn—thi seaut—n' Man, know thy Self-discover in you the Self, the God unknown to you! He will remain unknown as long as we would look for Him outside us.

Furthermore, others believe that the inscription in the temple conveyed by Peter was, actually, Agn—stai Theai' that is "to the Unknown Goddess'" which reveals the urge to discover within us the manifestation of the Divine Mother as the Kundalini. Afterwards, Origen maintained that the Christian ideal is "to become an inner unified man". However, the true union can be attained only through the Self Realization. When the Christian goes down into the depths of his own Self, he would be "transported in ecstasy above the intellect"

The human spiritual condition will not evolve to its climax (Self Realization) unless man's participation as the Qur'an stressed it: "God changes not what is in a people, until they change what is in themselves" (13.12), i.e. realize their inner Selves.

Also in Islam there is the saying: "Who so knoweth himself knoweth his Lord". The quest for the inner Self is compared with the circumambulation of Ka'ba seen as the Supreme Reality: "Circumambulating around Allah, you will soon forget yourself... You have been transformed into a particle that is gradually melting and disappearing. This is absolute love and its peak".

The Aquarian Gospel read: "God's meeting place with man is in the heart... And the people said: "Teach us to know the Holy One who speaks within the heart".

The Buddhist texts gathered by Notovitch under the title: The Life of Saint Issa (Jesus) showed that "Issa furthermore taught the pagans that they should not endeavor to see the eternal Spirit with their eyes, but to perceive Him with their hearts". The quotation appears again in the Tibetan manuscript seen by Roerich, in the variant: "Issa taught that men should not strive to behold the Eternal Spirit with one's own eyes but to feel it with the heart, and to become a pure and worthy soul".

The Gospel of Truth wrote: "in you dwells the light that does not fail". And the Gnostic teacher Monoimus stated in his letter to Theophrastus: "Omitting to seek after God... seek for Him from (out of) you, and learn who it is that absolutely appropriates unto Him, all things in thee... And learn from whence are sorrow, and joy, and love, and hatred...; and if you accurately investigate these (points), you will discover (God) Himself, in unity and in plurality, both in thyself". "Enter into yourself, and find there God, the angels, and the Kingdom", said the masters of the spiritual life".

Or between the midriff and the neck there is the heart' and the courage and the passion and love for combat against enemies define precisely the Anahat chakra.

Ancient Christian manuscripts found in Turfan (an ancient dialect) read: "If a man wants to see the manifestation of the one God, he has only to be pure in heart, for then he can see God. . . Indeed, this supreme goal aiming at uniting human being with its Creator is achieved through Self Realization (Yoga) that is the knowledge of the Self' or-since this is located in the heart - through the knowledge of the heart or "wisdom of the understanding heart". And a Gnostic text even wrote: "You are the children of the understanding heart".

Schuon explained: "In the teaching of every initiatory tradition, the organ of the spirit, or the main center of the spiritual life, is the heart". Also Lossky wrote that "For the ascetic tradition of the Christian East, the heart (kard'a, Greek.) is the centre of the human being... the point from which the whole of the spiritual life proceeds, and upon which it converges"

"The most personal part of man, the principle of his conscience and of his freedom, the spirit in human nature corresponds most nearly to the person. This is why the Greek Fathers are often ready to identify the nous with the image of God in man"

Jung mentioned the middle Ages concept about "the secrets of the heart, which are wholly hidden from all men's understanding". Johann Daniel Mylius believed that philosopher's stone (i. e. the Self) is located in punctum cordis (heart centre' Lat.). A hadith qudsi (direct revelation' in which God Himself talks through the Prophet) acknowledges God's presence in the heart:

"Heaven and earth cannot contain me, but the heart of my believing servant containeth me". The Prophet said: "Protect God in thy heart; then God shall protect thee". "O, happy man", sings Jami, "whose heart has been illumined by dhikr" (mantra). Consequently, the esoteric movement of Islam known as Sufism recognized the supremacy of the heart (qalb' Arab.).

In the 9th century, the Persian al-Bistami displayed an audacity that could have been deadly for him, when stating that he discovered God in his own heart. In Islam, the All becomes manifest in ourselves in "the eye of the heart" ('ayn al-qalb, Arab.), regarded in the Muslim esoterism as a spiritual organ and seat of the divine Uncreated.

The great Sufi master al-Hallaj said: "I saw my Lord with the eye of the heart. I said: Who art Thou? He answered: Thou". And ibn al-'Arabi added: "When you know yourself, your "I'" ness vanishes and you know that you and Allah are one and the same".

According to the Iranian Sufi Alaud-dawleh Semnani "the subtle organ of the heart (latifa qalbiya, Arab) contains the embryo of a mystical progeny which is in this latifa like a pearl in a conch; this pearl, or this progeny, is none other than the subtle organ which will be the real Self (latifa ana'iya, Arab.), i.e. the true personality".

The Sikh scripture read: "There is beautiful place within the cave of the heart" (Is gufaa mahi ik thaan suhaaiaa). "My beloved lives in the cave of my heart" (Pritam basat rid mahi khor). "Like the fragrance which remains in the flower, and like the reflection in the mirror, the Lord dwells deep within; search for Him within your own heart" (Puhap madh jiyu baas hai mukar mahi jaise shaayee).

"The Lord is in the soul, and the soul is in the Lord. This is realized through the Guru's Teachings" (Aatam mahi Ram ram mahi aatam cheenas Gur beechaaraa). "Through Self Realization, one dwells within the home of his inner being (heart); egotism and desire depart" (Aap pachhaanai ghar vasai haumai trisnaa jaai).

Guru Nanak also wrote: "A pure heart is the golden vessel to fill the Divine Nectar which is to be sucked from the Dasham Dwar through the two channels Ida and Pingala".

Meister Eckhart (c.1260-1328) wrote: "there is a something in the soul in which God dwells" [55]. Besides, he thought that this site

- centre of the being (light of the spirit)' uncreated and uncreatable (increatus et increabilis, Lat.) - is the place where man can realize union with God: The concept is ancient' since an Egyptian text from the time of the New Empire says that "man's heart is his God".

We would notice a possible connection between Atman (Self' Sanskrit.) and the Egyptian god Ammon' having also a close spelling. "The "dogmas" of the Theban theocracy, said: "Three are all the gods: Ammon' Ra and Path' that are matchless. (Their) name (that is the soul) is hidden as it is Ammon". Hidden is his name as Ammon' Ra belongs to him as face and Ptah is his body".

Amun actually means the Hidden One (amun' to hide' Egypt.). Leaving aside the god associated to the material body' we notice that the Theban theologians merged the other trinity members into the supreme divinity Ammon-Ra. Likewise it is worth noticing the identity Ammon-Amen... Ammon's paredre' Amaunet was depicted as the goddess of the wind, the sweet breeze (even God Himself).

Last but not least, in Iran people believed that Vohu Manah lived in man's heart. The Anahat chakra is located on the thymus level.

Chapter 4

Vishnu's Incarnations—The First Five

A study of the Vishnu Purana wherein the unmanifest Vishnu is beneath the water, standing as the first of the Trimurti, then the Lotus, standing as the second, and the opened Lotus showing Brahma, the third, the creative Mind.

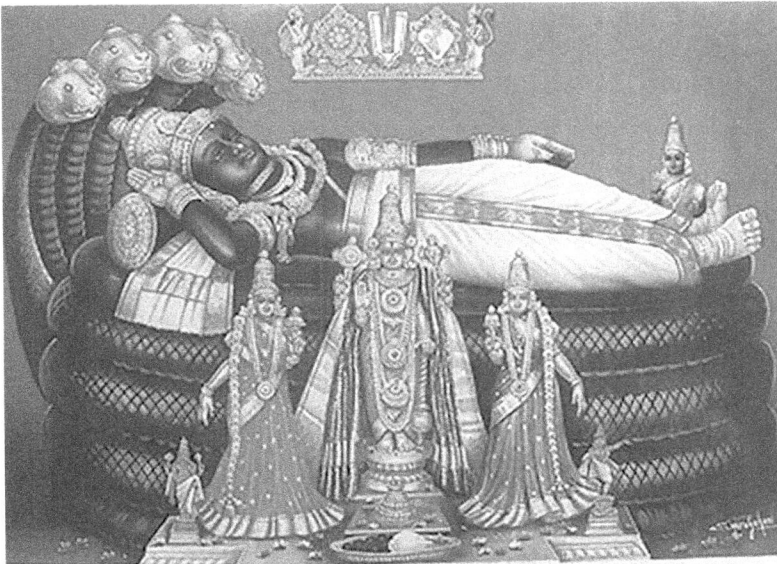

LORD SRI RANGANATHASWAMY SRIRANGAPATNA

SRI RANGANATHA SWAMY TEMPLE, SRIRANGAPATNA

The work of creation began with His activity which consisted in impregnating with His own life the matter of the solar system; that He gave His own life to build up form after form of atom, to make the great divisions in the Cosmos. He formed, one after another, the five tatwas or elements of earth, fire, water, space and ether. Then He meditated, and forms, as thoughts came forth. There His manifest work may be said to end, though He maintains ever the life of the atom.

As far as the active work of the Cosmos is concerned, He gives way to the next of the great forces that is to work, the force of Vishnu. His work is to gather together that matter that has been built, shaped, prepared, vivified, and build it into definite forms after the creative ideas are brought forth by the meditation of Brahma. He gives to matter a binding force; He gives to it those energies that hold form together. No form exists without Him, whether it is moving or unmoving.

As Shri Krishna, speaks in the Bhagavat Gita about the supremacy of Vishnu, saying, He is the life in every form; without it the form could not exist, without it, it would go back to its primeval elements and no longer live as form. He is the all-pervading life. The "Supporter of the Universe" is one of His names.

Mahadeva has a different function in the universe. He is the great Yogi; He is the great Teacher, the Mahaguru; He is sometimes called Jagadguru, the Teacher of the world. In the Gurugita we find Him as Teacher, to whom Parvati goes asking for instruction as to the nature of the Guru. He defines the Guru's work and the Guru's teaching. Every Guru on earth is a reflection of Mahadeva, and it is His life which he is commissioned to give out to the world. His function is mainly that of a Yogi immersed in contemplation, and always takes the ascetic form. When you see Him represented as the eternal Yogi, with the cord in His hand, sitting as an ascetic in contemplation, He is the supreme ideal of the ascetic life.

He does not manifest as an Avatar. Such manifestations come from Him who is the God, the Spirit, of evolution, who evolves all forms -that is from Vishnu. It is from Him that all Avatars come from. For it is He who by His infinite love dwells in every form that

260

He has made; with patience that nothing can exhaust, with love that nothing can tire, with quiet, calm endurance which no folly of man can shake from its eternal peace. He lives in every form, molding it as it will bear the molding, shaping it as it yields itself to His impulse, binding Himself, limiting Himself in order that His universe may grow. He is the Lord of eternal life and bliss, dwelling in every form.

Thus it is not difficult to see that from Him alone the Avataras come. Who else should take form save the One who gives form? Who else should work with this unending love save He, who, while the universe exists, binds Himself so that the universe may live and ultimately share His freedom? He is bound so that the Universe may be free. Who else should then come forth when special need arises?

Shri Mataji Nirmala Devi explains in one of her talks at Vishnu Puja, about how the creation of this world took place. She says, "The creation of this world took place in the Void (Bhavasagara) which surrounds the Adi Nabhi Chakra or navel centre in the body of the Primordial Being (Virat). Adi Vishnu, the Sustainer and Protector of evolution resides there. It was also there in the body of the Virat that Adi Brahmadeva started His creation. Anything that was to be born had to die, and was to be stored in a place on the Moon Channel (Adi Ida Nadi) of the Primordial Being called Parlok. This is the Primordial Being's Collective Subconscious expressed as subconscious mind in the human being. In the same fashion the Collective Supra-conscious was created on the Sun Channel (Adi Pingala Nadi) to accommodate the dead who sought joy through egotistical ambition."

Adi Vishnu protects and evolves the path of evolution. His Incarnations are like milestones in the progress of spiritual awareness, and develop, one by one, new dimensions of human perception. They show the light in the darkness of ignorance, and each Avatar adds a new boundless perception, a new fragrance, and a new color to the beauty of creation.

Matsya Avatar

Life had its first origin in water which was formed through the various combinations and permutations of the different cosmic essences (Tanmatras) of creation. It started as uni-cellular animals and evolved later on as multi-cellular.

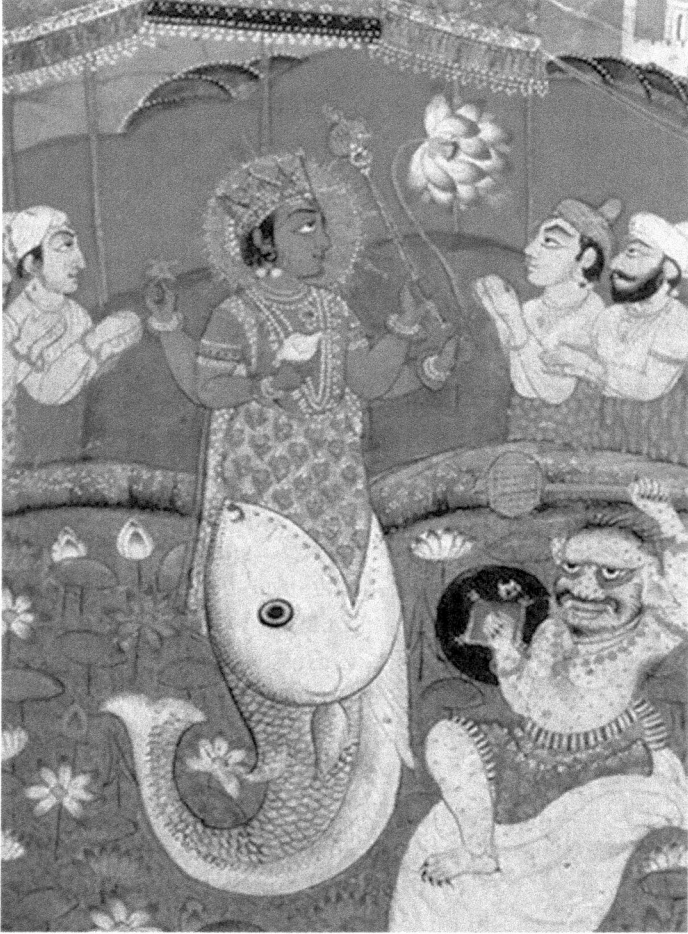

Fishes

The uni-cellular parasites that lived on higher types of fishes incarnated as big fishes with the awareness of the lower type. They became the source of satanic force. As they grew bigger and bigger they were eaten by other fish who were even larger and mightier. They were particularly destructive to other fish who were trying to make the evolutionary transition from water to land. To destroy these evil incarnations Adi Vishnu took the form of a fish becoming the leader of the fishes who wanted to come ashore. This was His first Incarnation known as Matsya avatar (Fish Incarnation).

The story goes that the great Manu, Vaivaswat Manu, the Root Manu, as we call Him--that is, a Manu not of one race only, but of a whole vast round of Cosmic evolution, presiding over the seven globes that are linked for the evolution of the world--that mighty Manu, sitting one day immersed in contemplation, saw a tiny fish gasping for water; and moved by compassion, He took the little fish and put it in a bowl, and the fish grew till it filled the bowl; and He placed it in a water vessel and it grew to the size of the vessel; then He took it out of that vessel and put it into a bigger one; afterwards into a tank, a pond, a river, the sea, and still the marvelous fish grew and grew and grew.

The time came when a vast change was impending; one of those changes called a minor pralay, and it was necessary that the seeds of life should be carried over that pralaya to the next Manvantara.

That would be a minor parlay and a minor Manvantara. What does that mean? It means a passage of the seeds of life from one globe to another; from what we call the globe preceding our own to our own earth. It is the function of the Root Manu, with the help and the guidance of the Divine, to transfer the seeds of life from one globe to the next, so as to plant them in a new soil where further growth is possible.

As waters rose, waters of matter submerging the globe which was passing into pralay, an ark, a vessel appeared; into this vessel stepped the great Rishi with others, and the seeds of life were carried by The Ark. As they went forth upon the waters a mighty fish appeared and to the horn of that fish the vessel was fastened by a rope. It conveyed the whole to safely land to the solid ground where the Manu resumes His work.

This story tells the history of the world, where in the vast surging ocean of matter, we see the Root Manu and the great Initiates gathering up the seeds of life from the world whose work is over, carrying them under the guidance of Vishnu to the new globe where new impulse is to be given to the life; and the reason why the fish form was chosen was simply because in the building up again of the world, it was at first covered with water, and only that form of life was originally possible.

You have in that first stage what the geologists call the Silurian Age, the age of fishes, when the great Divine manifestation was of all these forms of life. The Purana rightly starts in the previous Kalpa, with the manifestation in the form of the fish, to lead the fishes out of the water of the Ocean of Illusion to become reptiles.

Kurma Avatar

Then we find, tracing it onward, that this great age passes, and the world begins to rise out of the waters. How then shall types be brought forth in order that evolution may go on? The next great type is to be fitted either for land or for water; for the next stage of the earth shows the waters draining gradually away, and the land appearing, and the creatures that are the marked characteristic of the age must exist partially on land and partially in water. Here again there must be manifestation of the type of life, we call the reptile type; the tortoise is chosen as the typical creature, and while the tortoise typifies the type to be evolved, reptiles, amphibious creatures of every description swarm over the earth, becoming more and more landlike in their character as the proportion of land to water increases.

There is meanwhile going on, in the "imperishable sacred land," a preparation for further evolution where the great Rishis gather together. The type of the evolution that then took place was the Tortoise.

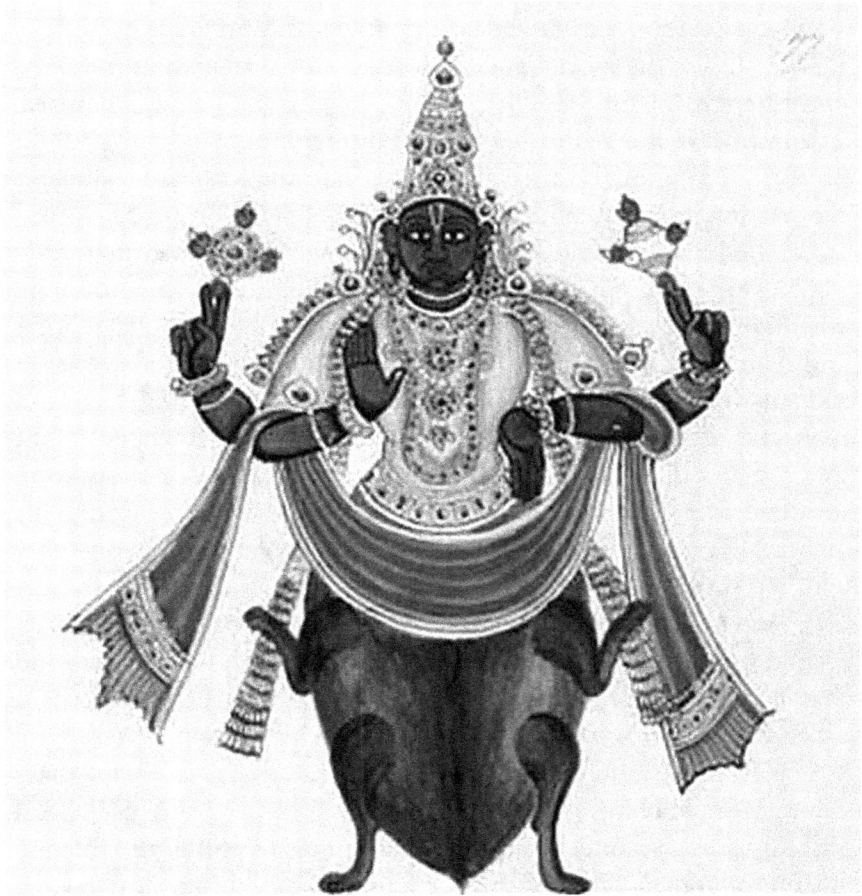

Kurma Avatar

An ark was tied to His tail while his hard back was used for churning the Kshirsagara (Samudra Manthan) which brought forth fourteen gifts for humanity.

This Incarnation later helped guide Noah's (Manu) Ark across the great deluge during the time of the Great Flood (Maha Pralay). The tortoise with its curved shell as protection represents the curvature of the earth. It teaches the reptiles to develop a protective shield.

As it emerged from the sea, it needed no other protection to survive. It was the most suitable form of animal to exist at that level of awareness. Firstly the development of physical being is ensured. The impulsive fear of death generates the beginning of the search for protection by animals - their first quest. The quest for survival marks the starting point of collective organization among animals.

The Divine in that form, makes Himself the base of the revolving axis of evolution. That is typified by Manthara, the mountain which, placed on the tortoise, is made to revolve by the hosts of Suras and Asuras, one pulling at the head of the serpent, and the other at the tail—the positive and negative forces. So the churning begins in matter, evolving types of life. The species that are generated in the lower world; these are the archetypes, always produced in preparation for the forward stretch of evolution. There came forth one by one the archetypes, the elephant, the horse, the woman, and so on, one after another, showing the track along which evolution was to go.

And most important of all, Amrita, nectar of immortality, comes forth, symbol of the one life which passes through every form--and that life appears above the waters the taking of which is necessary in order that every form may live.

Coming ashore and feeling the land beneath them these fish started crawling on land, creating reptiles. At this point Adi Vishnu took a second Incarnation coming as a reptile, the tortoise (Kurmavatara), to destroy the demons obstructing the progress of evolution.

Varaha Avatar

Then comes the third Avatar, the Varaha.

No earth is to be seen; the waters of the flood have overwhelmed it. The types that are to be produced on earth are waiting in the higher region for a place on which to manifest. How shall the earth be brought up from the waters which have overwhelmed it?

Now once again the great Helper is needed, the God, the Protector of Evolution. Then in the form of a mighty Boar, whose form filled the heaven, plunging down into the waters that He alone could separate, the Great One descends.

He brings up the earth from the lower region where it was lying awaiting His coming; and the land rises up again from below the surface of the flood, and the vast Lemurian continent on the earth in those ages surfaces.

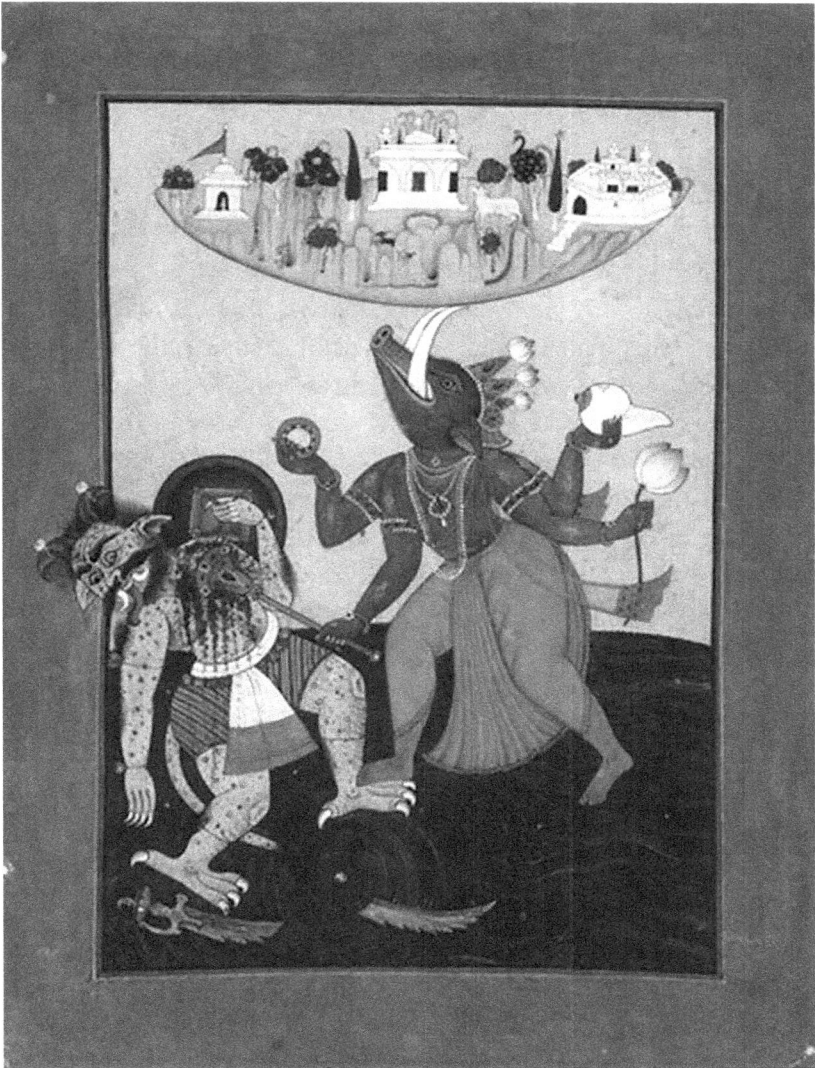

At the mammal stage in His third Incarnation as the wild boar (Varaha Avatar), the instinctual drive for protection expresses itself in more sophisticated patterns of behavior. At this stage, protective measures by herds of four-legged animals were exhibited. The boar also suggests further evolution into the four-legged animal stage (quadruped) from reptile.

On the Lemurian continent were developed many types of life, and there the mammals first made their appearance. When the Boar, the great type of the mammal, plunged into the waters to bring up the earth, then was started the mammalian evolution, and the continent thus rescued from the waters was crowded with the forms of the mammalian kingdom.

Just as the Fish had typified the Silurian epoch, just as the Tortoise had started on its way the great amphibian evolution, so did the Boar, that typical mammal, start the mammalian evolution, and we come to the Lemurian continent with its wonderful variety of forms of mammalian life. As animals died their spirits went into this Paraloka. They were born again on this earth where they learned through experiences. They were also guided towards evolution by different Incarnations (Avataras).

Narasimha Avatar

Then we come to a strange incarnation on this Lemurian continent: where frightful conflicts existed; and man as man had not yet quite come to birth. Strange forms were seen, half human and half animal, wholly monstrous; terrible struggles took place between these monstrous forms born from the slime as it is said--from the remains of former creations--and the newer and higher life in which the future evolution was enshrined.

These forms are represented in the Puranas as those of the race of Daityas, who ruled the earth, who struggled against the Deva manifestations, who conquered the Devas from time to time, who subjected them, who ruled over earth and heaven alike, bringing everything under their sway. There was the frightful conflict of forms, the forms of the past, monstrous in their strength and in their outline, against whom the Sons of Light were battling, against whom the great Lords of the Flame came down. One of these conflicts, the greatest of all, is given in the story of the Avatara when Shri Vishnu took His fourth Incarnation as Narasimha, half man with the upper part half lion.

It is the story of Prahlad. In him we have typified the dawning spirituality which is to show in the higher races of Daityas as they pass on into definite human evolution, and their form gives way that the sexual man may be born. Prahlad was an ardent devotee of Vishnu. His Daitya father strove to kill him because the name of Hari was ever on his lips.

He strove to slay him, with a sword, but the sword fell broken from the neck of the child; he then tried to poison him, and Vishnu appeared and ate first of the poisoned rice, so that the boy might eat it with the name of Hari on his lips; His father then strove to slay him by the furious elephant, by the fang of the serpent, by throwing him over a precipice, and by crushing him under a stone.

But ever the cry of "Hari, Hari," brought deliverance, for in the elephant, in the fang of the serpent, in the precipice, and in the stone, Hari was ever present, and his devotee was safe in that presence. Finally when the father, challenging the omnipresence of the Deity, pointed to the stone pillar and said in mocking language: "Is your Hari also in the pillar?"

"Hari, Hari," cried the boy, and the pillar burst asunder, and the mighty form of half lion and half man came forth and slew the Daitya that doubted, in order that he might learn the omnipresence of the Supreme.

At this point in evolution, man achieves a self-conscious domination over animals and natural forces. This Incarnation also expressed an intermediary step in evolution between the animal and the human stages. Narasimha role was to kill a major devil called Hiranya Kashipu.

Before man came into being he existed at the monkey stage. Monkeys had also been struggling in their evolutionary process. To assist them, the Primordial Preconscious Mind of the Virat Itself took incarnation as Hanuman, the Monkey God, and the devotee of

Shri Vishnu. Hanuman led the monkeys who were half human - 'the missing link' as Darwin called it in human evolution. Thus monkeys were helped to evolve into human beings.

Vamana Avatar

In His fifth Incarnation Shri Vishnu appeared for the first time as a human being. He took the form of the Short Man (Vamana avatar) who came on this earth to give leadership to people seeking God. Vamana was enlightened with the idea that he could capture the three worlds (Triloka) consisting of earth, heaven and hell. When man as man began to evolve, the Supreme came in human form, as Vamana, the Dwarf.

For man was yet a dwarf in the truly human stature, although vast in outer appearance. He came as the inner man, small, yet stronger than the outer form; against him was Bali, the mighty, showing the outer form, while Vamana, the Dwarf, showed the man that should be. And when Bali had offered a great sacrifice, the Dwarf as a Brahmana came to beg.

When we once come to the human Avataras, they are mostly Kshatriyas, but in two cases, they are Brahmanas, and this is one of them; for He was going to beg, and Kshatriya does not beg. Only a Brahmana to whom the earth's wealth was nothing, who had no store of wealth to hold, to whom gold and earth were one, only he could go with begging bowl in hand, to beg of the king.

Now Bali was a pious ruler, on the side of the evolution that was passing away, and gladly gave a boon. "Brahmana, take thy boon," said he. "Three steps of earth alone I ask for," said the Dwarf. Of that little man surely three steps would not cover much, and the great king with his world-wide dominion might well give three steps of earth to the short and puny Dwarf. But one step covered earth, and the next step covered sky. Where the third step could be planted so that the gift might be made complete?

Nothing was left for Bali to give except himself; nothing to make his gift complete. His word if broken it would only save his own body, nothing else. So, recognizing the Lord of all, he threw himself before Him, and the third step, planted on his body, fulfilled the promise of the king and made him the ruler of the lower regions, of Patala.

How full of significance is this inner man! So small at that stage but really so mighty, who was to rule alike the earth and heaven! He could find no place for his third step to put his foot upon save his own lower nature! He was to go forward and forward ever! That is hinted in the third step that was taken. What a graphic picture of the evolution that lay in front, the wondrous evolution that now was to begin.

When we enter the Treta Yuga, we come to another manifestation--that of Parashuram. His sixth form was as the Strong Man (Parashuram). He brought forth the powers achieved by self-control (Tapobala). When they were fully evolved, human beings developed their 'I-ness' and felt a need to seek the unknown within themselves.

They began to think about God, and became aware of the strengths of spiritual life, and started a new search of the inner life. The search was an individual one, and the seeker absolutely secluded him from society. Many renounced the world and went into complete retreat in the forests and jungles in search of the ultimate reality, often pursuing their quest day and night for years on end, and often for life after life. Parashuram was the founder of Hatha and Raja Yoga which were practiced all alone under the guidance of a Guru.

The Yuga had now gone far and the Kshatriya caste had risen and was ruling, mighty in its power, and great in its authority. The duty of the ruler is essentially protection: but they used their power not to protect, but to plunder, not to help but to oppress.

The first great lesson was given to the kings of the earth, the rulers of men, and a lesson that had to be repeated over and over again, and is not yet completely learnt. A divine manifestation came in order that, that lesson might be taught. The story goes that food was given to two Kshatriya women, each of whom was to bear a son.

The husband of one of them was a Brahmana. The two women exchanged the food, and that meant to bring forth a Kshatriya son was taken by the woman with the Brahmana husband. The food which was full of Kshatriya energy thus went into the Brahmana family. Thus was born Parashuram.

But while Parashuram was still in the body, a greater Avatara came forth to show what a Kshatriya king should be. The Kshatriyas abusing their place and their power were swept away by Parashuram. So that we have the strange phenomenon of the Brahmana coming with an axe to slay the Kshatriya, and twenty one times that axe was raised in slaughter, cutting the Kshatriya trunk off from the surface of the earth. So in corollary, this Incarnation brought forth the idea in the human mind that man can overpower all three worlds.

Thus it should be understood that Adi Vishnu's Incarnations, the line of evolution, lead the way towards higher, deeper and wider spiritual awareness which is the true index by which the development of the Creation can be measured. First the individual evolution is achieved and then the collective assimilation by the masses was experienced.

Chapter 5

Rama Avatar

The boy Rama was born, the ideal ruler, the utterly perfect king. While a boy He went forth with the great teacher Visvamitra, in order to protect the Yogi's sacrifice. Although just a boy, almost a child he was able to drive away the Rakshasas that interfered with the sacrifice, and then He and His beloved brother Lakshmana and the Yogi went on to the court of king Janaka.

There, at the court, was a great bow, which had belonged to Mahadeva Himself. To bend and string that bow was the task for the man who would wed Sita. Sita who was the incarnation of Shri Laxmi, a child of marvelous birth, the maiden who had sprung from the earth, had no physical father or mother. Who should wed the peerless maiden, the incarnation of Shri Laxmi, and the consort of Vishnu? Who should wed her save the Avatar of Vishnu Himself?

So the mighty bow remained unstrung, until the boy Rama came. He took it up with boyish carelessness, and bends it so strongly that it breaks in half, the crash echoing through earth and sky. He weds Sita,, and goes forth with Her, and with His brother Lakshmana and his bride, and with His father who had come to the bridal, in a vast procession, wending their way back to their own town Ayodhya.

This breaking of Mahadeva bow rung through the earth, shaking all the worlds, and all, both men and Devas, knew that the bow had been broken. Among the devotees of Mahadeva, Parashuram heard the clang of the broken bow, the bow of the One He worshipped; and proud with the might of His strength, still with the energy of Vishnu in Him. He went to meet this insolent boy, who had dared to break the bow that no other arm could bend. He challenged Him, and handing His own bow bid Him to try what He could do with that.

Could He shoot an arrow from its string? Rama took this offered bow, strung it, and set an arrow on the string. Then He stopped, for in front of Him there was the body of a Brahmana; should He draw an arrow against that form? As the two Rama stood face to face, the energy of the elder, it is written, passed into the younger; the energy of Vishnu, the energy of the Supreme, left the form in which it had been dwelling and entered the higher manifestation of the same divine life.

The bow was stretched and the arrow waiting to be shot, but Rama would not shoot it forth until He had pacified His antagonist; then feeling that energy pass, Parashuram bowed before Rama, diviner than Himself, hailed Him as the Supreme Lord of the worlds, bent in reverence before Him, and went away. That Avatar was over, although the form in which the energy had dwelt yet persisted.

Thus here there was the incarnation whose energy was taken aback by the Giver and put into a new vessel in which new work is to be done.

And so in other Avataras, He limits Himself for men's sake. Take the great king, Shri Rama. What did he come to show? The ideal Kshatriya, in every relation of the Kshatriya life; as son—a perfect son to a loving father as well as to a jealous and for the time unkind step-mother. For when the father's wife who was not His own mother bade him go forth to the forest on the very eve of His coronation as heir, His gentle answer was: "Mother, I shall go."

Perfect as son; perfect as husband; if He had not limited Himself by His own will how could he show what husband should be to wife, when Sita had been taken away by Ravan when they were in exile in the forest, how could He have shown the grief, have uttered the piteous lamentations, which have drawn tears from thousands of eyes, as He calls on plants and trees, animals and birds, on Gods and men, to tell Him where His wife, His other self, the life of His life, had gone? How could he have taught men what wife should be to a husband's heart unless He had limited Himself? The consciously Omnipresent Deity could not seek and search for His beloved who had disappeared.

And then as king; he was as perfect a king as could be. When the welfare of His subjects was concerned, when the safety of the kingdom was to be thought of, when He remembered that He as king stood for God and must be perfect in the eyes of His subjects, so that they might give the obedience and the loyalty, which men can only give to one whom they know as greater than themselves.

Then even when His wife was put to the test of fire for, Sita, the unsullied and the suffering; then she must pass through it to show that no sin or pollution had come upon her by the foul touch of Ravan, the Rakshasa. Then the demand that to win her husband's heart She must come forth pure as woman; and all this, because He was king as well as husband, and on the throne the people honored as Divine there must only be purity, spotless as driven snow. Those limitations were needed in order that a perfect example might be given to man, and man might learn to climb by reproducing virtues, made small in order that his small grasp might hold them.

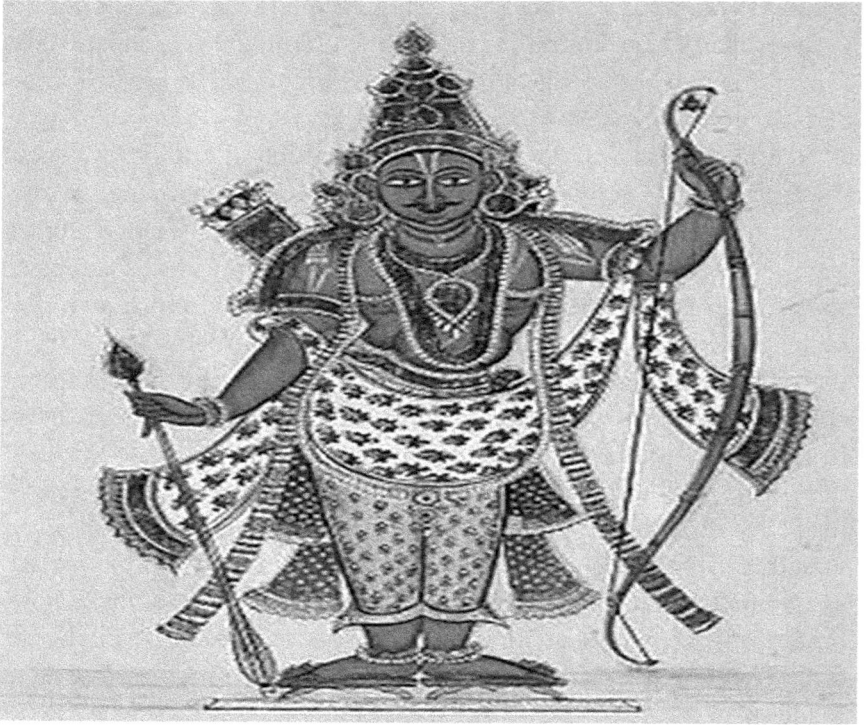

Adi Vishnu Himself took His seventh Incarnation during the Treta Yuga as Lord Rama, a human being who crossed the Ocean of Illusion and touched a new dimension of awareness. As Shri Rama, Adi Vishnu came to enlighten human, social and political consciousness as the true model of what Plato, thousands of years later, would call 'the philosopher King'.

He settled for human beings the rules of socio-political correct action (Samaj Tatha Rajkaran Dharma). He also expressed God's aspect of majesty and order within kingship and institutions, and led a life of an ideal human king (Mariada Purushottama). This was witnessed by multitudes, resulting in a mass awareness for the first time among human beings. Shri Rama was the ideal King for all Kings, and Ramrajya, His kingdom, was the ideal kingdom.

He reached a point in the Primordial Heart Chakra (Adi Anahat Chakra) crossing the Void along the central path (Adi

Sushumna Nadi). His wife Sita was an Incarnation of Adi Shakti. "The Ramayana", the epic about Lord Rama's exploits written by Valmiki tells how Lord Rama was made to forget by design that he was a Divine Incarnation for much of His life. It was decided that He should act completely as a human being to make human beings absolutely follow Him in His human ways. Later on, when Sita disappeared back into the Mother Earth, Lord Rama recalled His divinity.

At the time of Rama's Incarnation Adi Shakti existed in three persons:

- in Sita, his wife, as Mahalaxshmi;
- in Sati Anusuya who recreated Dattatreya, the Primordial Master, as Mahasaraswati;
- In Mandodari, the wife of Ravan, as Mahakali.

Earlier as Sita, although formally married to Rama in a wedding ceremony that was collectively sanctioned, she was still condemned by society. Krishna's love and adoration of Radha brought her glory without marriage, while Sita was denied that public acceptance even though she was the legal wife of Rama.

Sita was married to Rama in a very traditional way. When He went into exile, Ravan the Rakshasa, Satan disguised as an ascetic, appeared before her and took her away to the capital of his kingdom in Lanka. Rama fought a war with Ravan to rescue His wife, who was secluded by Ravan in the core of his island kingdom. Rama defeated His enemy and brought Sita back to His kingdom, Ayodhya.

Ravan was the mighty intelligence, the Rakshasa, who called forth the coming of Shri Rama. He was in his past life the keeper of Vishnu's heaven, door-keeper of the mighty Lord, devotee, and Bhakta, absolutely devoted to the Lord. It was he who cast his head into the fire in order that Mahadeva might be served. It is he in whose name have been written some of the most exquisite Stotras, breathing the spirit of complete devotion; it is in the mouth of Ravan words are put appealing to Mahadeva; and, describing Him as surrounded by the most repellent and undesirable, Pishachas and Bhuta, forms from which all beauty is withdrawn, he cries out in a passion of love: "Better wear pisacha-form, so we ever more are near and wait on Thee.

How did he then come to be the ravisher of Sita and the enemy of God?

Through lack of intuition, through the lack of power to recognize the meaning of an order, not following the words of the spirit, he refused to open the door of heaven when Sanat Kumara came and demanded entrance. He came under the curse of Sanat Kumara in order that his mistake might be compensated for.

He was asked: "Will you have seven incarnations friendly to Vishnu, or three in which you will be His enemy and oppose Him?" And because he was a true Bhakta, and because every moment of absence from his Lord meant to him hell of torture, he chose three of enmity, which would let him go back sooner to the Feet of the Beloved, rather than the seven of happiness, of friendliness. Better a short time of utter enmity than a longer remaining away with apparent happiness. It was love not hatred that made him choose the form of a Rakshasa rather than the form of a Rishi.

Hence having taken the form of a Rakshasa, he had to do his duty as a Rakshasa. He was not a weak man to be swayed by momentary thought or by transient objects. He had all the learning of the Vedas. He knew his duty. What was his duty? To put forward every force in his mighty nature to check evolution, to gather round him all the forces which were opposing evolution; to make himself the centre to every force that was setting itself against the will of the Lord; to gather them together as it were into one head, so that when their apparent triumph made the cry of the earth go up to Vishnu, the answer might come in Rama's Avatar and they be destroyed, so that the life-wave might go on.

Nobly he did the work, thoroughly he discharged his duty. It is said that even sages are confused about Dharma. His Dharma was the Dharma of a Rakshasa, to lead the whole forces of evil against one, whom in his inner soul, which at that time was clouded, yet whom he loved. When Shri Rama came, when He was wandering in the forest, how could he sting Him into leaving the life of His life, His beloved Sita?

By taking away from Him the one thing to which He clung, by taking away from Him the wife whom He loved as His very Self, by placing her in the spot where all the forces of evil were gathered together, he made one head responsible for destruction, which the arrow of Shri Rama might destroy.

Then the mighty battle began the struggle with all the forces of his great nature, ending when the arrow of Shri Rama that struck off the head of Ravan who was then the enemy. And from the corpse of the Rakshasa that fell upon the field near Lanka, the devotee went up to Goloka (a name for one of the heavens) to sit at the feet of the Beloved, and rest for awhile till the third incarnation had to be lived out.

Although she was the purest of the pure and the holiest of the holy, Sita was treated with suspicion by the citizens of Ayodhya, Rama's capital city. They would not accept her as queen, blaming her for having been abducted by force by Ravan. The suspicious citizens questioned her chastity, and committed collective sin by rejecting her. Although she was pregnant Rama was forced to forsake her.

She lived with the Saint Valmiki in the jungles of Bihar State where she gave birth to twin boys, Lava and Kusha. They were absolutely human personalities but of very great spiritual heritage from previous births. Sita taught them the Divine way of life. They were later born again in Bihar as Gautama, known as Lord Buddha, and as Shri Mahavir, the leader of the great religion, Jainism. This all happened 500 years before the birth of Christ. Internally they reached a very great height through these births.

They preached the doctrine of non-violence (Ahimsa) which was later developed into an extreme form of vegetarianism. They took birth in the Warrior Caste (Kshatriya) in order to keep away from the extremes of vegetarian abstinences, and to stay more balanced. Still their disciples carried their teachings to the extreme of abstinence and vegetarianism. They confused inner asceticism (Sanyasa) with organized institutions of asceticism, and non-violence with vegetarianism.

The great reign of Rama lasted ten thousand years in the Dwapara Yuga, the Yuga at the close of which Shri Krishna came.

Chapter 6

Krishna Avatar

Adi Vishnu's eighth incarnation was as Shri Krishna during the Dwapara Yuga, which perhaps is the most glorified of all the divine manifestations. Shri Krishna is the God of the household, the God of family life, the God whose manifestations attract in every phase of His Self-revelation; He is human to the very core. Born in humanity, He acts as a man.

As a child, He is a real child, full of playfulness, fun, and winsome grace. Growing up into boyhood, into manhood, He exercises the same human fascination over the hearts of men, women, and children; the God in whose presence there is always joy, the God in whose presence there is continual laughter and music. When we think of Shri Krishna we seem to hear the ripple of the river, the rustling of the leaves in the forest, the bellowing of the cows in the pasture, the laughter of happy children playing round their parents' knees.

He is so fundamentally the God who is human in everything; who bends in human sympathy over the cradle of the babe, who sympathizes with the play of the youth, who is the friend of the lover, the one who blesses the bridegroom and the bride, who smiles on the young mother when her first-born lies in her arms--everywhere the God of love and of human happiness. It is no wonder that His winsome grace has fascinated the hearts of men!

Because of the extremely complicated nature of the Avatar of Shri Krishna, and the vast range that He covered as regards His manifestations, in dealing with His life, we shall take it in stages -we shall see one great type of the teaching in each one, which the world is meant to learn from the playing of this drama before the eyes of men. To some extent the stages correspond with marked periods in the life, and may overlap each other; but they reveal a great deal about the purpose of this Avatar.

- First act of the great drama was to stand forth as the Object of devotion, and to show the love with which God regards His devotees. This was a very significant stage in the life of Shri Krishna.
- Then the second act of the drama may be said to be His character as the destroyer of the opposing forces that retard evolution and that runs through the whole of His life.
- The third act is that of the statesman, the wise, politically diplomatic, and intellectual actor on the world's stage of history, the guiding force of the nation by His wondrous policy and intelligence, standing forth not as king but rather as statesman.
- Then we have Him as friend, the human friend, especially of the Pandavas and Arjuna.
- The next act is that of Shri Krishna as Teacher, the world-teacher, not the teacher of one race alone.
- Then we see Him in the strange and wondrous aspect of the Searcher of the hearts of men, the Trier and tester of human nature.
- Finally, we may regard Him in His manifestation as the Supreme, the all-pervading life of the universe, who looks on nothing as outside Himself, and one who embraces evil as well as good, darkness and light, treating nothing alien to Himself.

The life-history of our own minds may be divided into these seven acts as it were. One aspect will attract one man, another aspect will attract another; all the aspects are worthy of study, all are provocative of devotion.

Devotion, is the earliest stage of His life, inspiring and full of benediction, those early years of the Lord as infant, as a child, as a young boy, when He is dwelling in Vraja, in the forest of Brindavan, living with the cowherds and their wives and children, the marvelous child who stole the hearts of men. It is noticeable that Shri Krishna chose to show Himself as the great object of devotion, as the lover of the devotee, in the form of a child, not in that of a man.

Before that birth took place upon earth, the deities had been to Vishnu in the higher regions, and had asked Him to interfere in order that earth might be lightened of her load, that the oppression of the incarnate Daityas might be slayed; and then Vishnu said to the Gods: "Go and incarnate yourselves in portions among men, go and take birth amidst humanity."

Great Rishis also took birth in the place where Vishnu Himself was to be born, so that when He came, the surroundings of the drama were, as it were, made in the place of His coming, and those that we speak of as the cowherds of Vraja, Nanda and the Gopis and all the inhabitants of that wondrously blessed spot, were, it is written looked like "God-like persons".

They were "the Protectors of the worlds" who were born as men for the progress of the world. Gods themselves had come down and taken birth as men. All that took place throughout the wonderful childhood of the Shri Krishna Lila all those who played and enacted the drama were no ordinary men, or women; they were the Protectors of the worlds incarnated as cowherds round Him.

And the Gopis, the graceful wives of the shepherds, they were the Rishis of ancient days, who by devotion to Vishnu had gained the blessing of being incarnated as Gopis, in order that they might surround His childhood, and pour out their love at the tiny feet of the boy they worshipped as Supreme.

When all these preparations were made for the coming of the child, the child was born. He was born in His four-armed form, shining out for the moment in the dungeon, which before His birth had been irradiated by Him through His mother's body, who was said to be like an alabaster vase--so pure was she. Her womb like the alabaster vase which was as a lamp containing Him, the world's light, so that the glory illuminated the darkness of the dungeon where she lay.

At His birth he came as Vishnu, for the moment showing Himself with all the signs of the Deity on Him, with the discus, the conch, the shrivatsa on His breast, with all the recognized emblems of the Lord. But that form quickly vanished, and only the human child lay before His parents' eyes. And the father, taking Him up, passed through the huge locked doors which miraculously opened before him, carried Him in safety into his brother's house, where He was to dwell, in the place prepared for His coming.

Shri Krishna who was the greatest expression of God the Father, incarnated to open another horizon in human understanding the power of Divine Love to watch the play of God's power as a witness. By His Incarnation, human imagination was to become aware of the witnessing powers of Almighty God. The Great Primordial Being (Virat) was actually expressed through Him. His advent enabled poets and philosophers to enter the intuitive realm of metaphysical perceptions. He employed the method, of Divine Diplomacy to explain the true nature of reality to people.

The beauty of Divine Diplomacy is to achieve the spiritual betterment of people. Its' essence is to guide ignorant and foolish people towards the path of righteousness and religion by diplomatic ways, by clever handling or by illusion. In short such people must be brought to the shores of Divine Love ' by hook or by crook'. Shri Krishna's life was spent with the masses, and thus His Incarnation gave rise to a mass spiritual movement. He appeared before Arjuna as the Virat, and for the first time human eyes got a glimpse of the Primordial Being Himself

As a babe He showed forth the power that was in Him, the destroyer of the forces of evil. And as He grows up He begins wandering through the fields and the forests, and the notes of His wondrous flute are heard all over all the plains. As a child of five He wandered with His magic flute in His hands, charming the hearts of all those who heard him.

The boys left tending the cattle and followed the music of the flute; the women left their household tasks and followed where the flute was playing; the men ceased their labors that they might feast their ears on the music of the flute. It was not only the men, the women and children, but the cows, it is said, stopped their grazing to listen as the notes fell on their ears, the calves ceased suckling as the music floated towards them, the river rippled up so that it might hear better, the trees bowed down their branches so that they might not lose a note, the birds felt silent lest their music should make a discord in the melody, as the wondrous child wandered over the country, and the music of heaven flowed from His magic flute.

And thus while He lived, played and sported, he won the hearts of all. Not only the hearts of the cowherds but the hearts of their wives and daughters too went out to that marvelous child. He played with them and loved them, and they would take Him up and place His baby feet on their bosoms, and would sing to Him as the Lord of all, the Supreme, and the mighty One. They recognized the Deity in the child that played round their homes, and many lessons that He taught them.

One day as a child of six, while he was wandering along, a number of the Gopis were bathing nude in the river, having cast aside their clothes-

-as they should not have done, that being against the law and showing carelessness of womanly modesty. Leaving their garments on the bank they had plunged into the river.

The child of six saw this with the eye of insight; He gathered up their clothes and climbed up a tree nearby, threw them round His own shoulders and waited to see what would happen. The water was bitterly cold and the Gopis were shivering; but they did not want to come out of it before the clear steady eyes of the child. And He called them to come and get the garments they had thrown off.

As they hesitated, the baby lips told them that they had sinned against God by immodestly casting aside the garments that should have been worn, and must therefore expiate their sin by coming and taking from His hands that which they had cast aside. They came and worshipped, and He gave them back their robes.

This story of Krishna as a child of six has often been the subject of criticism and discussion. It is spoken of as though he were a full grown man, insulting the modesty of women. The Gopis were Rishis, and the Lord, the Supreme, as a babe is teaching them a lesson. But there is more than that; there is a profound occult lesson behind the story. It is that when the soul is approaching the supreme Lord at one great stage of initiation, it has to pass through a great ordeal; stripped of everything on which it has hitherto relied, stripped of everything that is not of its inner Self, deprived of all external aid, external protection, or covering, the soul must stand naked and alone with nothing to rely on, save the life of the Self within it. If it flinches before the ordeal, if it clings to anything to which hitherto it has looked for help, if in that supreme hour it cries out for friend or even for the Guru himself, the soul fails in that ordeal. Naked and alone it must go forth, with absolutely none to aid it, save the divinity within itself. And it is that nakedness of the soul as it approaches the supreme goal that is told of in that story of Shri Krishna, the child, and the Gopis.

In their early days, Radha and Krishna played a game of Rasa (Ra + Sa - meaning "with energy"). Rasa is the play which manifests identification with the power of God. It was the play of Sahaja Yoga, of the divine circuit of vibrations. All Shri Krishna's playmates were innocent, simple cow herders (Gopis and Gopas). They did not know that he was trying to manifest the working of Sahaja Yoga (spontaneous growth of the inner self) through the play (Leela) of Rasa. This was the essence as told to us by Shri Mataji Nirmala Devi during Krishna Puja.

When Radha filled pitchers of water from the Yamuna River She automatically vibrated that water with Pranava as she was Adi Shakti and was carrying the water on her head. When Shri Krishna broke the pitchers the vibrated water was meant to fall on the soil of Brindavan where Krishna and Radha lived, vibrating it. Similarly when Radha placed her feet in the Yamuna River, the waters of the river became vibrated. So when Gopis and their husbands, the simple folk of Brindavan, carried water from the river in earthenware pitchers, Krishna broke the pitchers so that the vibrated water would fall from their heads onto their spinal cord. Their Kundalini would thus be awakened and raised, and they would get their Self-realization through the spontaneous awakening of Sahaja Yoga.

It was sportive and playful baptism, but all these tricks or designs of Krishna do not completely and immediately work out the whole manifestation of Sahaja Yoga. He sowed the seed of Sahaja Yoga, as His name Krishna meaning 'the one who sows' (Krishi). The Gopis and Gopas did get Kundalini awakening which was a great achievement. The awakened state of their Kundalini made the finite nature of human beings enlightened and enlarged their consciousness, but they still could not pierce into the infinite. That was left to be done after Krishna's time, and thus awakened their Kundalini needed many years of effort or many lives' experience to become receptive to Sahaja Yoga.

Then we learn more details of His play with the Gopis as a child of seven: how He wandered into the forest and disappeared and all went after Him seeking Him; how they tried to imitate His own play, in order to fill up the void that was left by His absence.

The child of seven, that He was at this time, disappeared for a while, but came back to those who loved Him, as God ever does with His Bhaktas. And then takes place that wondrous dance, the Rasa of Shri Krishna, part of His Lila, when He multiplied Himself so that every pair of Gopis found Him standing between them; amidst the ring of women the child was there between each pair of them, giving a hand to each; and so the mystic dance was danced.

This is another of those points of attack which are made by ignorant minds. It is as though He kept the child form in the Lila, in order that He might breathe harmlessly into men's blind unclean hearts the lesson He wanted to give.

There was also the other incident when He, He who is the Feeder of the worlds, sent for food and some of His Brahmin friends refused to give it. They sent away the boys who came to ask for food. When the men refused, He sent them back to the women, to see if they too would refuse the food which their husbands had declined to give.

And the women, who have ever loved the Lord, brought up the food from every part of their houses where they could find it and went out, bringing food for Him. All tried to stop them, but no, they pleaded; they must go to Him, to their Lover, to Shri Krishna. They did not want that the child of their love should be hungry. The implication always is that their love was purely physical love, as though that were possible with a child of seven.

There is not a religion in the world that has not taught that when the Supreme calls, all else must be cast aside. Jesus of Nazareth has also said "He that loved father or mother more than me, is not worthy of me; and he that loved son or daughter more than me is not worthy of me." "And every one that hath forsaken houses, or brethren, or sisters, or father, or mother, or wife, or children, or lands, for my name's sake, shall receive an hundred fold, and shall inherit everlasting life."

It is the same teaching in every other religion of the world. The terms of physical love are used to describe the relation between the soul and God.

Take the "Song of Solomon." If you take the Christian Bible, you will see "The Love of Christ for His Church"; and also will find the most passionate of love songs, a description of the exquisite female form in all the details of its attractive beauty; the cry of the lover to the beloved to come to him that they might take their fill of love.

So also in the songs of the Sufis, the mystics of the faith of Islam, woman's love is ever used as the best symbol of love between the soul and God. In all ages the love between husband and wife has been the symbol of union between the Supreme and His devotees; the closest of all earthly ties, the most intimate of all earthly unions, the merging of heart and body of twain into one. Where will you find a better image of the merging of the soul in its God?

Ever has the object of devotion been symbolized as the lover or husband, ever the devotee as wife or mistress? This symbology is universal, because it is fundamentally true. The absolute surrender of the wife to the husband upon earth is that of the absolute surrender of the soul to God. That is the justification of the Rasa of Shri Krishna; that is the explanation of the story of His life in Vraja.

Whilst Dattatraya's incarnation was created in the Void, Shri Krishna's was at a much higher point, higher than even the Primordial

Heart Chakra on which Lord Rama took incarnation. Shri Krishna's seat in the body of the Virat is the Adi Vishuddhi Chakra, and is placed at the base of the neck inside the spinal cord. Shri Krishna was in fact the complete incarnation of the Virat whose form (Swarup) He showed in a vision to His disciple Arjuna, during his discourse on the battlefield as spelt out in the "Shrimad Bhagawad Gita".

As the embodiment of the witness state He killed many Rakshasas and Rakshasis, as did Lord Rama. These entities have to be killed and destroyed again and again whenever they come in the way of human evolution.

Adi Shakti's incarnations are mostly to kill demons too. The incarnations of Radha show how the ideas of human beings gradually changed. The life as Radha was definitely a peg above in social advancement in the dogmatic thinking of society since the time of Sita. She was not married to Shri Krishna in a formal human way (Lowkika). Their wedding was divine

(Alowkika), and was performed spiritually and socially in the presence of many people by Brahmadeva.

In ancient times it was said that one should speak the truth (Satyam) which is pleasing (Priyam). Often to tell the truth can hurt another's feelings. This contradictory statement was later challenged by many intellectuals. Shri Krishna explained that if the object of the betterment of spirit (Hita) is inserted between telling the truth and pleasing or endearing, then it is possible to unobtrusively tell the truth. He meant that if truth is told for the betterment or upliftment of spirit, ultimately it becomes an endearment and pleases the spirit.

It is important to understand the incarnation of Shri Krishna. The word 'Krishna' comes from the word 'Krishi' – 'Krishi' means 'agriculture'. He had sown the seeds of spirituality. Shri Rama during his life time had created many maryadas or limitations or boundaries. People had begun binding themselves mentally; it was not spontaneous, it was not *Sahaja*. As a result people became extremely serious. They wouldn't talk much, they wouldn't laugh, and they wouldn't enjoy anything. So Shri Krishna decided to first free them from this conditioning in such as way that they could enjoy themselves.

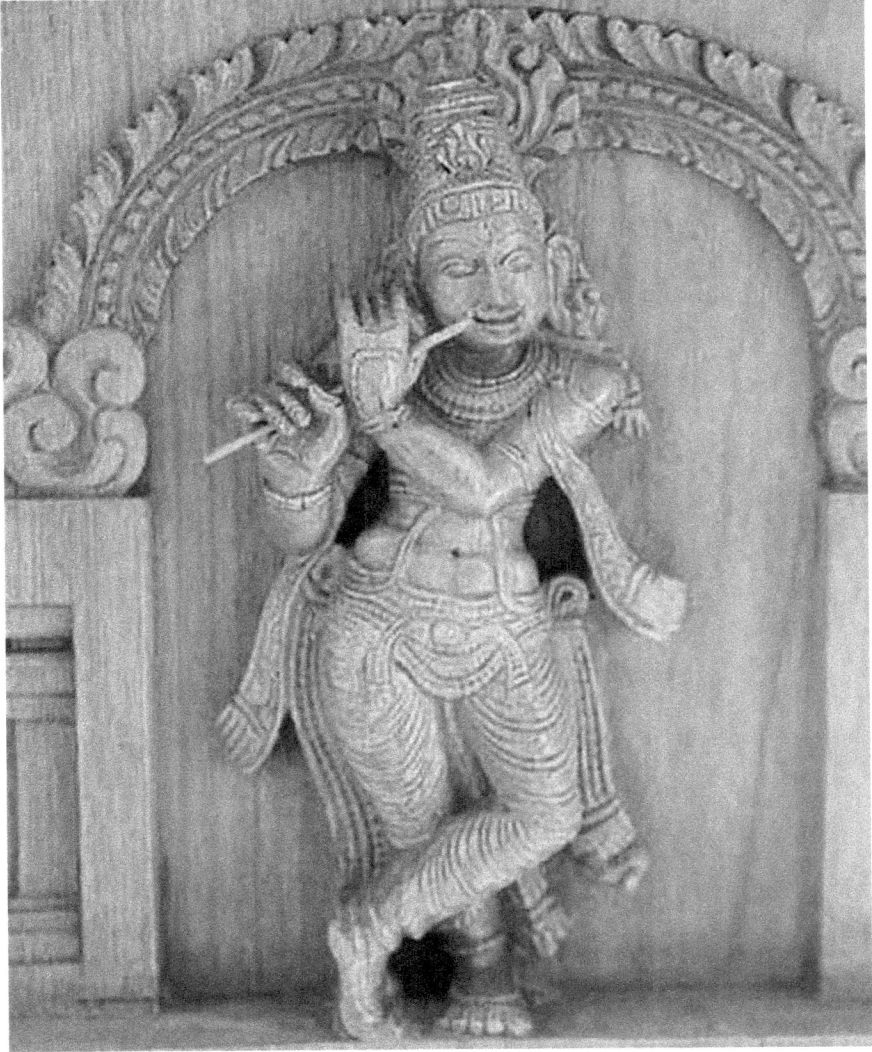

He discovered three methods for achieving this goal.

1. The first one was to become a Realised Soul – Sthita
    Pragnya – to go beyond all temptations, to go beyond ego
    and all kinds of conditioning. Sthita Pragnya is a state of
    detachment, where a person doesn't take to any grievances,

jealousies, and other petty tendencies. He however did not tell how that could be achieved.

The second thing he described was karma or that one had to do work and do that in such a manner so as to leave the fruit of the work at the Lotus Feet of God or the Divine Power.

He was aware of the human potential for misinterpretation and capacity to twist everything to suit their ego gratifications which makes it highly difficult to surrender anything at the feet of the Divine. Thus he made an impossible situation for the people. This was the way that he prepared the land.

2. Second thing is that 'Pushpam falam toya' 'Flowers, fruit and water – whatever you offer me, I will take it'. But when you do that, you must have *Ananya bhakti. Ananya* means completely single-minded *bhakti*, when there is not 'the other'. This is only possible after Realisation.

Only after Realisation you can put the fruits of your work at the Lotus Feet of the Divine, and only after Self Realisation you can have *Ananya Bhakti*, means a single pointed Devotion. He wanted the people to give up the absurd ideas about *bhakti* that people were engaged in. He wanted to neutralise the absurdities of human beings. *Ananya Bhakti* is only possible when you are a Realised Soul, when you are connected with the Divine and when there is not the other. This is how he tried to bring about a three-way transformation on human beings.

3. The third thing was to create discretion in people. At this juncture when we are faced with all sorts of challenges it is really very important to know through discretion what is good and what is bad. What may be good to some may not be so for others. But the Divine Discretion is very, different and it acts by itself.

Once you are in the realm of Divine Discretion, you cannot commit mistakes even if you want to do it. Sometimes it appears that in that Divine Discretion you may do something wrong or you have done something wrong. But if it is Divine, ultimately it will turn out to be good. This Divine Discretion gives us the real joy of our being. So the third point was for Him to make people joyous and happy.

In order to get the people free of the various maryadas and conditionings that they had built around themselves from the incarnation of Shri Rama, Shri Krishna devised several methods to make the people have joyous attitude to life. Even though it may look frivolous, there was joy expressed. All that he did was to give them a joyous attitude to life.

He spoke of detachment, of being joyful but detached". People found it difficult to understand this as their joy were all born out of attachment. Detachment meant giving up. But the truth is attachment creates more worry leading to creation of restrictions which in turn prevents one from actually enjoying.

People have created all sorts of restrictions, or maryadas, that of religion, of false values, of country, of nationality, social maryadas and so on. In this confusion, they no longer enjoyed anything. But if you have Divine Discretion, you will know with whom to talk, where to go, what to enjoy. Attachment prevents a holistic view. If you are detached you can see things from a broader perspective as you become thoughtlessly aware.

Even in the situation were Arjuna felt depressed that he had to fight his own brothers, relatives and friends, Shri Krishna tells Arjuna to fight as it was his Dharma. Besides those he was fighting against were people who did not live in Dharma, they were adharmis. The fighting was justified because they had been deceived, and not fighting would mean that they would become slaves of deception, which was against Divine discretion. Hence fighting was justified. Besides, after the fight, they got back what they deserved.

This was the Divine Discretion of Shri Krishna, instilled within us, as part and parcel of the Vishuddhi Chakra, where Shri Krishna resides. But when he rises to your Sahasrar, when he rises to that level, then he becomes Virat. So Virata's chakra is placed in the head above the Agnya. And this Virat is the form of Shri Krishna who has risen above the Agnya, i.e. the ego.

Once you rise above the ego you become the Virat, whose powers are tremendous. The power of Virat is it acts globally. The power of Virat is that it can penetrate into the subtle side of human beings in such a manner that we are connected with everything, we are not separate. We are connected with the whole universe.

We become cosmic citizens so to say and all the things with which we are connected also get our vibrations, our ideas, our ambitions – everything passes through that. And it works. It is the Virat Shakti that works, which to us seem like miracles. Once we enter the area of Virat the entire focus shifts, thinking then becomes a global thinking. One forgets his limited area of influence, that of position or family, that of status or wealth.

Shri Krishna was the Yogeshwara -the" God of Yoga". He was the Lord of our Union with the Divine.

He was Yogeshwara and a real Yogi is a person who gets this Yogeshwara awakened within him. The word "Yoga" that we understand is the union of our attention with the Divine. As soon as we become the spirit, we get the powers of "collective consciousness". It is the gift of Shri Krishna to start feeling the collectivity.

Your ego and superego are sucked in whereby, you get rid of your karmas and your conditionings and a sprouting of the new life of the new age starts... He is the Ishwara of all the Yogis and for Him everything is a play –a "Leela". Unlike Shri Rama, for whom life was not a play but a platform to demonstrate how to lead a very dharmic life as "Maryada Purushottama", Shri Krishna came up to show, that He is the "Leeladhara" - the one who plays the Leela,

Further the Yogeshwara Shri Krishna has said that: "Sarvam dharmam pari tajya mamekam sharanam vraja". Everybody's duties are called as dharmas because you are duty bound, they form your dharmas. Similarly there is "rashtra dharma"i.e. patriotism to your country, "samaj dharma" that is duty towards your society, "pati dharma", that is duties of husbands to their wives and that of wives to their husbands.

Dharma is also in relationship; the sister-brother relationships, "stridharma" etc. Shri Krishna said, "give up all these dharmas, give up all the duties, give up all your relationships, and just surrender yourself fully to Me" - sarwa dharmam pari tajya mama cam sharanam Vraja.". Because you have become the collective being, you become one with Him, and He looks after your dharmas, and relationships, and purifies them once you have surrendered yourself to Him fully.

There is a misunderstanding about the story of Shri Krishna having 16000 wives. The five wives that He married were the five principles or the five elements. He made them into women and married them.

Similarly the 16.000 women that he married were the 16.000 powers that he needed to channelize his work and energies. Hence those 16000 powers were born as women, whom he married through whom he worked out his Leelas. To Him it was not a relationship of man and wife, but a pure relationship where sex, temptations and perversions had no existence at all.

His powers as Yogeshwara are evident from the story of His five wives wanting to go and pray to a saint who stayed across the river Tapi. When they decided to go for worship after selecting an auspicious time and reached the river they found that the river was in a spate and could not cross it. So they went to Krishna and told Him about the situation.

He said: "Really? Just go and tell the river. If our husband, Shri Krishna, is "Yogeshwara", (that means one who never indulges into any sex activity) then please subside."

They went and told the river: "If He is the Yogeshwara, then please subside." The river subsided. They went to the other side, performed the pujas to their guru and returned. Again the river was in a spate and they could not cross. So they went to the guru. They said: "See, we cannot cross, the river is in spate."

He asked them: "Really, how did you come?"

They said: "Shri Krishna asked us to tell the river, "If I am the Yogeshwara, please go down, it will go down. We asked the question and the river subsided and we were able to come."

The guru then said: "All right, now you go and ask the question, that if I, the mute, that means if I have eaten all the food you've given me, but I've not enjoyed it, I've not indulged into it, then let the river subside."

They went and told the river, "Whatever food we offered to him, if he has not eaten any food, then you subside". And the river subsid!

Thus what is to be learnt from this is that we have to be connected to the vital that enables us to reach the state of collective consciousness or the Yogeshwara .Thus the incarnations are the light, which are enlightening the path, on which we are walking and they take us to realms where they are the Kings and Lords.

To worship Yogeshwara, we must know that our relationships with everyone in this world have to be pure. He wanted to break all the nonsensical shackles of traditions and false fanaticism. But He did it in a very beautiful manner keeping the relationships absolutely pure.

Once while answering to a question on whether Shri Krishna was married to Radha, Shri Mataji replied "He is eternally married to her and that He actually performed the marriage on the day He was born. He was brought by His father across the river and put down on the bank of the river. Then Shri Brahmadeva himself came on this earth. That's why He wears a yellow cloth to cover the lower half of his waist, given as a blessing from Brahmadeva. Brahmadeva, himself came, made Him into a grown up man and married Him to Radha. Then again He became a child, just to appear to be a child. Somebody may appear to be a child. To some of you, I appear to you to be a sixteen year old girl as you say, but I'm not. I may be according to some sixty years of age, but I'm not. My age is eternal. I can't say what age is mine. It could be two years old or it could be absolutely ageless, it could be anything. So in His whole life, whatever He did, He did with the purity of understanding. So Radhaji was married to Him first. And afterwards He came as a child."

During the incarnation of Shri Krishna, Adi Shakti took several forms:

1. Mahakali for a very short time as Vishnumaya the infant sister of Shri Krishna. She was actually born as the daughter of Yeshoda, Shri Krishna's foster mother, and was killed by Khamsa the demon.
2. She later took birth as Draupadi, wife of the Pandavas.
3. Yashoda was herself an Incarnation of Mahasaraswati.
4. As Mahalaxshmi she took two forms: as Radha and Rukmini. 'Ra' means power or energy; 'dha' means sustenance, so Radha meant the one who sustained the power. As Rukmini She became Queen to Shri Krishna as King.

Thus Shri Krishna's incarnation was that of Yogeshwara, come to remove the shackles of dharma and to rise above it, and also to worship him with a pure heart. He is our Ishwara, and we should purify our attention in order to be able to worship him.

Shri Krishna also has the Samhara-shakti, His power of destruction which is symbolized by the Sudarshan chakra in his hand. He is compassionate, He stands by His Bhaktas, and He comes on this earth to revive your dharma, to establish the holy state of human beings.

We come to the third stage of Statesman, a marvelously interesting feature in His life--the tact, the delicacy, the foresight, the skill in always putting the man opposed to Him in the wrong, and so winning His way and carrying others with Him. As you know, this part of His life is played out especially in connection with the Pandavas. He is the one who in every difficulty steps forward as ambassador; it is He who goes with Arjuna and Bhima to slay the giant king Jarasandha, who was going to make a human sacrifice to Mahadeva, a sacrifice that was put a stop to as it was blasphemous; it was He who went with them in order that the conflict might take place without transgressing the strictest rules of Kshatriya morality.

He, Arjuna and his brother enter into the city of the king. They did not go by the open gate, as it was the pathway of the friend. They wanted to show that they were enemies and hence they broke down a portion of the wall and entered. To show that they had come for the celebration of triumph and the fulfillment of a vow they entered wearing flowers and sandals so that they will not go undecorated. Offered food, the answer of the great ambassador was that they would not take food and they would first meet the king and explain their purpose.

When the time arrived He told the king in the most courteous but the clearest language that all these acts were done so that he may know that they had come not as friends but as foes to challenge him to battle.

So again when the question arises, after the thirteen years of exile, how shall the land be won back without struggle, without fight? He stood in the assembly of Pandavas and their friends with the wisest counsel how perchance war may be averted; you see Him offering to go as ambassador that all the magic of His golden tongue may be used for the preservation of peace. He went and called on Duryodhana as the courtesy demands, he never failed in the perfect duty of the ambassador, fulfilling every demand of politeness. He did not touch the food that would make a bond between Him and the one against whom He had come to struggle.

When in the assembly of hostile kings He tried to pacify and please. He apologized with the gentlest humility. To the great king, the blind king, He spoke in the name of the Pandavas as suppliant, not as outraged and indignant foe. With his soft words He tried to turn away words of wrath, and used every device of oratory to win their hearts and convince their judgments.

Again, when the battle of Kurukshetra was over, when all the sons of the blind king are slain, He once again went as ambassador to meet the childless father and, and even more bitter, the childless mother, so that the first anger may break itself on Him, and His words may charm away the wrath and soothe the grief of the bereft. Later on He still guided and advised till all the work was done, till His task was accomplished and His end was drawing near.

A statesman of marvelous ability; a politician of keenest tact and insight; as though to say to men of the world that when they are acting as men of the world they should be careful of righteousness, but also careful of discretion and of skill, that there is nothing alien to the truth of religion in the skill of the tongue and in the use of the keen intelligence of the brain.

Then again Shri Krishna's character is that of a Friend of the family. When they first meet in this life onwards, how constant His friendship, how ceaseless His protection, how careful His thought to guard their honor and their lives; and yet how wise; at every point where His presence would have frustrated the object of His coming, He went away.

He was not present at the great game of dice, for that was necessary for the working out of the divine purpose; He was away. He remained away, until Draupadi cried in her agony for help when her modesty was threatened; then he came with Dharma and clothed her with garments as they were dragged from her; but then the game was over, the dice were cast, and destiny had gone on its appointed road.

He came to bring about that battle on Kurukshetra. He came, in order to carry out that one object in preparation for the centuries that stretched in front; but in carrying that out, He would give every chance to men who were entangled in that evil by their own past, so that if one of them would answer to His pleading he might come over to the side, of light against the forces of darkness.

He never wavered in His object; yet He never left any means that man could use to prevent that object taking place. A lesson full of significance! The will of the Supreme must be done, but everything should be done within the scope that righteousness permits and what compassion suggests in order that men may choose light as against darkness, and only the resolutely obstinate may at last be, whelmed in the ruin that falls upon the land.

As Teacher who gave the Bhagavad-Gita between the contending armies on Kurukshetra. He was the Teacher not of Arjuna alone, not of India alone, but of every human heart which can listen to spiritual instruction, and understand a little of the profound wisdom that were clothed in the words of man.

He said: "I, O Arjuna, am the Teacher and the mind is my pupil;" the mind of every man who is willing to be taught; the mind of everyone who is ready to be instructed. Never does the spiritual teacher withhold knowledge because he grudges the giving. He is hampered in the giving by the want of receptivity in those to whom his message is addressed. It is not the withholding of the teacher but the closing of the heart of the hearer with the key of gold, and desires for fame, power, and the enjoyments of this world.

He tests the hearts of His beloved in order to see if within the heart one grain of evil still remains that will prevent their union with Him. They cannot enter there if even one sin is left in their nature. And so in tenderness and not in anger, in wisest love and not with a desire to mislead, the Lord of Love tries the hearts of His beloved, so that any evil that is in them may be wrung out by the grip that He places on them. Two or three occasions he tries them.

One time when the battle of Kurukshetra had been raging many a day; thousands and tens of thousands of the dead lay scattered on that terrible field, and every day when the sun rose Bhishma came forth, as head of the army, carrying before him everything, except where Arjuna barred his way; but Arjuna could not be everywhere; he was called away, with the horses guided by the Charioteer Shri Krishna sweeping across the field like a whirlwind, carrying victory in their course; and where the Charioteer and Arjuna were not there Bhishma had his way.

The hearts of the Pandavas sank low within them, and at last one night under their tents, resting before the next day's struggle, the bitter despondency of King Yudhishtir broke out in words, and he declared that until Bhishma was slain nothing could be done. Then came the test from the lips of the searcher of hearts. "Behold, I will go forth and slay him on the morrow." Would Yudhishtir consent? A promise stood in his way.

Again, when Duryodhana and Arjuna had gone to Shri Krishna who lay sleeping, the question arose as to what each should take. Alone, unarmed, Shri Krishna would go with one, He would not fight; a mighty battalion of troops He would give to the other. Arjuna chose the unarmed Krishna; Duryodhana, on the other hand chose the mighty army ready to fight; so the word of the Avatar was pledged that He would not fight. Unarmed He went into the battle,

clad in his yellow silken robe, and only with the whip of the charioteer in His hand; twice, in order to stimulate Arjuna into combat,
He had sprung down from the chariot and gone forth with His whip
in His hand as though He would attack Bhishma and slay him where
he fought.

Each time Arjuna stopped Him, reminding Him of His words.
Now came the trial for the blameless King, as he is often called;
should Shri Krishna break His word to give him victory? He stood
firm. "Thy promise is given," was his answer; "that promise may not
be broken." He passed the trial; he stood the test.

But still one weakness was left in that noble heart; one underlying weakness that threatened to keep him away from his Lord. The
lack of power to stand absolutely alone in the moment of trial, ever
clinging to someone stronger than himself, in order that his own
decision might be upheld. That last weakness had to be burnt out as
by fire.

In a critical moment of the battle the word came that the success of Drona was succeeding continuously and cannot be resisted
and the only way to slay him was to spread the report that his son was
dead, and then he would no longer fight. Bhima slew an elephant of
the same name as Drona's son, and he said in the hearing of Drona:
"Ashvatthama is dead."

But Drona would not believe unless King Yudhishtir said so.
Then the test came. Will he tell a practical lie but a nominal truth,
in order to win the battle? He refused; not for his brother's pleadings
would he do it. Would he stand firm by truth quite alone when all
the revered seemed to be on the other side? The great One said: "Say
that Ashvatthama is slain."

Ought he to have done it because Shri Krishna, told him to do
so? Ought he to have told the lie because the revered One counseled
it? Neither for the voice of God nor man, may the human soul do a
thing which he knows to be against God and His law. He must stand
in the universe alone, rather than sin against right.

When the lie was told under cover of that excuse, Yudhishtir
doing what he wished in his heart under cover of the command from
one he revered, he fell from his chariot, descended to the ground, and

suffering and misery followed him from that day till the day of his ending, until in the face of the King of the celestials he stood alone, holding the duty of protection- even to a dog higher than divine command and joy of heaven. And then he showed that the lesson had worked out in his purification, and that the heart was clean from the slightest taint of weakness.

Oh, but men say, Shri Krishna counseled the telling of a lie! What is there in this world that the Supreme does not do? There is no life but His, no Self but His, nothing save His life through His entire universe; and every act is His act, when you go back to the ultimate. He had warned themof that truth. "I" He said, "am the gambling of the cheat," as well as the chants of the Veda.

Strange lesson, and hard to learn, and yet true. For at every stage of evolution there is a lesson to be learnt. He teaches all the lessons; at each point of growth the next step is to be taken, and very often that step is the experiencing of evil, in order that suffering may burn the desire for evil out of the very heart.

Just as the knife of the surgeon is different from the knife of the murderer, although both may pierce the human flesh, the one cutting to cure, the other to slay; so is the sharp knife of the Supreme, when by experience of evil and consequent pain He purifies the man, different, because the motive is other than the doing of evil to gratify passion, the stepping aside from righteousness in order to please the lower nature.

Chapter 7

Avatar of Adi Shakti

When evolution reached the human stage, freedom was granted to human beings at the time of Adam and Eve, to choose between the evolutionary process of life and destruction, the anti-life process. Choosing evolution was the only way individuals could mature into evolved and realized souls.

Some human beings however chose the anti-life process, developing methods of destruction. From the Collective Subconscious and Collective Supra-conscious they came again and again on this earth to lead anti-life and anti-Divine activities. They spawned the creation of evil forces of hatred, and when they came on this earth they became malignant, and were thrown into hell. From hell these satanic forces emerged and rose up into the Void.

Shri Mataji speaks of the wrath of Shri Ganesha, and says, "Hell's gates are located in front of the Mooladhar Chakra where Shri Ganesha's trunk trumpets angry waves of wrath. With the trumpeting of his temper he throws these evil spirits back into hell. He hurls them into their assigned level of hell where they remain for ages. They pass through punishments and again are re-born on this earth where they continue their venture of destruction."

This spiritual awakening in man grew very strong and was again challenged by the evil forces that descended in incarnation to disturb their search through penance (Yagna). At this time, much before the sixth Incarnation of Shri Vishnu as Lord Rama, the Primordial

Mother incarnated as the Goddess Durga, Mother of the Universe. She incarnated from the Primordial Heart Centre (Adi Anahat Chakra) called the Sacred Heart in the Virat. There have been one hundred and eight major Incarnations of the Goddess Durga to save seekers from the evil of satanic forces.

Many were killed by Durga, the ferocious Avatar of Adi Shakti, and some were cursed to remain as lower animals in hell. Hell has seven layers which have been described in many ancient scriptures. Though many of these devils were destroyed physically many times some of them take human rebirth before the advent of every Incarnation. So in this age of Kaliyuga they are once again back in the flesh, but this time they have come in the garb of religion as false gurus and fake yogis. They will all be exposed one by one through their own ill-doing by Adi Shakti Herself who has incarnated as Mahamaya (the Great Illusion).

Mahesha (Shiva), Vishnu and Brahmadeva form the trinity who incarnated as one teacher God, the Primordial Master (Dattatreya). He came onto this earth to teach people the secrets of the Divine, to reveal God, and to help them cross the Ocean of Illusion themselves within their own identity. Evolution could not go further in the hands of human beings who were in the bondage of ignorance, so they were given guidance through this incarnation of the Primordial Master (Adi Guru) again and again in different lives.

He was created as the three-headed child, Dattatreya, by Adi Shakti who appeared on earth during the Treta Yuga as Sati Anusuya, wife of the Sage Aatreya. He was born as Adi Nath who founded Jainism - one of the oldest religions. Then he was born as Raja Janaka, father of Janaki also called Sita, Rama's wife. She was an Incarnation of Adi Shakti.

He was also born as Macchinder Nath, and again as Zoroaster who was worshipped by the ancient Persians, and still revered by Parsees. Earlier He had taken birth as Abraham and later as Moses, the Fathers of Judaism. In China He was born as Confucius and as Lao Tzu, and in Greece as Socrates.

He took a very significant Incarnation as Mohammed Sahib, the Messenger (Paigamber) and founder of Islam, whose daughter

Fatima was Sita reborn, an Incarnation of Adi Shakti. Yet again he took birth as Guru Nanak, founder of the Sikh religion whose sister was Nanaki (Janaki, Sita, Fatima). Most recently he was born as Shri Sai Baba of Shirdi in the Indian State of Maharashtra where he died just over a 100 years ago. Altogether there were ten major Avataras of Dattatreya.

Later they were born in Arabia as Hassan and Husain, the two sons of Fatima, daughter of Mohammed Sahib. They were murdered in a very violent war at Karbala. Their death signifies a great sacrifice in the name of religion. It is an indication how people who are extreme in nature take to fanaticism and, in their blindness, kill the very essence of religion which is nothing but the life lived by the Divine born in flesh and blood as an Incarnation. This awakening gave a rude shock to the mass of religious human beings of the land, and there ensued a phenomenon of mass repentance.

In this way people were made to realize that there can be no attachment to war for a realized soul. Violence and non-violence are attributes of mind but awareness is beyond these extremes. In defense of righteousness one has to go to war, but when one becomes the witness one only sees the play of war without taking any credit or discredit for it, or being disturbed by its aggression.

After Fatima, the reincarnation of Sita died, sectarian war broke out among the Muslims. One side, the Shiva sect, was founded by her, for, in Indian dialect Sita is pronounced Shiya. They are known today as Shiites. Shiya women are regarded as fair, innocent and beautiful because of their motherly expressions; in the same way the women of Janakapur, Sita's birthplace in India, are similarly blessed by Mahalaxshmi.

After her incarnation as Sita, She was born and lived in China as Kuan Yin, the Mother of Mercy, as a virgin. Adi Shakti took her first Incarnation in Nepal where still today the Goddess is the presiding national Deity. Most of Her births were on the Himalayas near Nepal where people have mixed Indian and Chinese features. The women of Nepal are mostly fair and soft skinned, and are known to be very serene and beautiful. Because of their high cheek bones they look very young all the time. Adi Shaktis facial expression is very much in this mould; to be precise she looks Nepali.

The fourth human birth of Adi Shakti was as the Virgin Mary, Mother of Christ. She incarnated in the Middle Eastern kingdom of Judea. Unlike Radha who had created her only son, Maha Vishnu, in the body of the Virat in the Vaikuntha stage but did not manifest Him in a body on this earth, it was as a virgin that Mary conceived Jesus Christ, the ninth Incarnation of Adi Vishnu. The greatness of this Incarnation cannot be adequately described in words but in the "Devi Bhagawad" there is a passage about Christ. It tells how He was born in heaven to Radha as Maha Vishnu, the only Son of the Virat.

He is none other than Shri Ganesha, the symbol of eternal child-hood. His body was constructed from the body of Shri Kartikeya, the only brother of Shri Ganesha. The body was created by Brahma Himself, and was conceived by one-sixteenth part of Shri Krishna, the Virat, who was His Father.

As Maha Vishnu He was the sustainer (Ashraya) of the whole world. A father always wants his son to be greater than himself, so Shri Krishna gave His son a boon making Maha Vishnu a million times greater than Himself and promising to place Him even higher than Himself. His Being would contain unlimited Brahma, Vishnu and Mahesha (Shiva), and from His forehead eleven Puthras (Christ's disciples) would be created.

Radha in Mary's Incarnation wanted to give Her Son the name of Her Lord, Krishna. Krishna comes from 'krishi' + 'na'. 'Krishi' means farming, 'na' means the one who carries. So the name 'Christ' came from the 'krishi' in Krishna. The name Jesus was derived from Jasoda, a form of Yeshoda, foster mother of Shri Krishna. Radha also wanted to give Yeshoda's name to Her Son because of Yeshoda's devotion and worship of Her in Brindavan and Gokul. The abbreviation of Yeshoda was Jesu or Yesu, so Radha/Mary named Her Son Jesus Christ.

In the life of Jesus Christ, the highest expression of the essence of spiritual innocence as God the Son came onto earth. Human beings witnessed the sacrifice of the dearest and Only Son of the Father (Virat) for humanity's sake. This allowed a deeper human perception of God's great love for the human race. The crucifixion of Christ happened at a time when people knew about God the Father, but did not know how to crucify their human self to allow the spiritual self to express itself.

This is the real meaning of the resurrection of Christ: that man could be the physical witness of the immortality of the Spirit which does not suffer and never perishes. For the first time, human awareness registered the truth of the immortality of Spirit which Shri Krishna had preached in His lifetime which is recorded in the 'Bhagavat Gita' written by the poet Vyasa.

When one takes the name of Shri Krishna one has to take the name of Radha first, so a seeker recites the mantra to the Virat as Radha-Krishna. Similarly Sita's name has to be taken before Rama's for the mantra Sita- Rama. Even the Virgin Mary (Kanya) who was so quiet and potential at the time of Christ was recognized later on by His disciples as the power behind Him.

She was worshipped for many years after her death by early Christians. In modern times human beings who are satanic personalities are challenging the validity of the Primordial Mother's virginity and the Virgin Birth in particular. Mary has clearly shown the power of virginity that can raise a mother to such an exalted powerful position that she can conceive a child by desire alone. She had reached that high stage of evolution when by Her Divine Will, She could immaculately conceive.

There are other such instances in Hindu Pauranic literature when Kunti, by the wish of the Mantra, gave birth to the Pandavas and to Karna immaculately.

Radha had created Her Only Son, Maha Vishnu, in the Vaikuntha stage but as Radha She could not conceive a child because she was unmarried. As Mary though, she conceived her child outside marriage in complete virginity. This is an expression of the power of virginity, the sinless Immaculate Conception.

In Mary's life the greatest advancement in social consciousness regarding the power of chastity came about, and society went through yet another evolution. Though a virgin She was raised to such an exalted position by the birth of Christ that She was acceptable to public opinion as the Mother of God not just then but still today.

Through a deeper understanding of Sahaja Yoga the reader will grasp the simplicity of the Immaculate Conception. Mary proved she was the Primordial Mother by conceiving the child in Her Sacred Heart (Primordial Heart Chakra). The Sacred Heart is the place where the Mother of the Universe (Jagadamba) exists.

In the same way that she conceived the universe she also conceived Jesus Christ and moved it through the Adi Sushumna Nadi into the Adi Swadishtan Chakra which controls the Primordial Uterus (Kumbha) to give Him human birth as a baby. In that divine heaven of creativity the Immaculate Conception took the form of a zygote egg (Andam). It remained in that state for many ages (Kalpas) until Adi Shakti took birth as Mary. She then manifested it as Jesus Christ. It was not difficult for Adi Shakti to do that. Unfortunately the greatness of her powers was only recognized after she departed from the earth.

A seeker gets his re-birth in exactly the same way through Sahaja Yoga. Adi Shakti wants to give second birth to all seekers. She conceives the subtle body (Sukshma Sharira) of the seeker in her heart. Her attention raises the Kundalini in the seeker's subtle body. She blesses his soul (Jivatman) which has been raised to her heart, and brings the soul to the limbic area of the brain by her attention. There she causes it to pass through all the chakras of the brain until it is born through the Brahmarandra, the hole in the fontanel bone on top of the skull. This is how every soul gets rebirth as a Sahaja Yogi.

The tenth and last Incarnation of Adi Vishnu will be created on the Primordial Brain (Sahasrar) and will be known as Shri Kalki. This will be a Collective Being created through Sahaja Yoga during the Kaliyuga by the Incarnation of Adi Shakti as the Great Illusion (Mahamaya). She will take a human birth with all her powers to promote the entry of humanity into the Golden Age or Age of Aquarius (Satya Yuga). This is the Age in which the Kingdom of God is to be established on earth.

Through Her compassionate action within this world, the Collective Being is already beginning to emerge today, formed by all the realized souls who collectively are merging themselves into God's consciousness. The power of Kalki is known as Mahamaya because she is a great illusion. She is absolutely humane, but expresses the three integrated powers of Mahakali, Mahalaxshmi and Mahasaraswati.

She exhibits her powers to the masses by giving mass Self-realization, by which seekers enter the realm of collective consciousness. This can be said to be the most significant event in the history of spiritual evolution because, in it, the whole creation, under the guidance of Divine Love, begins to return to its source which is Divine Love.

The awakening of Kalki began the day this Incarnation of Adi Shakti took human form. Individuals poured onto the earth as souls in search of reality: people who were affluent started abandoning materialism; many gave up all old ideas of luxury and comfort, and took to a simpler lifestyle.

Those who get their Self-realization in this Age will be the white-robed horsemen who will enter the Kingdom of God as promised in scriptures of many faiths. The rest will be destroyed. Thus a new world of living collective consciousness will be born.

Lord Vishnu takes all these Incarnations to be the leader of evolutionary process in different stages. His Power, Mahalaxshmi, also incarnates with Him, and evolves Her Incarnations in various evolutionary processes. Until the human stage, evolution takes place without the subject being aware of it.

Only in the last and final stage of Kalki, when Adi Shakti Herself incarnates, will human beings jump into a higher awareness of collective consciousness, and in their lifetime, be fully aware of their 'new birth.

Chapter 8

Incarnation of Jesus Christ

Mataji speaks of Christ as having taken birth on this earth as a human being to perform the task of enlightening the human awareness and establishing within their conscious knowing that they are not this body, but they are the spirit. The message of Christ was His resurrection by which he showed that we are the spirit and not the body. He ascended into the realm of spirit, as He was 'Pranava'.

Christ was born in a stable to a very ordinary carpenter, not in a palace or to a king. He was kept in the dry grass to indicate that all the worldly things are just like dry grass, 'Tranavat'. At a very young age He was crucified. He went through the crucifixion as He had to perform the task of opening the Agnya Chakra.

He was here to save human beings, but His greater purpose was to create the passage between, the Vishuddhi and the Sahasrar, that is the Agnya in the Primordial being, the Virat. In the evolutionary trajectory every incarnation came on this Earth to open a door within us, to create an opening that will enlighten our awareness, a little more.

Christ came precisely to open this small little door, which is constricted, by our ego and our super-ego. Ego and super-ego are the two by-products of our thought process -one being the product of thoughts of the past and the other being the product of thoughts of the future. He came to enable us to cross that gap and in the process He sacrificed Himself, His body, when He was crucified on the cross.

He accepted the ordeal of dying on the cross in order that the constriction at the Agnya Chakra of humanity may be opened.

The resurrection had become necessary as human beings, had lost all control over themselves and at the level of consciousness, we were a lost people. We had no balance of any kind in life and were totally under the sway of the mind which often became uncontrollable and there was no wisdom in its judgments. Human beings are conditioned in many ways, like being ritualistic even in their spirituality.

Being egoistic is another conditioning which blinds a person from discriminating between right and wrong. Nations have warred, thousands killed, tortured and butchered because of the ego of a few people. People were not even aware of their own cruelty and violence. Even the poorest of the poor are fighting for nonsensical things.

Affluence in some countries on the other hand has also made them blind to the evil effects of materialism. Greed for money and aggrandizement has made man to cheat against one another with utter disregard to values and self-dignity.

Jesus came in those days when people had no idea about spirituality at all. Christ was an incarnation of Shri Ganesha. Two great powers are combined in Jesus Christ. The first power is that of Shri Ganesh, who is recognised as his original power; and the other is that of Shri Kartikeya. Because of this, the incarnation of Jesus Christ is of complete "Brahman Tatwa" or "Aum kar". Shri Krishna being the father of Jesus Christ bestowed a number of boons on Jesus Christ prior to his birth.

One of these boons was that, " You (Jesus Christ) would dwell on a plane higher than that of mine." This could be explained to mean, that while the plane of Shri Krishna is the Vishuddhi Chakra, located at the base of our neck, the plane of Jesus is Agnya Chakra, which is located at the junction of the optic thalamus (pineal and pituitary glands).

The second boon granted by Shri Krishna was that, "You (Christ) would be the support of the whole universe".

The third boon was that, "You would be the first to receive one-sixteenth part of all the offerings made to me in Puja".

In this way, after bestowing a number of boons, Shri Krishna permitted Shri Jesus Christ to incarnate on the earth.

If we look at Christ and His life we find that He didn't fight anyone. He didn't argue with anyone and He accepted everything. He accepted the death on the cross. He accepted it because He knew that it is for not only His resurrection, but that of the whole world.

The life of Christ was that of a simple, poor son of a carpenter for whom money was nothing. In His life, Christ did not marry. To Him, Spirit was everything. He was preaching and telling people to get their spiritual awakening. He tried to impress upon them the need to use this life to prepare for the life beyond.

He was very intelligent and even as a small boy he could discuss very deeply on spiritual matters. He was a person created by the Divine for fulfilment of a purpose in the human evolution. He was Shri Ganesh who had for the first time incarnated on this Earth. He was Pranava, the Om, or the pure vibration of knowledge itself. Despite that, nobody recognised Him because they could not recognise or understand the Truth. Their own wrong doings, evil thinking, greed and aggression made them blind, and ultimately they crucified Him.

Even when on the Cross, Christ said, "Forgive them for they know not what they do." Such was the life of Christ who sacrificed His life for the betterment of Humanity, for helping them evolve. They could go through the suffering because of the power of love, their love for human beings. When you love others, then you start thinking about 'what is the best you can do for them?' Your enjoyment only comes through your capacity to love. That's what Christ has taught us.

He had love for all human beings and He wanted to prepare them for their Resurrection.

It's a very difficult task that He performed. People at that point of time were absolutely ignorant about spirituality but He kept talking and through tales and parables He communicated that resurrection is the most important thing that they should try to achieve. He knew that when resurrection takes place, the Kundalini rises and connects you to the Divine Power, which is all-pervading.

Then the person starts understanding that there's a life beyond-a higher type of life which connects you to the Divine Power, a power that gives you the Absolute Truth. If your third eye is to be opened, it means Christ consciousness is to be awakened on your Agnya Chakra.

When the Agnya Chakra is awakened, a witness state is created within you. You become the witness of the whole drama. It is a state of thoughtless awareness, where you are able to silently witness the whole drama, even while you are enacting it.

Once the Agnya Chakra becomes clearer and there is no domination by the ego or the mind and its conditionings then you become the channel for creating peace. Wherever you are you can create peace. It may look like you are suffering, but you are not. You are doing it for others, for surroundings, friends, neighbours, and may be even for the countrymen.

When you have crossed the passage at the Agnya Chakra you become a channel for the Divine Force that can work out anything. It can change and transform people. It has happened to many people individually before. Christ did it to bring peace on this Earth. If there is no peace within there cannot be peace on the outside.

Many countries talk of peace but they are engaged in war and fighting. The only solution is to transform them by dissolving the ego and its conditionings through the crossing of the passage at the Agnya Chakra. The Divine discretion will make people see the truth as it is and not make them justify their wrong doings thereby shielding the aggressive forces which is the cause of ruining of the peace of the world.

Jesus tried to neutralise the problems of the ego and make man a milder personality devoid of aggression caused due to dominating ego. The ego tries to cover up things and makes a person to show him superior to others. This kind of mischief of the ego is very harmful and damaging. It makes man to lose control over him and leads people in the wrong direction.

Spirituality makes a person very humble. His heart becomes mild and in that humility things work. His humility makes him glorified. Ego makes a person conditioned which prevents individual and collective enjoyment. This creates disharmony needing correction, just like the stock markets correct themselves when there is a bullish sway of a few stocks.

Similarly nature corrects itself through earthquakes, floods and volcanic eruptions. So also, racialism and its conditionings has created rift among people and an undercurrent of hate and jealousy has crept in into normal life. This world is one and egoist and racial conditioning of one community thinking them to be greater is a very bad conditioning. You become conscious of your defects when the Agnya gets crossed over.

When you understand your own value, you'll understand you should know yourself by your own self. Christ sacrificed his life for bringing this resurrection into play so that we get our Divine discretion. The path that He created makes the ordeal of passing through our ego and our conditionings very easy, which otherwise was a great struggle.

Shri Mataji Nirmala Devi, in her address at the Hinduja Auditorium, Bombay, on the 26th September 1979, on the subject "Shri Kundalini Shakti and Shri Jesus Christ" She said that it is altogether a new subject for the common people because nobody has at any time before, attempted to establish any connection between Jesus Christ and Shri Kundalini Shakti. On the Virat tree of religion, saints of various kinds bloomed as flowers in many countries and languages. It is only at the level of the Virat or the level of cosmic consciousness that one can understand the relation between these great saints and the sweet fragrance of the message that they were trying to convey through their religion. If one would see the principle behind all this it is clear that all these saints are like many flowers on the same tree of religion and are connected with each other because of the one and the same power.

The Bible says "I will come to thee as tongues of flames". Israeli people explained this to mean that, "When the Lord would incarnate, He would be emitting flames of fire and therefore, they would not be able to witness Him". The real meaning of this is that "you would witness the Kundalini Shakti in the Sahasrar Chakra". There are several such references to the Kundalini Shakti and Sahasrar in the Bible.

The "Markandeya Purana" written by Markandeya Rishi, explained a number of such subtler points. In the same Purana, there is a graphic description of Shri Mahavishnu which if meditated upon will correspond with the description of Jesus Christ. The word, 'Christ', has been derived from the word, 'Krishna'. As a matter of fact, the father of Jesus Christ is Shri Krishna. That is why He is called 'Christ'. The mother of Shri Krishna, Shri Yashoda Mata; was addressed as ''Yesu''. Even today in northern Indian the word ''Yeshu'' is pronounced as ''Jesu''. It is therefore, clear that from 'Yashoda' came the word 'Yeshu' and then further became the word ''Jesu'' and finally the name 'Jesus Christ'.

The stories narrated by Jesus Christ about His Father were actually those about Shri Krishna and the Virata. Although, Shri Krishna did not reincarnate during the period when Jesus Christ lived on the Earth, his teachings centred round the theme as to how the seekers should know the 'Virat-Purusha' or God Almighty. The Mother of Jesus Christ, Mother Mary was none other than the Goddess Maha Laxmi. She is the Adi Shakti the Primordial Mother. Therefore, Jesus Christ used to address his Mother as the ''Holy Ghost''.

Jesus Christ possessed all powers of Ekadashi Rudra that is eleven powers of destruction. These powers have their centres located around the cranium of our head. When the incarnation of Kalki takes place, all these eleven powers perform the work of destruction. Out of these eleven powers one is that of Shri Hanuman, the other is of Shri Bhairava. In the Bible, these two powers are named as Saint Gabriel and Saint Michael respectively. After Self-realization in Sahaja Yoga one can awaken these powers by addressing them in Sanskrit, Marathi or even in English. The Nadi on our right side, which is known as 'Pingala-Nadi', is activated by the power of Shri Hanuman by chanting the mantra of Shri Hanuman. Similarly, by chanting the name of Saint Michael one would experience relief in the Ida-Nadi located on our left side and manifest the power of Saint Michael or Shri Bhairava.

The awakening of the Kundalini very much depends on the condition of the Agnya Chakra of the seeker. In the present age, many persons have highly inflated egos which are mainly because we lead an extremely egocentric life. This egoistic thinking and, working together with beliefs based on them, keeps man entangled in a web of his own creation and prevents his ascent. Jesus Christ has given three weapons to break free from this entanglement.

The first among these weapons is "forgiveness". It operates as the "Purusha, form in Shri Ganesha principle" which manifests itself in the form of 'forgiveness' in human principle. In fact forgiveness is a very powerful weapon. It protects man against the ego. If somebody hurts us, troubles or insults us, our mind is engrossed in contemplating on him and gets disturbed. Continuous thinking of those events further aggravates the mental entanglements. To overcome such troubles forgiveness is a very powerful weapon given by Jesus Christ to get rid of troubles caused by others.

The Agnya Chakra, which is the Jesus principle in us, becomes active only after awakening of the Kundalini and this Chakra is a very subtle one. There is a very subtle door or a narrow pathway for facilitating the Kundalini energy to rise and go beyond this Chakra. That is why Jesus Christ said, "I am the door". Jesus Christ incarnated on this earth for facilitating the passage through this door, and he himself was the first to pass through it. People crucified Jesus Christ because of their ego. Their intellectual pride prevented them from accepting Jesus Christ, as an incarnation of God. Jesus had done nothing wrong except to have preached the Truth, talked about good things, taught about how to lead a cultured way of life, preached Love and cured people of their ailments. In spite of this, the people tortured him. God Almighty sent His beloved Son, Jesus Christ, on this earth to uplift them from their ignorance but the people crucified him. It is therefore necessary to understand the meaning of the "SELF". Jesus Christ tried to awaken the Kundalini, but with great difficulty could give realization to some twenty one persons.

The Kundalini, that is Mother Gauri, created Shri Ganesha by Her will- power, tapasya and noble deeds. It was when Shri Ganesha prepared himself for incarnation that Jesus Christ was born. There are many things in this world for which man has no satisfactory explanation like how does a seed sprout? How do we breathe? How do we make movements? Where from does the power in our brain originate? How you came into this world? Can any man satisfactorily explain these things? We say that earth has gravitational force. But where from did this force come? A number of such things, which are the cause of our wonderment, remain unexplained because of our existence under the influence of an illusion. This illusion unless blown up will restrict or prevent the spiritual evolution of man.

At every stage of evolution, the incarnations have appeared to give that push in his evolution that left to himself man on his own would not be capable of. It is the Divine desire that incarnates to assist man to take the next step in his evolution. But every age has tortured and treated the Saints who advocated these steps in evolution very badly. But now the Satya Yuga has commenced. Jesus Christ, who had caused the opening of the Agnya Chakra of the Cosmos, has set in motion the Ekadashi Rudras, the mighty destructive powers that will strike anything that goes against Truth.

If one great lesson is to be learnt from the life of Jesus Christ, it is that you have to remain contented in the state in which the Almighty has placed you. Jesus did not change his mission. He did not separate himself from the society, but actively involved with all norms of the society. He attended marriage ceremonies and even made the arrangements.

He never showed his helplessness. He was much more dynamic than most kings. He was not afraid of anyone. Whatever He had to say he said it. He was not afraid of crucifixion or of any such so-called punishment. It is only the human beings who have these false ideas about life and want to impose them on God. God is not concept at all because concept is a thought.

Jesus Christ came on this earth not only to save us, to give us happiness but also to give us joy, because human beings in their ignorance, are unnecessarily beating themselves, and destroying themselves. Man by his own wayward ways like drinking, gambling, and wrong beliefs was involuntarily seeking their own destruction. He came like a morning flower to make us happy. To be Christ like is to open up one's Heart as He did to all the people around. He went and talked to multitudes opening up His heart to give them happiness. He wanted each one to be born again, which is not going through the ritual of baptism but to enlighten our awareness at the point it had reached. So be joyous that here at Agnya Chakra again Christ is born within us and He is there. We can know him there and can ask for His help always. The time has come for us all to get all that is promised in the scriptures, not only in the Bible but all the scriptures of the world. The time has come to become a Christian, Brahmin, and a pir, through our Kundalini awakening.

Jesus Christ incarnated to open the Agnya Chakra and to dissolve our ego you have to rise beyond thought at a higher level into thoughtless awareness where you are not in thought, but you are in the center of thought in the sense that one thought rises and falls and there is a place in between. Another thought rises and falls. You are in the center of these thoughts, the 'Vilamba' as we call it...

In this Kaliyuga, all those who are seeking God shall find Him and millions of people will be able to do so. Sahaja Yoga is the Last Judgement. This is described in the Bible. You are judged only after you come to Sahaja Yoga. For that purpose you, however, have to surrender yourself completely after coming to Sahaja Yoga. It is only when you stabilise in Sahaja Yoga, that the state of thoughtless awareness is established. So long as the Kundalini power does not pass through the Agnya Chakra, the stage of thoughtless awareness is not reached. This is the first step in the way of thoughtless awareness of the seeker. As soon as the Kundalini crosses the Agnya Chakra, the thoughtless awareness is established.

It is the power of Jesus Christ which is instrumental in opening the subtle door located above the Agnya Chakra. For that purpose you are to recite the 'Lord's prayer' composed by Jesus Christ. After crossing this door, the Kundalini power enters the limbic area of the brain. It is after the Kundalini enters this area, which is also termed as the Kingdom of God, that the state of thoughtless awareness is established. In the limbic area of the brain there are Chakras which activate the seven main Chakras and also the secondary Chakras in the body.

Now, let us consider the reasons why the Agnya Chakra is spoiled. One of the main reasons of this deterioration is your eyes. You should take great care of the eyes, as they are very important. Then the Agnya Chakra is also spoiled on account of bowing before or touching one's head at the feet of an unauthorised Guru. That is why Jesus Christ has told not to bow one's head before every person or place, because by doing so, you unknowingly lose everything that you have gained and your Agnya Chakra will get constricted.

In order to keep the Agnya Chakra in proper order, one should always read the scriptures and the sacred texts. One should never read unholy literature. Many people may say, 'What does that matter? On account of our profession, we have to do certain things which may not be strictly proper". But then, by doing such unholy activities the eyes get spoiled. Even by looking at any unchaste and filthy man the Agnya Chakra may get constricted.

Jesus Christ firmly told, "Thou shall not commit adultery which means thou shall not have adulterous eyes". Thus, it again comes to the eyes. If your eyes are unholy, you have eye troubles and your eyes get weakened. This does not mean that if you have to use spectacles, you become an unholy or improper person. It is the law of life that you have to use spectacles at an advanced age.

The eyes are spoiled because you do not keep them steady, and are always moving them from one place to another. So also the attention of some people is constantly shifting from one object to another. These people are not even aware that such action spoils the eyes. The other reason of deterioration of the Agnya Chakra lies in the manner in which you work. If you overwork then you become work- conscious.

The work that you are doing may be good, but even then, if it is beyond the normal level, be it over-reading, overstitching or over-thinking, it will spoil the Agnya Chakra. The reason is that while you overwork, you forget God. During the course of such work, God-consciousness does to stabilize in you.

The Kundalini is the Truth. When you will merge into the Truth, when you will get absorbed in it, only then you would under-stand that you are but an instrument of God. If the Agnya Chakra of any person does not open, Kundalini would not rise, because the Mooladhar Chakra would also remain constricted till the Agnya Chakra remains constricted.

If a person's Agnya Chakra is too much constricted, the Kundalini power would not rise, whatever efforts you may make. For removing the catch on the Agnya Chakra, we apply "Kumkum". This has the effect of reducing the troubles of the ego as also other troubles.

When the "Kumkum' is applied on the forehead above the Agnya Chakra, the Chakra is opened and Kundalini rises. Such is the intimate connection between Jesus Christ and the Kundalini Power. Shri Ganesha, who is stationed at the Mooladhar, and protects the modesty of Shri Kundalini, also opens the door at the Agnya Chakra, for the Kundalini to pass through it.

What is it that we have to do for maintaining the Agnya Chakra in order?

The ways are many. Extremity in every action spoils the society, and therefore excessiveness in any walk of life is not proper and should be avoided. Maintaining the balance enables our eyes to get rest. There are many exercises for the eyes which help to keep the Agnya Chakra in a healthy condition. One of these is to watch your own ego and yourself as if you are observing your own image in a mirror.

If you do this, the strain on the eyes due to ego will be minimised. The other area which is very important is that part of the back of the head that is exactly behind the forehead. It is in the area which is at a distance of about the thickness of eight fingers (about 5 inches) above the base of the neck, and is known as the area of Shri Maha Ganesha. Shri Ganesha incarnated as Maha Ganesha and the same incarnation is of Jesus Christ.

Shri Christ's place is in the centre of the forehead and is surrounded by the kingdom of the Ekadasha Rudras. Jesus Christ is the Master of that kingdom. The Ekadashi Rudras comprise of Shri Maha Ganesha, as also Shri Shanmugam (The Lord with six faces). If you open your eyes, after awakening of the 'Kundalini' you would experience that your vision is somewhat dimmed or blurred. This is so because when the 'Kundalini' awakens, the pupils of your eyes are dilated and get cooled. This happens on account of the action of para-sympathetic nervous system. Even mere thinking of Shri Jesus Christ, contemplating or meditating on Him would relieve Agnya Chakra.

Yoga is a science that advocates control of the mind, concentration or focused attention, and walking on the path of Truth. The second birth or Upanayana among the Hindus, or the Baptism amongst the Christians is nothing but the re-establishment of the connection with the Divine. This is possible only by the awakening of the Kundalini energy which after it rises, passes through the six energy centres and piercing the Sahasrar Chakra, establishes the union with the all-pervading power of God.

Jesus Christ healed many with the power of love flowing through him. Jesus Christ came to save and liberate the whole mankind. He was 'Aum kar' incarnate, the 'Pranava' and the 'Truth'. The bodies of the other incarnations were made up of "earth principle", whereas the body of Jesus was made of the 'soul principle' which was why He was resurrected after death. It was only through the resurrection that His disciples could know that He was no other than God Himself.

If we recognize that God incarnated as Jesus Christ we can grow in spirituality which will enlighten the soul spreading happiness and bliss everywhere.

Chapter 9

Incarnation of Lord Buddha

We come to the ninth Avatara as it is called, that of the Lord Buddha. A theory exists that the Lord Buddha, though an incarnation of Vishnu, came to lead astray those who did not believe the Vedas, came to spread confusion upon earth. Vishnu is the Lord of order, not of disorder; the Lord of love, not the Lord of hatred; the Lord of compassion, who only slays to help the life onward when the form has become an obstruction.

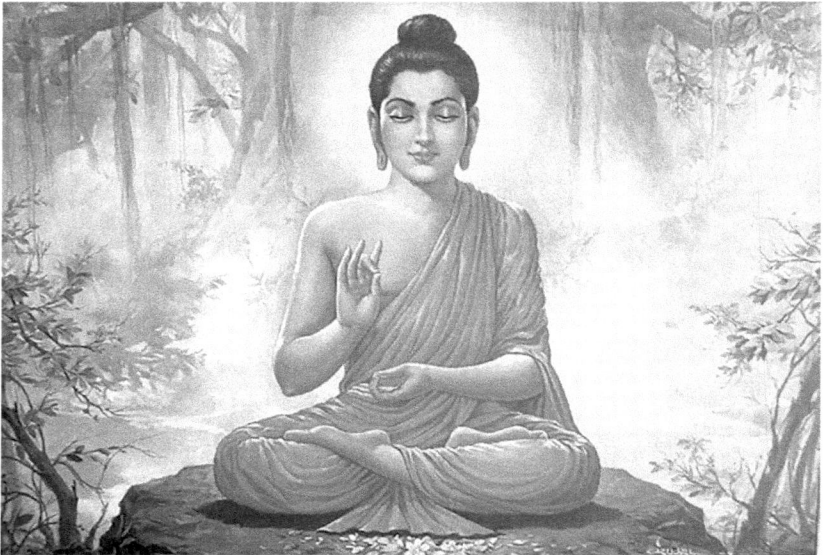

And they blaspheme who speak of an incarnation of the Supreme, as coming to mislead the world that He has made. But there is another point in regard to The Lord Buddha, in the sense of the word that he may not be as per our definition of an Avatar.

He was the first of our own humanity who climbed upwards to that point, and there merged with the Divine and received full illumination. His was not a body taken by the Divine for the purpose of revealing Himself, but was the last in myriads of births through which he had climbed to merge in Isvara at last. That is not what is normally spoken of as an Avatar.

In the case of the Avatar, the evolving births are in previous kalpas, and the Avatar comes after the man has merged in the Divine, and the body is taken for the purpose of revelation. But he who became Gautama Buddha had climbed through birth after birth in our own kalpa, as well as in the kalpas that went before; and he was incarnated many times and rose onward to take the office of the Buddha; for the Buddha is the title of an office, not of a particular man.

Finally by his own struggles, the very first of our race, he was able to reach that great function in the world. What is the function? - That of the Teacher of Gods and men. The previous Buddhas had been Buddhas who came from another planet. Humanity had not lived long enough here to evolve its own son to that height. Gautama Buddha was human-born. After birth in India He had completed His course and took His final body in Aryavarta, to make the proclamation of the law to men.

But the proclamation was not made primarily for India. It was given in India because India is the place whence the great religious revelations go forth by the will of the Supreme. Therefore He was born in India, but His law was specially meant for nations beyond the boundaries of Aryavarta, that they might learn a pure morality, a noble ethic, all of which had become much disjoined, because of the darkness of the age.

Peace you find in the teachings of the Lord Buddha two great divisions; one a philosophy meant for the learned, and another one – an ethic disjoined from the philosophy, which was noble, pure and great, yet easy to be grasped for the masses. It was necessary to give a teaching of morality fitted for a more materialistic age, so that even if nations would not believe in the Gods they might still practice morality and obey the teachings of the Lord.

In order that India itself might not lose its subtle metaphysical teachings and the widespread belief among all classes of people in the existence of the Gods and their part in the affairs of men, the work of the great Lord Buddha was done. He left morality built upon a basis that could not be shaken by any change of faith, and, having done His work, passed away.

Looking back at the life of Lord Buddha, he was born as Gautama, in a royal family and then he became an aesthetic because he was very much hurt to see three types of problems from which human beings suffered and he came to the conclusion, that all these three types of problems are because we have desires. So he said that if you become desire less then there will be no problems. He studied the Vedas, the Tuprichadas, and all kinds of things; he went to many saints; he could not get his realization.

An incarnation also has to reach a point of realization in a different way, like the whole potential has to open out, the incarnation has tremendous potential and that expresses itself once the door is opened outward. Buddha realized the greatest problem of human beings is his ego, in his ego he goes to the extremes, from one end to another, and so he worked throughout on the Pingala Nadi for us and stationed himself on our ego to control it. On the Agnya Chakra Christ in the center, Buddha is on the left and Mahaveera, is on the right.

All of them are called as Lords, because they are the rulers of these three areas around the Agnya chakra which is the area of Tapas, or penance. They have done the penance that allows the rest of humanity to progress on the path of evolution without having to go through all the efforts, sacrifice and hardships that they went through. We, at this stage of evolution need not have to go into the jungles, run away from society, endanger one's life, and do penance.

Buddha in his lifetime, although he said there was no need for austerities, he himself went through those austerities. At that point in time, they needed people who would go all out for propagation of his ideas. Hence he never believed in any austerities. Moreover he was also not a vegetarian.

In fact once on going to a village as he was hungry, he asked one of the hunters, called as Kirakas for food. He said that that morning he had killed a wild boar but it would take some time as it was of very hot blood. He did not wait for the red meat of the wild boar to get cooled down, but ate it and died. That is the reason why The Buddhists became vegetarians, because Buddha died eating hot meat.

He tried to control the people with him in a very loving and affectionate way. Once a boy came to him and asked him to be initiated. He said, "My child, only the Brahmins can be initiated, (meaning the realized souls), what is your birth?" The boy said, "I don't know my birth." He went back to his mother and asked her what his birth, who was my father, was?

She said, "My child I was a very poor woman and I didn't know how to exist so I had many lords. I don't know who your father is." When he went back to Buddha and Lord asked him about his caste, he told Buddha that his mother told him that as she had many lords, and didn't know from whom he was born, he didn't have any caste. Buddha embraced, the boy and said "you are a Brahmin, because you have told the truth."

The essence of his life is truth. First we have to be honest to ourselves. Many times people, in a bid to escape from the truth give arguments and explanations. There is no need to give explanation to the spirit which is residing within you, as it is enlightened in your attention.

Buddha's teachings were essentially centered on to getting rid of the ego. Hence he said get rid of everything- your hair, even your eyelashes, anything that can be shaved off from your hands and feet. He then asked his disciples to wear a Kashia, means saffron clothes, with everything shaved, and the ladies could only wear two dresses, one - the blouse and one a sari - whether you are a queen, or a sweeper.

Buddha always praised people who were natural. Buddha preached Brahmacharya or celibacy, because if you go too much to the right side our Mooladhar is lost. Mooladhar is like brakes - the right side is the accelerator and the left is the Mooladhar which is the brake. Buddha looked after all the people who came to him, saw to it that they were celibate and he was the one who gave them balance and managed them. Once you start going on the right side, you end up automatically being egoistic and very unnaturally speedy, and uncontrollable. Buddha helped restore chastity.

Thus the first message of Buddha is honesty to you, honesty in your chastity, and complete sacrifice of everything. His teaching was in the transcendence of the ego and to be truthful through attention to life's passage, moment to moment. His teachings were to be applied to oneself first and through meditation to purify one's life for the work of God.

Buddha said,

"Buddham Sharanam Gachami,	I bow to all those who are realized souls.
Dharmam Sharanam Gachami,	I bow myself, to my
Dharma, Sangam Sharanam Gachami,	I bow to collectivity."

In these three things he has solved the problems of all three types of people - first is the Buddham, the one who is a realized soul, all the realized souls are to be respected, to be surrendered to, Buddham Sharanam Gachami, I surrender myself to all the Buddhas, whether he is black, white or of blue race, whether he is from Spain, Italy, India, or from any other place, whether he is a Jew, Muslim, or from any religion, whether he's a legitimate child or illegitimate, whether he is aristocratic or from the poorest of poor, whether he has money or no money, whether he's unwell or alright, whether he had a very bad past, or not - everything had to be forgotten, all the Buddhas must be respected and surrendered to.

Then the second is Dharmam Sharanam Gachami, whether it is money, house, or any possession, any kind of labour, any sort of work has all to be respected and surrendered. So this depravity of the ego you can see in the life of Buddha who was light, who was enlightenment, who was compassion, who was knowledge, who was joy. In his life he never criticized anyone, he just took an easier course, and he just left things alone. He's the one who taught detachment from within. Today we are able to bathe in the light of His hard work, compassion, dedication, sacrifice and steadfastness to truth.

The third was Sangam Sharanam Gachami, surrender to the collective, to the group, to the society. He taught that while growth was individual, one had to do one's own sadhana for getting rid of one's ego; it was the Sanga that would provide the platform, the right atmosphere and the right environment for that growth, for that evolution to take place.

Then was sent another great One, overshadowed by the power of Mahadeva, Shri Shankaracharya, in order that by His teaching He might give, the Advaita Vedanta, the philosophy which would do intellectually what morally the Buddha had done. His works intellectually guarded spirituality and allowed a materialistic age to break its teeth on the hard nut of a flawless philosophy.

Thus in India metaphysical religion triumphed, while the teaching of the Blessed One passed from the Indian soil, to do its noble work in lands other than the land of Aryavarta, which must keep unshaken its belief in the Gods, and where highest and lowest alike must bow before their power. That is the real truth about this much disputed question as to the teaching of the ninth Avatar; the fact was that His teaching was not meant for His birthplace, but was meant for other younger nations that were rising up around, who did not follow the Vedas, but who yet needed instruction in the path of righteousness. His teachings were given not to mislead them but to guide them.

But, the rich knowledge and secrets of the Vedas and the Upanishads were preserved by the coming of the great Teacher of the Advaita. Shri Adi Shankaracharya who, bestowed with the power of Mahadeva was born a few years after the passing away of the Buddha. As the records of the Dwarka Math show plainly, Adi Shankaracharya was born within 60 or 70 years of the passing away of the Buddha.

Chapter 10

PREDICTIONS about Shri Mataji's Incarnation

These words of H. H. Mataji were recorded at Sholapur in January 1982, when she spoke about predictions done long ago, about Her Advent and Sahaja Yoga, particularly by Acharya Kaka Bhujandar Satwacharya, in his book "NADI GRANTH".

She spoke of how what was predicted 14,000 years back through astrology is coming true today. About 2000 years ago an astrologer from Karnataka had predicted that this Great Yogi will come on this earth on Pisces and how gradually we will start seeing some miracles from 1964 to 1966. He says that initially it may be little bit but real change in the age (MANVANTAR), the new age will start from 1970 and by 1980 it will take its grip. That time, by this new method, new age will be formed, the old one (VAIVASTA) will be over.

He then says that one of the Yugas will be over i.e. KALI YUGA, will be over and from 1970. A new age of active divinity will start i. e. the Krita Yuga. That time the Sun will rule in a new way. The axis of earth will be reduced and the speed of the earth will be reduced gradually. And at that time a great MAHAYOGI will be born who will be completely PARABRAHMA and he will possess all the powers to do or not to do.

As per the predictions, this Mahayogi would bring a new method which will make the pure power of your Chakras to rise, as a result of the awakening of the KUNDALINI SHAKTI and the Sadhak or devotee will get his enlightenment. ACHARYA KAKA BHUJANDER TATWACHARY had made this prediction about 2000 years ago. He further had written that this new method of MAHAYOGA will enable one to experience the joy of Self-realization in this very life time.

Prior to this age, people who wanted Moksha or liberation would get into BHAKTI (devotion) or GYANA through reading of PATANJALI Yoga sutras and then they would get their Moksha or liberation. In the ancient times to attain this state many people including great saints sacrificed their body, lived in caves, shut them off from society and even died. They sat in a state of Samadhi meditating for hours and days together to such an extent that sometimes even ants would grow upon them making ant hills. They would still persist in their sadhana until they got their realization.

That will not be necessary with this new method. You won't die either. Those who achieve Atma Sakshat kar by this new method will have BRAHMANANDA, or the joy of BRAHMA, without going into SAMADHI. They will have the joy of BRAHMA which was the SAHAJA- SAMADHI according to him.

Here it may be recollected that Shri Mataji Nirmala Devi was born on March 23rd 1923 on the cusp of Pisces and Aries on the day of Summer Equinox. The prediction of a Maha Yogi to be a Parabrahma having all powers of doing or being in a witness state is suggestive of the powers of Mahakali, Mahasaraswati and Mahalaxmi, which Shri Mataji Nirmala Devi has, and who has also taught all of us how to activate those powers in us, who is the Mahayogi predicted 2000 years ago.

Amongst millions, first one will get realization and who will be able to give self-realization to others. Then all the human race can get over their death i.e. destruction, through this Yoga. You will have to lead a normal life, married or not but lead the life of a normal householder and living in the society. All the diseases will disappear through this Yoga; people can be cured by merely touching. This yoga will be for human beings like the making of ARDHNARINATESHWARA (SHIVA). The old age will disappear, their body will remain as it is and they will have a body which is divine. The body will become more subtle and they can enter into the body of others to get them cured. They will not be touched by the fire or weapons. These subtle things can be seen with your own eyes and this will happen all over the world.

India is a country of great PUNYAS. That is why there are powers which will look after the afflictions of this country and this country will gradually rise. He further says they may go for the Third World War and will have to suffer for it. After that this Great Incarnation will interfere and all the countries will come together, with an understanding of collective oneness and they will understand that war is so horrible. A conference of all the countries will be held in a big city. There, not the politicians but the yogis will direct them. Because of China's aggressive policies and the Third World War we will have to bear lots of problems and will have to fill the gaps. But through prayers, we will be able to unite all the countries.

By the new inventions of Science, the divine knowledge and the science will become one. With the science we will be able to establish the existence of God and death. That is how there will be coordination, there will be co-relationship between the science and the spirit or the divine knowledge.

Then he says that because of MAYA, yogis had to suffer a lot and do a lot of penance to become collectively conscious - BRAHMIT i.e. to feel the BRAHMA but the new yoga, the Maha Yoga will make it all very "SAHAJA". The new Yoga system, when it will manifest in the different countries in the new age, the administration will be governed by people with varying degrees of power depending on their depth and quality of practice of the yoga. They will be able to create a society which will completely fulfill their desires and necessities and people won't need to accumulate loads of money. Poverty and sickness will be completely finished and in their absence the country, the SAMAJ, (the society) will be healthy and restful and without any anger.

Besides this prediction by the Indian astrologer, an American lady by the name of Jacqueline Murray had predicted about a great personality, a lady, who will be born in India, a lady; around 1924, and Shri Mataji was born in 1923. Cheerio, the great numerologist had also said about 1980 the new Advent will start a new age. There is a difference of 10 years.

Another lady called Alice Bailey, in a state of supra-consciousness has said that since Indians have all their attention on Yoga, a new Yoga will come by which the people will be connected to Holy Ghost. She also has said that there is a danger of Third World War which may be inevitable but can be avoided if people develop love for each other with this Yoga.

Then, again Saint Dnyaneshwar, the saint from Maharashtra who lived in late 17th century wrote extensively about the coming of the new age, where people will live in harmony and with love towards each other after becoming realized through Kundalini awakening.

Shri Mataji writes in her book "Meta Modern Era", when I was born, I saw people taking to a new course all over the world not to believe in God or spirituality, but to believe in money or power. At this juncture, I must say, my father, who was another great evolved soul, came to my help and he told me: 'You know what your mission in this life is'. I said: "I know that." Then he said: "You are standing on the seventh floor of a building. From there you see many who are on the ground floor. How will they believe that you are on the seventh floor? If you could raise them even up to the first or second floor, then they may start thinking that there is a higher state which they have to achieve. So the first slab of physical achievement is over, the second slab of the emotional is over and the third, the mental, also will be over. But now they have to go beyond this mental and, that too, not individually but collectively." I knew my mission very well of collective awakening, but I was born in such a blind world.

My Father continued: "Any discovery which is individual has to be brought to the collective otherwise it has no meaning, it does not serve any purpose." I told him: "I know my job is to find out a method by which we can really give en-masse Realization." He was overjoyed to hear that, and so I started working on many human beings. My life with my Father was full - with a lot of social contacts because he was a great freedom fighter and later on he became a member of our constituent assembly, the central assembly.

I met lots of his friends, their wives, children, and I could see, through my own subtle ways, what 'problem was responsible for their static state. I started working and finding out, researching what the problem of human beings is.

At the end of 1946, I reached the conclusion that I had to do it in a very deep silent way, and through the inner movement of my being I had to find out what was so problematic about human centers and their three channels.

Ultimately in the year of 1947 I had to go to a seminar of one of the so-called masters because he requested my husband, who had his friend staying in that place, who arranged my visit. I was amazed to see this man, who was ten years younger than me, looking at least twenty years older than me. But he mesmerized all the people and they shouted and screamed and some barked like dogs. Just by mesmerizing, he was taking them to their past.

This really shocked me. I was sitting under a tree to watch what he was doing. At night I went alone to the seashore, sat there alone meditating about how, somehow or other, I could use my own Kundalini for the en-masse realization of people. That was the moment when it worked, and it clicked. I was surprised, that with a little deeper penetration, I could work it out.

The experience was like this. I saw my Kundalini rising very fast like a telescope opening out and it was a beautiful color that you see when the iron is heated up, a red, rose color, but extremely cooling and soothing. The Kundalini went through my fontanel bone area (Brahmarandra) which was open from my childhood and was pouring out Divine vibrations (Purnabrahma). But this new experience gave me a new dimension of understanding of my Divine force. It came like a very promising reality that it was time for me to start my collective work. I found that the whole of my being was filled with great peace and joy.

I opened my eyes, went to this false master and told him: "Now the last centre can be opened for everyone". I was amazed to see that he had no idea about the centers, or about the three channels which I knew from my very childhood. I found out that there were so many of them who were very false masters and were just money-oriented, working through mesmerism by encouraging anti-Christ activities of immorality or by saying that this world is coming to an end.

I started my work with one person and I was amazed how she reached her fourth dimension in no time. She was a very old but a very nice religious lady who achieved this state in no time. Another one was younger lady who also was very easy and in seconds she received her ascent. Since that day she has got her vibrations. Then I took some twenty five people to the same seashore and I was surprised that twelve out of them felt the self- realization. From that day this work started working en-masse. Of course now even if there are 18,000 to 20,000 people almost all can get their Self-Realization, especially in Russia.

So many people have been cured in these conferences. I must confess that I am lucky. I am being used as the desire of the God Almighty to emit these forceful holy vibrations to give realization to thousands and thousands of people very happily that I in my life, to my amazement, the time has come, the blossom time, where there are so many flowers on this earth who are seekers of truth and they can easily become the fruits.

I had to move to London because my husband got elected to the post of Secretary General of the International Maritime Organization, and there I started my work with seven hippies who were very difficult people. I found that in their escape from the Western culture to anti-culture, they had become extremely arrogant, possessive and aggressive. I started to work on them and gradually they became aware that they were not in the fourth dimension (in which they always felt they were) and that they had no right to assert their so-called higher state existence on others.

After four years I could manage to get these seven hippies to come around. In between I kept coming to India and had a great response in my state of Maharashtra, where thousands of people started getting Realization.

Human beings evolution to the present status has been over a relatively short period of time as compared to the earlier species right from the stage of an amoeba.

The evolutionary process may be compared to the principles on which a spacecraft progresses to its destination. The spacecraft has several sections, one fitting into the next in a series. When a spacecraft is launched from the ground, after some time, the lowest or outermost section blasts the rest of the spacecraft which then acquires a much faster speed.

If the initial speed was say X miles per hour, then after the first blast it becomes X2 miles, per hour. Through a series of such accelerating blasts, the spacecraft goes outside the gravity of the earth and proceeds towards its object which may be the moon or Jupiter. Our evolution also takes place at a similar high speed. Life is first created at the stage of amoeba. After an explosion, life reaches another stage - that of ape or other intermediary stages. After a series of such explosions, human beings are created.

At the human state also, in the beginning, our attention is only on food and some protection from nature, like a house or a hut. After achieving that, once a certain stage of higher development is reached, we suddenly get exploded into a state where we become mentally very alert and intelligent. Thus we take to science and develop technology, by which we could go to the Moon or Jupiter. Then with some other blasting different from mental achievement, we develop an emotional state in our being.

When we see the whole world burning with hatred and competition, a new state is achieved and this is a state of hankering for compassion, love and peace. At this stage, or even earlier we start seeking something beyond human understanding. We then turn ourselves to another internal blasting, where after we take to religion and God. Soon people found that religious practices are mere rituals which do not touch, much less transform the inner self. It becomes apparent that we have to seek something beyond our minds.

When the seekers of truth start seeking honestly, and deliberately he rises to a realm, where he achieves the fourth dimension in his awareness (Turiya). Turiya stage is the state of total subtle awareness. We live in three dimensions normally. The saints achieved their fourth dimension and through this ascent, they reach a state of complete tranquility, complete integration and total awareness of reality. The three dimensions in which we normally exist are physical, mental and emotional, and the fourth dimension is spiritual. Now by intensely using the first three dimensions we come to realize the futility of our lives and we then start seeking the absolute truth, as we are not satisfied with whatever we know.

We had a saint called Markandeya, who they say lived fourteen thousand years ago. He has written about this fourth dimension and has described it as the blessing of the Primordial Mother. The second person, who was very well equipped with this knowledge, was Adi Shankaracharya who has written many books. The first book he wrote was Viveka Chudamani, in which he describes this fourth dimension and explains why we should try to attain this fourth dimension. He has written in praise of the Primordial Mother, especially in Saundarya Lahari, where he described all the Divine vibrations as 'the vibrations of the loving beauty of the Primordial Mother."

Then, in the Twelfth Century, came a great saint called Dnyaneshwar in Maharashtra. It was a tradition of his time that one master of Nath Panthis could give realization only to one disciple. This master was not supposed even to talk about the fourth dimension to normal people. They were only told that they should remember God and should sing the praise of God. But he, the great poet and a very great saint, Dnyaneshwar, felt that it was time that the subject of spiritual ascent should be made much more clear to people.

In Gita there is no description of the Kundalini or of the awakening, though Shri Krishna, at the very outset, has said that a person should achieve the state of Sthitapragya, which means, the one who is balanced, through enlightenment by Divine knowledge. All this was a description, but he did not talk about how it is brought about.

The Nath Panthis

It was Shri Dnyaneshwar who wrote a treatise on Gita called as Jnyaneshwari. In the sixth chapter he very sweetly described the nature of this fourth power, called the Kundalini which rests in the triangular bone and the way it is awakened by some great soul by which one gets his fourth state of awareness. He did not take permission from his guru to give realization to others but he only asked that he should be permitted to at least write about it.

Later on, this sixth chapter was not understood by the people who were in charge of religion (dharma-martandas). They said that this sixth chapter was not to be read (Nishiddha) and thus this great chapter was completely neglected by the people and they just tried to follow the path of Bhakti, which means devotion to God by chanting the names of God or singing the praise of God Almighty.

Later on, in the sixteenth century many saints existed who started talking and singing about Kundalini, the channels and the subtle centers. Some of the saints tried to give Self-Realization to their disciples but they actually gave it only to very few persons because they thought that the world was not yet ready to receive Self-Realization. As Kabira has written: "How am I to explain to these people, who are blind, about the light, mostly who are blind?"

The awakening of Kundalini was done by people who were very few in number because there were very few real seekers.

My job is to awaken your Kundalini power so that it could pierce your Sahasrar Chakra This work is of collective nature; I have therefore, to do it in the case of one and all. I want to tell you about Jesus Christ, Guru Nanaka, King Janaka and a number of other incarnations and the way they relate with the collectivity. Similarly, I wish to talk to you about incarnations of Shri Rama, Shri Krishna etc., and also about Shri Shiva because, all the powers of these Gods and deities are in us. Now, the time has come for collective consciousness to manifest."

Chapter 11

Shri Kalki Avatara

We come to the tenth Avatara, the future one, the Kalki. The word Kalki is actually an abbreviation of the word Nishkalank synonymous with Nirmala, which means something that is spotlessly clean. This incarnation has been described in many Puranas.

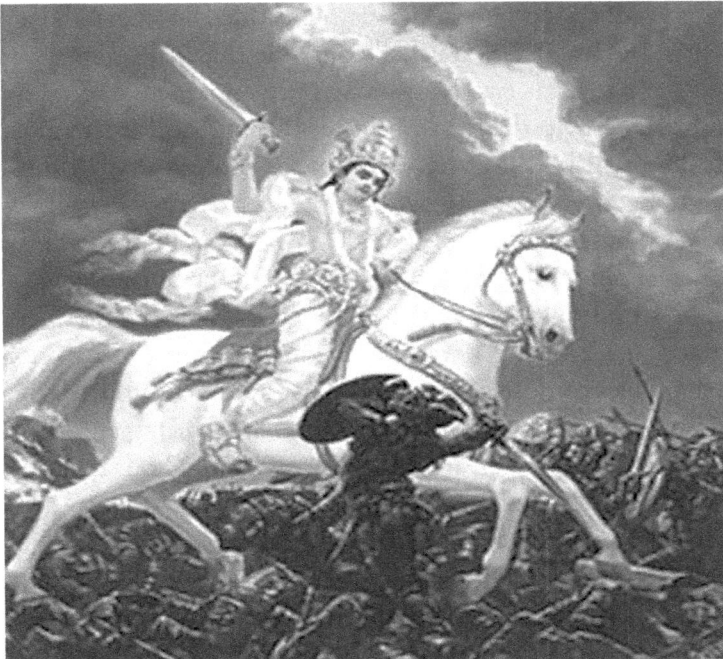

With the coming of Kalki it has been predicted that the Kali Yuga will pass away and there will be a brighter age consisting of a higher rate of men. He will come when the sixth Root Race will be born on the Earth. There will then be a great change in the world, a great manifestation of truth, and intuitive knowing and occultism will be more prevalent. It has been mentioned in the Kalki Purana, that in His coming the rule over the sixth Root Race will pass on to the hands of the two Kings – the ideal King and the ideal Priest.

As we look back at the times of all earlier incarnations and events in the stream of time we find over and over again the two great figures-the ideal King and the ideal Priest both of them always working together. The one rules, the other teaches; the one governs the nation, the other instructs it and such a pair of mighty ones come down in every age for each and every Race. Each Race has its own Teacher, the ideal Brahmana, called in the Buddhist language the Bodhisattva, the learned, full of wisdom and truth. Each has also its own ruler, the Manu.

The Manu in each race is the ideal King, the Brahmana in each race is the ideal Teacher; and it is mentioned in the Kalki Purana that when the Kalki Avatara shall come He shall call from the sacred village of Shamballa- two Kings who have remained throughout the age in order to help the world in its evolution. And the name of the Manu who will be the King of the next Race, is said in the Kalki Purana to be Moru; and the name of the ideal Brahmana who will be the Teacher of the next Race is said to be Devapi; and these two are King and Teacher for the sixth Race that is to be born.

The wondrous story of the past reveals that the choosing of the new Race, the evolving of it, the making of a new Root Race, is a thing that takes centuries, millenniums, sometimes hundreds of thousands of years; and that the two who are to be its King and Priest, the Manu and the Brahmana, are at Their work throughout the centuries, choosing the men who may be the seeds of the new Race.

Shri Mataji Nirmala Devi in her historic speech at Bombay on 28th September 1979 spoke extensively on the coming of Kalki. Referring to what has been said in the Puranas about the arrival of Kalki on this Earth riding a white horse, in a village of Sambhalpur,

She clarified that in the word Sambhal, 'Bhal' is the forehead. That means Kalki is situated on your Bal, meaning the forehead which is where he is going to be born. Between Christ and this destroying incarnation of Mahavishnu called Kalki, there is a time given to human beings to rectify them, for them to enter into the kingdom of God, which in the Bible is called as the Last Judgment.

The population of the world today is maximum, because all those who have aspirations to enter into the kingdom of God are either born in the modern times or are going to be born very soon. They are choosing one by one, trying and testing those who shall form the nucleus of the sixth Race. They are taking soul by soul, subjecting each to many a test, to many an ordeal, to see if there be the strength out of which a new Race can spring. This is the most important time because Sahaja Yoga is the last judgment.

In the modern times people are at different stages of evolution of their attentions or 'CHITTA'. There could be people who have too much of Tamasikvrutti, inertia, sluggishness or slow moving temperament. These when exaggerated make people to take to alcohol, drugs or some such addiction which take them away from reality and make them numb. On the other side, are the people who are extremely ambitious, want to win the whole world, be powerfully independent and do not want to have any relationship with God or the Divine who are on their own-malignant & cancerous. Thus in Kali-Yoga there are people who have either gone to an extremes of being too alcoholic or escapists, running away from reality, from awareness or from truth and beauty or to the other extreme of being ego-oriented and denying everything that is beautiful. So we have those who are super-ego oriented, very much conditioned, lethargic and absolutely revolting. On the other side are people who are extremely ambitious dominating and destroying each other by their ambition and competition.

When we talk of 'KALKI' we have to remember that between getting our realization and entering into the kingdom of God, we can falter very much. This is called as 'Yoga Brasht sthiti' people take to yoga, enter into the yoga, and are still enchanted by their Pravruttis e.g. a ego or money oriented man, who wants to dominate, may form groups and try to dominate them by his ideas. This is known as "Yoga-Bhrasta", where a person falls from his Yoga, comes down from his Yoga.

Sahaja Yoga takes its roots, very sweetly into the heart of all the seekers, who are simple hearted, less complicated and who are in the center and more balanced. It works very spontaneously, and effortlessly.

In Sahaja yoga each one grows and he has full freedom to do that. In order to grow it is necessary to keep to the mains, to the growth with the whole that is not restricted to one person here and there, or if one tries to overpower the rest. In Sahaja yoga as in Nature, nothing grows out of bounds. Everything is controlled. Yoga Bhrashta Sthiti is the worst thing that can happen which could take a human being down to lower evolved forms of being.

This is the power of Kalki which is secretly working behind Sahaja yoga. Kalki means there are eleven powers, which are guarding the beauty of Sahaja yoga. With the eleven destructive powers of Kalki having started working, one should be very careful and try not to trouble or harm any good and saintly person.

Shri Mataji Nirmala Devi, the incarnation of Mahamaya, had stated it in very explicit terms in her speech on the Kalki Avatar at Bombay on 28th September 1979, not only to the Sahaja yogis, but to the whole world today, 'that "Be careful". Do not try to harm others. Do not try to take advantage of others, and do not try to show off your own powers. Because if once this destruction starts in your life you won't know how to stop it. When you associate or live with evil minded people, you also suffer. The innocents suffer. This sort of life that we have been leading, of compromising, not understanding what the truth, accepting with blind faith, is widely prevalent all over the world.

Even in the name of God we are committing sins. Instead of clearing it out and understanding it through our developed brain we are easily carried away by people who have some sort of a Hypnotic and Charismatic influence. Innocent people who succumb to their charms, only end up giving the control of themselves into their hands. Such over dependence and lack of alertness will pull one into their influence and the 'Eleven Rudras' or destructive powers, of Kalki will not spare or compromise with such nonsensical people.

Hence Shri Mataji Nirmala Devi, who in Her Divine Vision was able to visualize the immensity of destruction that could fall if we invite the wrath of Shri Kalki, used to often warn not to play a fool with Him, and to not take it easy and compromise with these non-sensical people. Stick on to the right used to be her constant word of caution. Lack of reverence and absolute denial of the Supreme who created us has made some of us very ego-oriented, arrogant and to commit sins without regrets or repentance. This is extremely wrong and is against our Ascent. Ego-oriented and money-oriented actions will not stand the test of time and the test of truth. Amassing of wealth has never made man happy and one who has amassed wealth is able to gain respect only as long as he holds on to that money and power that gives him that money.

Sahaja yoga is the last judgment by which you will become cit-izens of God but this is possible only in an attitude of complete sur-render and understanding of divine love.

Hence the incarnation of Kalki is imminent, and he has been endowed with the Hanan Shakti or the destructive powers of Shri Krishna, Brahma Deva, the Tandav of Shiva, Bhairava's Khadaga Shri Ganesha's Parshu, Shri Hanuman's Gada and the Siddhis all of which are going to destroy are given to Him. Buddha's forgiveness and Mahavira's AHIMSA, are going to turn upside down. Kalki with all these eleven powers will be coming to finish all that are left out after the final sorting done on the basis of Sahaja Yoga.

It is not going to be ordinary Hanana, like even the Devi has done. Devi has killed all the Rakshasas, thousands of years ago, but they are back in the seat again. Now the problem is very different. The problem of Kali- Yuga is that the people are not pure or simple like a Sadhu or the other extreme like that of a Rakshasa. The Rakshasas have entered the brains of man in subtle form or vrittis and are doing all sorts of wrong things in the name of Religion, politics, progress and education. Once you have sided with them, then they are in your brains, they are within you. You may be a good person, but you may be destroyed because you are having them in your heads.

Hence it is really very difficult to say who is really a negative or a positive person. Only Sahaja Yoga is going to cleanse you and make you absolutely positive. This is the only way when your Ankura (Sprouting) can happen, when it starts giving your Self- Realization. After Self-Realization, you start enjoying that Self. When you start enjoying it, you give up all the things that make you compromise and make you a horribly mixed-up person. All this confusion will then go away. Hence it is essential to free yourselves of all the wrong doings.

The timing of the Kalki avatar as described in the Kalki Purana is to be understood as when the chakra of Kalki is caught up in our body. In the Kundalini awakening, we find that if the Mendhu or the head goes out of order, the Kundalini doesn't rise. The whole head become logged and the Kundalini doesn't rise above the Hamsa Chakra. At the most they might try to raise it up to Agnya, but then it drops down.

The influence of false gurus, too much thinking also create problem of the right side and one of the aspects of Kalki gets spoiled; and an imbalance is created . If the whole forehead is full of bumps, we must know that the Kalki Chakra is out of order and the person may be about to go through some sort of calamity. When the Kalki Chakra is caught up, all your fingers, palms and hands start burning. Catching of the Kalki Chakra is indicative of the person going down with a horrible decease like Cancer, leprosy or some sort of calamity. So the Kalki Chakra must be kept all right. There are at least eleven Sukshma Chakras in the Kalki Chakra at least some of which need to be kept clean, pure and alive, so that others can be restored. If all the eleven Chakras are ruined then it is very difficult to give Realization.

What is the thing that one should do to keep the Kalki alright?

To keep your Kalki Chakra all right you must have Awe for God, a reverence. If you are not afraid of God, then you will not be afraid of doing something wrong. When you have that Awe for God, who is all pervading, all powerful, He has the powers to raise us to the state of higher being and also to bestow all the blessings that He has. He is very compassionate. The most important thing as far as God is concerned is the relation you must establish, by first finding out your Self, your Atma, and then relating yourself to that.

Chapter 12

Sahaja Yoga-Today's Mahayoga

The meaning of 'Sahaja Yoga' can be better understood if we split it into its component parts: 'Saha' means 'with', 'ja' means 'born', and 'yoga' is 'the union' or 'the technique'. So Sahaja Yoga means that the technique of evolving is inborn in each of us. Just as we are born, without any effort on our part, with our hands, our feet and our human awareness so also we are born for our spontaneous union with the Divine which comes to us equally effortlessly.

Many find it hard to accept the truth that they can achieve Self-realization effortlessly. But as Sahaja Yoga is the process of evolution it cannot be achieved by any human effort. It is the working of life itself. When we plant a seed in the Earth it germinates by itself. It grows from a tiny seed with potentiality into a seedling and then develops into a big tree with a trunk, branches, roots and leaves. What human effort makes any difference to this spontaneous growth?

If Self-realization means identification with you no amount of human effort can achieve it. If a small particle of dust exists, it just exists. How much effort did the Himalayas put into being what they are? Animals take this fact for granted and they exist without making any effort to be themselves. The evolutionary process is the work of Mother Nature, and she does this work without any help from human effort or human intelligence. It is only man's ego that does not allow him to accept this simple truth.

The earth moves around the Sun with terrific speed but she holds us and sustains us in space with great love and understanding. The Sun shines to give us life, and goes at night to the other side of the world to let us sleep. The Moon also plays her own role here, and the stars have their place too. Such a beautifully organized stage has been created for human beings without man doing anything towards its creation. The harmonious working of the elements of the Creation clearly exhibits its universal theme of Divine Love.

In this unity of Creation universes revolve in complete harmony. The whole Creation is like a musical melody, and is the impassive witness to evolution and to the role of human beings in it. In his freedom and dignity, man has evolved just to learn the mastery of enjoying it. The Creator as conductor of this musical extravaganza has given His creatures freedom to choose their role, and to bring their instrument into tune with His Absolute instrument.

In the beginning when Creation came into being, the separation took place between Almighty God (Parabrahma) and His Power (Adi Shakti). The Divine Power, separated from God, created universe after universe in her journey back towards Him. In our universe she created the solar system, and the planet Earth to sustain life through the various phases of evolution, and finally created human beings. At this stage, for the first time, an inkling of the higher self (Atma) reflecting Almighty God Himself entered into the awareness of man. The union of these two identities, one human and finite the other Divine and infinite, is possible only in human awareness.

We can understand this more clearly by means of analogies. We can envisage God as the driver of His automobile pressing on the accelerator or the brake. By the use of these forces He ultimately creates the human being who, in time, rises to become a learner driver. When this happens God moves to the passenger's seat, and man drives the car under strict supervision.

At first as a learner driver he makes numerous errors, but one day he finally masters the art of driving. When this happens, God retires as instructor and lets human beings take His place in the driver's seat. From this vantage point the newly qualified driver, the Self-realized human being, witnesses the use of the brake and accelerator which are really part and parcel of his own being.

Another meaning of 'Sahaja' is 'simple and spontaneous'. The working of Sahaja Yoga is very simple although the operation of its mechanism within us is quite complicated.

Through Her infinite Divine Power (Pranava) Adi Shakti creates three finite personalities to perform Her three functions:

(1) As Mahakali She brings the creation into existence and also destroys it.
(2) As Mahasaraswati She creates universes, ultimately creating the Earth.
(3) As Mahalaxshmi She integrates these two forces and evolves to reveal her love.

She organizes through the co-ordination of combinations and permutations of her three powers, and ultimately evolves human beings as the epitome of her creation. These forces interact to create the physical, mental, emotional and spiritual bodies of human beings. The first three bodies are finite; the last one is for infinite happenings. These forces of evolution first of all give human beings the freedom of choice.

In human beings Almighty God is expressed as the subtle being (Sukshma), His infinite nature being reflected as Divine Spirit (Atma). The union or yoga of God as Divine Spirit (Atma) with the Divine Power (Kundalini) takes place in human beings through the residual power of the Kundalini whose nature is finite. The expression of this Divine Power in human beings creates the human attention which is made finer through Kundalini awakening. At the moment of Self-realization this attention pierces the infinite realm of collective consciousness.

In the evolutionary process one fish had to be the first to cross the threshold of the land before many others followed. The same principle is at work in mass Self-realization. In every major evolutionary leap of mankind an Incarnation takes birth to guide and lead the course of evolution. Incarnations represent different aspects of

God who take birth to guide humanity through different stages of life at different periods in time (Yugas). All these stages have been 'Sahaja' or spontaneous. As the last and most important stage, mass Self-realization and the unique discovery of Sahaja Yoga is the gift of modern times (Kaliyuga). They are the culmination of this communication between God and man.

The Unconscious is the awareness of Almighty God and a realized soul is like the light of a lamp. One realized soul has to enlighten another just as one lamp can enlighten another. Through Sahaja Yoga a soul gets his Self- realization to begin with, and then learns how to give realization to others. Only through Sahaja Yoga can this sacred knowledge of the Kundalini science be fully learned.

Sahaja Yoga has some very simple rules as Shri Mataji was once comparing it to subscribing to a telephone service:

- if you are not connected you should get connected
- if you are not connected do not behave as if you are connected
- if you are not connected and you continually try to dial someone on a disconnected phone, you may spoil your instrument
- If you are not connected, or have no appointment with a VIP (Almighty God), you will annoy Him greatly by persistently dialing His number.

In Sahaja Yoga real seekers are judged differently from false ones. Reading about God and becoming identified with the words of the book and actually experiencing God are two different things altogether. God has to be felt as a personal experience. Merely knowing the scriptures does not guarantee Self-realization. On the contrary, those who feel at the end of their intellectual search, and who find no joy any longer in studying or reading about God, they are the ones who jump effortlessly into the unknown realm of collective consciousness. Describing the great unconscious stage which we have to occupy is not the same as occupying it. This will only happen when the human mind gets its priorities right. All that is really important is done by Almighty God.

Many people put tremendous effort into achieving God. They recite His name, and seek His blessings and attention as a birthright, as if God owes them something or is indebted to them in some way. They suffer from some form of superiority complex. Unwilling to recognize Divine Incarnations in their lifetime they crucify or kill them, later build temples and churches to them, and sing their glory. Such people's egos prevent them from recognizing a being higher than themselves in human form or because it does not fit into their acquired artificial ideas.

A rich person, for instance, might not accept an Incarnation born in poor circumstances. The chances of an intellectual accepting anyone as an Incarnation are pretty bleak. Intelligence is the greatest hurdle to acceptance because human beings depend on it throughout their objective search. They are not willing to abandon this instrument of intelligence with which they have so extensively experimented.

Moreover seekers have fixed ideas about Self-realization, God and Incarnations, How can the Divine fit into the mould which humans have designed for Him? He is what He is, and cannot be made to order just to suit human notions which are so varied and so vague.

Today, spiritual shopping or shopping for God has become the norm and people are attracted to them easily. Both kinds are the victims of ignorance. It is exceedingly difficult to raise the Kundalini of people who through effort or ignorance have access to the realm of the collective subconscious or the collective supra-conscious in their awareness. They are not aware that the apparent powers which they enjoy belong to other entities. These entities dominate the true self and reality is tucked away in ignorance. It is not easy to convince people who believe they are powerful and who use these extra-sensory personalities. Unless and until they get attacked by their so-called associates from the collective subconscious and supra- conscious realms they will not believe.

The followers of such people are also bound to be affected. When the light finally dawns and they realize how they have been duped and cheated, such victims need special help and attention by Sahaja Yogis. If they do not wholeheartedly surrender then the Unconscious loses its interest in them.

Alcoholics and addicts of all kinds are also stuck in the subconscious strata, and having become slaves of their habits, cannot crawl out of the mire. One strength given by Sahaja Yoga is that of non-involvement, and after becoming Sahaja Yogis many have cast off the chains of their slavery by observing their own condition.

Sahaja Yoga does not respect men and women who have no respect for their own chastity. Those who torture their bodies in the name of religion and subsequently suffer, or those who pamper themselves endlessly and succeed in their aim of developing beautiful bodies, get little respect too. The quality of their life does not change and they are very superficial individuals. Sahaja Yoga teaches how to love and adore the human body as the temple of Almighty God.

THE CREATION OF KUNDALINI IN HUMAN BEINGS

The Kundalini is the harp on which the Divine plays the melody of its Love. She is the ladder by which the seeker steps across the threshold into the fathomless Unconscious. She is the jumping board that allows one to soar from finite to infinite in the ocean of freedom, peace and bliss. Kundalini is the goal of that long-promised abode, the Kingdom of Almighty God.

Ancient sages who meditated and achieved great heights of awareness, have written a lot about Kundalini. Living away from the public in forest dwellings they saw the working of Kundalini within themselves during meditation. Apart from descriptions in ancient Indian scriptures, Kundalini has also been described in religious books like the Throats' Bible and the Koran as 'the fire tree'. In those books there are many references couched in secretive language which few would have understood. The Bible tells of the first meeting of all the disciples with the Virgin Mary after the Crucifixion. The closed room they met in "was filled with a great wind, and there appeared above their heads, as it were, separate tongues of fire, and they were filled with the Holy Ghost." This is a description of a vision of Kundalini.

Various Chinese philosophers have also described the Kundalini in their writings, and Greek mythology has catalogued the same Gods and Goddesses as mentioned earlier. The Zen Buddhist religion teaches very clearly that the basis of Buddhist meditation is the science of Kundalini. The name 'Kundalini' was bestowed by Indian sages. God has never given a name to anything He has created. It is the feminine form of the word 'Kaunda' which means 'rings' or 'coils' in Sanskrit.

Although written in secretive language, the description of Kundalini in those ancient scriptures is easily intelligible to a Sahaja Yogi. Realized souls can visualize and understand the subtle implication behind the meanings of gross sentences. In every religion, the flame of truth burns on the wick of Kundalini. She is a universal identity in every human being. Knowledge of Kundalini is mostly described in Sanskrit texts, but Shri Mataji Nirmala Devi has brought that great ancient knowledge and explained it using scientific terminology to suit the modern need.

One should not, even for a moment, be obsessed with the idea that knowledge can be contained or expressed only through one language. Nor does the expression of truth, expressed through one language, make other languages in any way less important.

THE ENTRY OF THE KUNDALINI INTO THE HUMAN FETUS

Two divine happenings take place in the human being when he exists as a fetus in his mother's womb:

1) The Spirit (Atma) enters the fetus's heart which then starts to pulsate. The waves of this pulsation move in 3 1/2 coils
2) Simultaneously the Divine Power (Pranava) enters the fetus through the brain.

Encased by the skull the human brain is conical in shape. At the very top, in the area of the fontanel bone, it has an apex, as well as a base and three sides like a prism. These three layers of the brain are made of different material and have different densities. The brain therefore acts like a prism with a quality of refraction. When the Divine Power enters the brain it is divided into three channels, as the prism-like brain has three sides to it like a pyramid.

Of these three channels, two enter through two of the sides of the brain, and one from its apex. They pass over the primary coil, created by the heart's throbbing (Ishwari Power), interact on each other and create seven chakras. At a later date these subtle centers manifest as gross physical centers outside the spinal cord. They are:

1) Sahasrar Chakra in the brain
2) Agnya Chakra at the crossing point of the optic nerve
3) Vishuddhi Chakra manifests the cervical plexus
4) Ana hat or Hridhaya Chakra manifests the cardiac plexus
5) Nabhi or Manipur Chakra manifests the solar plexus
6) Swadishtan Chakra manifests the aortic plexus
7) Mooladhar Chakra manifests the pelvic plexus -

These are the body's major plexuses which are gross in nature, but each has sub-plexuses .When the Kundalini enters the apex of the brain, the fontanel bone (Brahmarandra - 'Brahma' means 'the Divine', 'Randra' means 'a hole'), She descends straight down through the brain into the spinal cord. From the two sides of the brain the Divine Power flows within. These undergo refraction at two major points and, in accord with the parallelogram of forces; the rays falling on the sloping side of the brain get divided into two components. One pair that goes out of the body; the other pair which enter the spinal cord. This latter pair forms the left and right channels in the spinal cord known as Ida and Pingala Nadis. These two subtle channels later manifest as the left and right sympathetic nervous system.

It is at the back of the brain that the Divine Power enters and goes down into the spinal cord as 'A' Stream. It is also from the back of the fetus that the Divine Power enters the spinal cord as 'B' Stream.

These two streams of divinity combine to form the central nervous system. The 'A' Stream allows human beings to perform voluntary actions; by the 'B' Stream they perform involuntary actions.

From the brain's apex the Divine Power (Pranava) enters and settles down as three powers in the human being. The lowest one is the Mahakali Power, the second one is the Mahasaraswati Power, and the topmost one is the Mahalaxshmi Power. These three Powers create three pairs of Deities and their respective Powers. Firstly Mahakali creates Shri Ganesha, and then all the other Deities are created. They are:

1. Shiva + Parvati (Durga)
2. Brahma + Saraswati
3. Vishnu + Laxmi These Deities also manifest Shri Krishna with His Power Radha, and the Lord Jesus Christ whose Power is His Mother Mary (Mahalaxshmi Herself). These two Deities are the evolved human Incarnations of Shri Vishnu and Shri Ganesha respectively.

After this activity the Pranava which has divided into three enters the spinal cord. Its lowest strand (Mahakali or Gauri Power) disappears into the coccyx as Kundalini.

From the coil of Kundalini Shri Ganesha is placed on the Mooladhar Chakra which lies outside her abode of Mooladhar. He rests on that chakra guarding the chastity of His Mother Kundalini. Each human being has an individual Kundalini which is his mother, and he is her only son. She is Gauri who resides in a dormant state waiting for the opportune moment to give her only child 'second birth' (Dina) or Self-realization. The other Deities remain on their different centers:

1) Sahasrar Chakra -   Adi Shakti Herself
2) Agnya Chakra -   Jesus Christ + His Mother Mary
3) Vishuddhi Chakra -   Shri Krishna + Shri Radha
4) Ana hat Chakra -   Shri Rama + Shri Sita (right side)

	Shri Shiva + Shri Parvati (left side) Shri Jagadamba (Durga) in the centre
5) Nabhi Chakra -	Shri Vishnu + Shri Laxmi
6) Swadishtan Chakra -	Shri Brahmadeva + Shri Saraswati
7) Mooladhar Chakra -	Shri Ganesha + Shri Gauri

Through the primary coil of Kundalini in the heart these Powers create a new transforming mechanism called Hridyakash. This is the light of the cardiac centre popularly known as the Sacred Heart, and is reflected around the heart as seven auras. It receives information on the state or mood of the Divine Spirit, and whether or not the Spirit is pleased with the play of the Primordial Mother (Adi Shakti). It is an interwoven system and is more elaborately explained at a later point.

The middle strand (Mahasaraswati Power) oozes out into the vacuum or Void created by Kundalini disappearance into the coccyx. The topmost strand (Mahalaxshmi Power) remains as the upper section of the Sushumna Nadi, and manifests as the parasympathetic nervous system, while the lower section of this central channel remains as a part of the Void.

With the descent of Prana all the Deities settle down in their respective chakras with the exception of Shri Shiva. Shri Shiva identifies with the Divine Spirit (Atma) which He accompanies into the fetus in the case of non-realized beings. His Power Parvati identifies with the Mahakali Power of Adi Shakti. This is the basic difference between man and the Primordial Being in their spiritual blueprint. The separation of Shiva and Shakti (Parvati) thus occurs; when they meet again the yoga is said to take place.

1. As the fetus welcomes the Spirit into the heart the first throb in the heart region can be heard. Shiva settles down in the heart of non- realized souls. Parvati manifests as the Deity Durga, independent of Her Lord, just for the creation of the physical body of each human being. She

moves into the central chamber of the heart chakra called the Sacred Heart.

2. Lord Vishnu settles down with His Power and Consort Laxmi in the navel centre. From His navel issues a lotus-like centre which dangles around the Nabhi Chakra.

3. This is the Swadishtan Chakra, and Lord Brahmadeva and His Power Saraswati take their places as presiding Deities of this centre.

4. The dangling chakra moves in a circle around the Nabhi Chakra creating an area called the Ocean of Illusion (Bhavasagara) or the Void. Lord Vishnu, through His ten Incarnations which represent the ten stages of the evolution of the Primordial Being (Virat), crosses this Void.

5. His seventh Incarnation was as Shri Rama who resides on the right side of the heart chakra with His Power, Shri Sita. Rama incarnated as the representation of a personality who was the perfect male human being (Mariyada Purushottama).

6. Lord Vishnu's eighth Incarnation was as Shri Krishna who, with His Power Radha, resides on the Vishuddhi Chakra. Shri Krishna was the ultimate expression of the Primordial Being (Virat) in human form, and taught us to regard the Creation as a play (Leela) of the Divine Power.

7. In the brain above the Vishuddhi, where the optic nerves cross each other, is the Agnya Chakra where Lord Jesus Christ resides in every human being. He is the complete manifestation of the Son God principle. His body was formed from Shri Kartikeya, only brother of Shri Ganesha and a Divine personality. Although He came as a human being His resurrection was made possible by the Divine substance of His human body. In the Vaikuntha stage He was created as Maha Vishnu, the only son of Krishna and Radha. As the ninth Incarnation of Vishnu he was called Boudda or 'the mild Incarnation'.

8. The Sahasrar Chakra (the limbic area of the brain) is governed by Adi Shakti in a form called the Great Illusion

who recently incarnated as Shri Mataji Nirmala Devi in our own times and created the environment conducive for the coming of Shri Kalki. She is the Power of the tenth and final Incarnation of Vishnu, Shri Kalki the Collective Being, who is yet to come.

The parasympathetic nervous system is the gross expression of the Mahalaxshmi Power, which first manifests in the limbic area of the Sahasrar Chakra, and which goes on to become the vagus nerve. After this nerve a Void is created in the central channel (Sushumna Nadi) of each human being, when the Kundalini enters the triangular bone. In this Void is placed the Primordial Master (Adi Guru) formed from Brahma, Vishnu and Mahesha (Shiva).

This Primordial Master is also known as Dattatreya. He has taken many human births as a prophet and teacher such as Raja Janaka, Adi Nath, Macchinder Nath, Zoroaster, Guru Nanaka, and Sai Nath of Shirdi. This Deity helps human beings to seek their salvation by crossing the Void or Ocean of Illusion within themselves.

The chakras are created from the five elements (earth, water, air, fire and ether) which are transformed by five kinds of material power. The primary coil of Kundalini, the Ishwari Power, and the three Powers of Mahakali, Mahasaraswati and Mahalaxshmi create a structure which looks like a bulbous bell-shaped flower. The left and right sympathetic nervous systems manifest from the subtle Ida and Pingala Nadis outside the spinal cord. These systems lie along the spinal cord, outside the vertebrae, and form a bulbous ganglionic chain. They run along to the coccyx at the base of the spinal cord. A little way below the end of the coccyx they meet each other forming a circle around the Mooladhar Chakra. This is the lowest centre and the only one placed outside the spinal cord or the cranial bones. All the centers are controlled by their presiding Deities, and in the gross are expressed as ganglions. All organs appear to be controlled through the ganglions.

The term "parasympathetic and sympathetic nervous systems", both branches of the autonomous nervous system are scientific terms which when sublimated to include the working of the Divine power through them gives an altogether different interpretation of our body structure and its role in evolution as expressed to us by Shri Mataji Nirmala Devi.

THE AUTONOMOUS NERVOUS SYSTEM

Functionally the autonomous nervous system must be understood by their Divine nature. They are the gross channels to express the subtle energy of Divine Love, and ultimately to bestow Self-realization. When the Primordial Mother wants to fill a human being with Her Power (Prana), she releases it through parasympathetic activity for his use. When humans use this Prana for some effort or extra emergency requirements, it is a sympathetic activity function. Someone can increase their heart rate, for example, by running for a short time. In that case the Prana is used for a need in a state of emergency. But reducing the heart rate cannot be done, as this can only happen through parasympathetic activity. Only Adi Shakti, residing in the brain, can bring down the heart rate.

We must clearly understand how and why chemicals like adrenalin or acetylcholine work in different ways. Depending on the circumstances, either of them can relax or constrict (augment) a particular organ. If, through sympathetic nervous system activity, the coronary blood vessels get dilated, due to the same activity the arteries generally get constricted from the adrenalin secreted by the sympathetic nervous system. While there is constriction in the bronchial muscles by the parasympathetic nervous system, there is dilation of the muscles on the whole.

The mode of action seems contradictory, but if the two different functions of these two systems are understood in terms of the aim or the purpose of their activity, they can be easily understood. The sympathetic nervous system sends one kind of nerve impulse, while the parasympathetic sends different nerve impulses. These impulses may constrict or dilate, may increase or decrease the activity, but the purpose or the expression of these two systems is either to divert or to act. They pour energy into the organs, or use the energy already present in the organs. The sympathetic activity is brought into play by the human effort of conscious activity, and also for any extraordinary action.

Although the parasympathetic nervous system seems to be acting on its own, the decisions whether to augment or constrict an organ are actually taken by the Deities, who are responsible for looking after the needs of every organ.

Medical science, like all other sciences, is an objective knowledge hence it is partial knowledge, and to a great extent is vague about these systems. It is very hard to show the energies of the Divine Power that flow along the spinal cord because they are subtle and invisible to the naked eye. They can only be perceived when one has developed the eyes of the Divine Spirit (Atma).

This may sound all very abstruse. However, in our experiments with Sahaja Yoga many people have clearly seen the Kundalini pulsating in the triangular bone called the coccyx. Moreover one can see her upward movement with the naked eye. With a stethoscope it is even possible to record the pulsations although they are feeble. At the top of the head, a seeker himself feels the throb of the Kundalini. There are many such physical proofs which people have seen with their own eyes, even non- realized people. The pupils of the eyes of those whose Kundalini has been raised dilate like the pupils of small children, suggesting parasympathetic activity.

In the case of eyes, dilated pupils are a controversial subject for medical science to decide whether it is parasympathetic or sympathetic activity. In childhood, when the ego and superego are not fully developed, and when the fontanel bone is still quite soft, the pupils dilate because of parasympathetic activity. As the child grows, ego and superego develop fully, and then dilation of the pupils becomes sympathetic activity as they adjust to darkness. Even constriction of the pupils is sympathetic because the optic nerves are using the Divine Energy (Pranava).

Broadly speaking, it is the sympathetic nervous system, human in nature, which brings about whatever normal or extra activity human beings are involved in, and can perform by their conscious or subconscious mind. Whenever the supply of energy is spontaneous it is Divine in nature, and the parasympathetic nervous system is brought into play.

DEVELOPMENT OF EGO AND SUPEREGO

The brain is triangular in shape, and the rays of the Divine Power, which fall on the inclined plane of its two sides, undergo two physical phenomena:

1) Firstly, because they fall straight on the inclined plane and enter the brain, these rays divide with the result that one component force enters the brain and the other component force exits the brain. The same phenomenon re-occurs later when these two lines of force cross each other in the brain at the Agnya Chakra. The crossing takes place as a result of the refraction in the brain due to its different densities at different levels.

2) The two components which go out of the brain take the human attention outside the body, as it reacts to outside impulses. Ego and superego are created as a reaction. When a child is born, the mother starts nursing her baby by impulse, just as an animal does. The child sucks on the mother's breast and feels unity with joy. When the mother moves the child from one breast to the other the child feels hurt and unhappy. The reaction mounts up in the child's brain in opposite directions.

In this way ego is gradually inflated in the brain like a balloon. After this resistant behavior by the child, the mother scolds or rebukes this assertion of ego which creates conditioning in the child's mind. This conditioning creates the superego, and a balloon-like structure starts developing on the left side of the brain. The ego on the right side of the brain and the superego on the left side grow until they cover the soft bone (fontanel) on top of the head. The fontanel bone becomes fully calcified at the age of five or six years.

The ego and superego are controlled by the Agnya Chakra. This subtle centre is placed at the meeting point of all three forces where the optic nerves cross. The balloons of ego and superego start growing from the Vishuddhi Chakra. When the ego is fully developed it spreads on the right side of the head in line with the ear and moves towards the front side of the brain. This development takes place because of thinking and planning.

The size and shape of the brain in the forehead of a human being differs substantially from that of a monkey. A monkey's brain is slanting and smaller in size because the ego development is very rudimentary. The activities of thinking and planning by the preconscious mind create fumes of waste products which accumulate as ego.

The superego stores all that conditions the mind, and develops behind the left ear and grows backwards over the head covering the whole back of the brain. All one's experiences, good and bad, are stored in the subconscious mind, while all the waste fumes of these emotional and feelings-related activities create the superego. Thus the preconscious mind (Mana) and the subconscious mind (Suptamana) use the Divine Power from the Sun Channel (Pingala) and the Moon Channel (Ida) respectively.

The activity of the whole sympathetic nervous system is supplied by the Divine Energy that flows in the right and left channels. The right channel starts on the left of the brain, and the left channel starts on the right side of the brain. The Agnya Chakra is placed at their crossing point, and controls the pituitary and pineal bodies in the gross. Thus the pituitary controls the ego and the pineal controls the superego. The pineal which controls the superego is over-developed in animals. In human beings there is balance between the ego and superego, by which both the ego and superego come to the centre on top of the brain near the fontanel bone.

The complete covering of the brain and the calcification of the fontanel bone separates human beings from the All-pervading Divine Power. In this way humans develop their "I-ness" or own identity. When both ego and superego are balanced by the temperate life of devotion of a householder, the Kundalini awakened through Sahaja Yoga, breaks through the centre of the brain. She takes the attention of the seeker into the All-pervading Power, the Universal Unconscious.

His attention moves onto the left or the right side of the system according to the nature of his activity. Any energy that is needed for this activity comes from the Ida or Pingala Nadis, and the Deities which are placed at the centre of the chakras decide the appropriate mode of action. The two parabolae of energy emerge from the two sides on the Pingala and Ida Nadis, one in a clockwise direction, the other in an anti-clockwise direction. The energy needed is transformed by the Deities. They are in contact with the seats of the subtle centers (Peethas) in the brain, and also with the auras of the Spirit that encircle the Divine Spirit (Atma) in the heart.

SUPRACONSCIOUS ACTIVITY

Most of the expositions about Kundalini have come to us so far through the Sages who practiced Hatha Yoga. The word 'Hatha' itself was derived from 'Ha' meaning 'Sun', and 'Tha' meaning 'Moon', clearly indicating that both sympathetic channels were used. The system of Hatha Yoga did not only relate to the working of conscious effort, but also to subconscious effort. Patanjali, very clearly wrote in his 'Sciences of Practices' that those wanting to practice this system of enlightenment must shun the forest dwellers. Through the various methods of abstinence (conscious effort) it was possible to control the organs (Indriyas).

It was equally necessary to pay attention to the working of the subconscious (subconscious effort), which is responsible for the suppression of reflexes caused by conditioning, or the forceful control of desires. For example, we can abstain from telling lies by controlling the tongue, but only by controlling the subconscious itself can we nip the thought of telling lies in the bud.

Abstinence is the way to master the preconscious mind, and love is the medicine to cure the subconscious mind. It is unfortunate that most of the modern yogis have lost the real meaning of Hatha Yoga. There is no place for love in their precepts and practices. For most of them acquiring mastery over physical powers like karate or acupuncture is their reason for becoming Hatha Yogis.

Even in ancient times, yogis who were initially mild-mannered individuals became extremely hot-tempered people after following Hatha Yoga for some time. They developed a supra-conscious personality because this right channel connects the mind with the supra-conscious realm, and with their attention, they grappled with the supernatural and material powers, and gained mastery over them. Such a yogi can overcome the force of gravity, and can fly in the air by stopping or arresting the workings of his sympathetic system. He can even stop the beating of his heart for a while. He can live in water for months on end but he has no love within him. He becomes an overpowering egoistic personality, and like the sun, he burns anyone who annoys him, reducing that individual to a heap of ashes (Bhasmisat).

In ancient scriptures the prowess of these so-called 'spiritual yogis' was well known. There are innumerable historical instances of yogis possessed with such a cruel nature. They are able to focus their attention on the Agnya Chakra through the Ida Nadi, through the use of power concentration, or finally by controlling their sex lives.

Until you are able to understand the meaning of the Self, the physical body would remain imperfect and would be unable to verify the truth. But once the physical instrument is connected with truth you are able to verify the Truth. It follows therefore, that first you have to accept Sahaja Yoga and get Self-realization. After Self realization, the vibrations of 'Chaitanya' begin to flow from your hands. The flow of these vibrations or Chaitanya helps to discriminate whether a particular event, situation, person or thing is true or not. If a particular matter is true, then waves of cool vibrations start flowing into the palms while if it untrue, hot vibrations is felt.

It is very important to understand that until the animal stage there was no need for animals to solve the problem of life as animals were under the complete command of God. At the human stage, however, as we learn from the story of Adam and Eve, they were given the choice and freedom to solve the problem of life itself. That was how evolution was to go a step further. Without such freedom human beings were not equipped to learn the secrets of Divine Power.

Chapter 13

Conclusion

Only in proportion as His spirit enters into us, can we in our little measure be helpers in the universe of which He is the one life. Until we, in all our doings and speaking, place ourselves within the Cosmic whole, feeling as He feels, thinking as He thinks, knowing for the time as He knows, we cannot be co-creators in the evolution as human being.

It is not that a man in past universes has climbed upward and has become one with Isvara; but it is that a man has climbed so far as to become so great, so perfect in his manhood, and so full of love and devotion to God and man, that God is able to permeate him with a portion of His own influence, His own power, His own knowledge, and send him forth into the world as a superhuman manifestation of Himself. The individual Ego remains; that is the great distinction. The man is there, though the power that is acting is the manifested God.

Therefore the manifestation will be colored by the special characteristics of the one over whom this overshadowing is made; and you will be able to trace in the thoughts of this inspired teacher, the characteristics of the race, of the individual, of the form of knowledge which belongs to that man in the incarnation in which the great overshadowing takes place.

That is the fundamental difference.

Divine power comes down, illuminates and irradiates the man for the moment, and he speaks for the time with authority, with knowledge, which in his normal state he will be unable probably to compass. Such are the prophets who have illuminated the world age after age; such were in ancient days the Brahmanas who were the mouth of God.

They come to the world to give a new impulse to spiritual truth. But there is a general inspiration like when you may be drawn away for a moment into higher, more peaceful realms, when you have come across something of beauty, of art, of the wonders of science, of the grandeur of philosophy, when you have for a time lost sight of the pettiness's of earth, of trivial troubles, of small worries and annoyances, and felt yourself lifted into a calmer region, into a light that is not the light of common earth, when you stood before some wondrous picture wherein the palette of the painter has been taxed to light the canvas with all the hues of beauteous color that art can give to human sight.

Or when you saw in some wondrous sculpture, the gracious living curves that the chisel has freed from the roughness of the marble, Or when you listened while the diviner spell of music has lifted you, step by step, till you seem to hear the Gandharvas singing and almost the divine flute is being played and echoing in the lower world, Or when you stood on the mountain peak with the snows around you, and felt the grandeur of the unmoving nature that shows out God as well as the human spirit.

If you have known any of these peaceful spots in life's desert, then you know how all-pervading is inspiration; how wondrous the beauty and the power of God shown forth in man and in the world; then you know, the truth of that great proclamation of Shri Krishna the beloved: "Whatever is royal, good, beautiful, and mighty, understand thou that to go forth from My Splendor"; all is the reflection of that Tejas, which is His and His alone. For as there is nothing in the universe without His love and life, so there is no beauty that is not His beauty, that is not a ray of the illimitable splendor, one little beam from the unfailing source of life."

And so we find that if we try to expand ourselves beyond the limits of our own system, we can commune with the One Existence, the Para-Brahma, whom sages revere in silence. The more ignorant the man, the more he thinks he can grasp. The less he understands, the more he resents being told that there are some things beyond the grasp of his intellect, existences so mighty that he cannot even dream of the lowest of the attributes that mark them out. And for me, many an age must pass before I shall be able to think of dealing with these profounder problems. Therefore, I say to you frankly that these mighty Ones whom we worship are the Gods of our system; beyond them there stretch mightier Ones yet, whom, perhaps, myriads of kalpas hence, we may begin to understand and worship.

There He gives the law of these appearances: "When, O son of Pritha, I live in the order of the deities, and then I act in every respect as a deity. When I live in the order of the Gandharvas, then I act in every respect as a Gandharva. When I live in the order of the Nags, I act as a Naga. When I live in the order of the Yakshas, or that of the Rakshasas, I act after the manner of that order. Born now in the order of humanity, I must act as a human being" - A profound truth, a truth that few in modern times recognize and understand. Every type in the universe, in its own place, is good; every type in the universe, in its own place, is necessary. There is no life save His life; how could any type then come into existence apart from the universal life?

We speak of good and evil forms as regards our own evolution. But from the wider standpoint of the Cosmos, good and evil are relative terms, and everything is very good in the sight of the Supreme who lives in every one. How can a type come into existence in which He cannot live? How can anything live and move, save as it has its being in Him? Each type has its work; each type has its place; the Rakshasa as much as the Deva, of the Asura as much as of the Sura.

Our world is one of the links in this chain, and you and I pass round this chain in successive incarnations in the great stages of life. The world--our present world--is the midway globe of one such chain. You have read perhaps of the seven-leaved lotus, the Saptaparnapadma; looked at with the higher sight, gazed at with the open vision of the seer, that mighty group of creative and directing

Beings looks like the lotus with its seven leaves and the great Ones are at the heart of the lotus. It is as though you could see a vast lotus-flower spread out in space, the tips of the seven leaves being the mighty Intelligences presiding over the evolution of the chains of worlds.

That lotus symbol is not merely a symbol but a high reality. And because the great Rishis of old saw with the open eye of knowledge, saw the lotus- flower spread in space, they took it as the symbol of Cosmos, the lotus with its seven leaves, each one a mighty Deva presiding over a separate line of evolution. We are primarily concerned with our own planetary Deva and through Him with the great Devas of the solar system.

But when He is working for the building of this world He must work within the limitations and conditions of those very materials that make this world. These being influenced by the ceaseless interplay of Sattva, Rajas, and Tamas, Tamas has the ascendancy, aided and, as it were, worked by Rajas, so that they predominate over Sattva in the foreseen evolution, when the two combining overpower the third, when the force of Rajas and the inertia and stubbornness of Tamas, binding themselves together, check the action, the harmony, the pleasure-giving qualities of Sattwa.

Then comes one of the conditions in which the Lord comes forth to restore that which had been disturbed of the balanced interworking of the three gunas. To regain such balance between them so as to enable evolution to go forward smoothly He re-establishes the balance of power which gives orderly motion. In these fundamental attributes of matter, the three gunas, lies the first reason of the need for Avataras.

The second need has to do with man himself. When He came to deal with the evolution of man He had a harder task to perform than in the evolution of the lower forms of life – whether in the mineral, vegetable or the animal kingdom. On them the law is imposed and they must obey its impulse. But with man it is not so.

In man Isvara sets himself to produce an image of Him, which is not the case in the lower kingdoms. As life has evolved, one force after another has come out, and in man there begins to come out the central life. The time has arrived for the evolution of the sovereign power of will, the self-initiated motion which is part of the life of the Supreme. There is only one will in the universe, the will of Isvara, and all must conform itself to that will. All is conditioned by that will, and must move according to that will, and that will marks out the straight line of evolution. There may be swerving neither to the right hand nor to the left. There is but one Self and that Self is yours and mine as much as His.

There must evolve at one stage of this wondrous evolution that royal power of will which is seen in Him. And from the Atma within us, which is He in us, there flows forth the sovereign will into the sheaths in which the Atma is held.

But what happens is this: the force that goes out through the sheaths and gives them some of its own nature, and each sheath begins to set up a reflection of the will on its own account, and you get the "I" of the body which wants to go this way, and the "I" of passion or emotion which wants to go that way, and the "I" of the mind which wants to go a third way, and none of these ways is the way of the Atma, the Supreme.

These are the illusory wills of man. Each of them is determined in its direction by external attraction; the man's body wants to move in a particular way because something attracts it, or repels it: it moves to what it likes or what is congenial to it, and moves away from that which it dislikes, from that from which it feels itself repelled. But that motion of the body is but motion determined by the Cosmos around and not by the Self within.

Similarly the emotions or passions are drawn this way or that by the objects of the senses, and so also the mind lets the senses run after objects as a horse that has broken its reins flies away with the unskilled driver. These forces reinforce the Rajasic guna and help to bring about the predominance of reckless desires that are not according to the one will.

Otherwise how would one learn right if you knew not wrong? How would you choose well if you knew not evil? How would you recognize the light if there were no darkness? How would you move if there were no resistance? The forces that are called dark, the forces of the Rakshasas, of the Asuras, of all that seem to be working against Isvara--these are the forces that call out the inner strength of the Self in man. The evolution of force can only be made by struggle, by combat, by effort, by exercise, and it is by pulling against their strength, that the outer manifestation begins to unfold itself.

In the seed the life is hidden, and in order that it sprouts we need to plant the seed in the ground, so that the forces in the ground press on it, the rays of the sun from outside make vibrations that work on it, and the water from the rain comes through the soil into it and forces it to swell, making the seed to grow. It begins to grow by pushing the ground with the roots downwards, and against the opposition of the ground, the growing plant mounts upward.

When the little plant appears above the soil, the wind comes, blows and tries to drag it away, and, in order to live and not perish, it strikes its roots deeper to get a better hold against the battering force of the wind. Thus the tree grows against the forces which try to tear it out. If these forces were not there, the root would not have grown.

And so it is with the root of Isvara, the life within us. If everything around us was smooth and easy, we would remain supine, lethargic, and indifferent. It is the whip of pain, suffering, and disappointment, that drives us harder and brings out the forces of our internal life which otherwise would remain undeveloped. If a man has to grow then sitting on a couch with pillows and comforts at hand will not help. But exposing him to difficulties will make a man grow into a man and not into a log.

That is why there are forces, but it sometimes comes in the guise of evil. These forces are necessary. They test evolution; they strengthen evolution, so that it does not take the next step onward till it has strength enough to hold its own. One step is made firm by opposition before the next is taken.

But when, by the conflicting wills of men, the forces that work for retardation are so reinforced by men's unruly wishes that they threaten progress, and then there is reinforcement from the other side. The presence of the Avatar of the forces that threaten evolution calls forth the presence of the Avataras that leads to the progress of humanity.

We come to the third cause. The Avataras does not come without a call. When the earth, is very heavy with its load of evil, "Save us, O supreme Lord," the Devas cry. In answer to that cry the Lord comes forth. By the will of the one Supreme, there is one incarnated in form who gathers up together the forces that make for retardation, in order that, they may be destroyed by the opposing force of good, and thus the balance may be re-established and evolution go on along its appointed road. Devas work for joy, the reward of Heaven. Rakshasas also serve Him, first for rule on earth, and enjoy as they will in this lower world. Both sides serve for reward, and are moved by the things that please.

Though all powers are His, the Rakshasas, the Asura as much as Sura; for your evolution you must be on the side of good, and struggle to the utmost against evil. Just because evil is relative, because it exists by the one will, because Rakshasa is His as much as Deva, do not think that you can go on their side and walk along their path. It is not so. If you yield to ambition, and pride, if you set yourselves against the will of Isvara, if you struggle for the separated self, if you identify yourself with the past instead of with the future towards which you should be directing your steps, then, if your Karma be at a certain stage, you pass into the ranks of those who work as enemies, because you have chosen that fate for yourself, at the promptings of the lower nature. Then with bitter inner pain and sorrow, you will have to work out your own will against the will of the Lord, and feel the anguish of the rending that separates the inner from the outer life.

The will of the Divine for you is evolution. These forces are made to help your evolution only if you strive against them. If you yield to them, you only strengthen them. Therefore, Krishna says, "O Arjuna, stand up and fight. Do not be supine; do not yield yourself to the forces; they are there to call out your energies by opposition and you must not sink down on the floor of the chariot.

SHRI BRAHMADEVA SARASWATI-Shri

Brahmadeva Saraswati!

Om Shri Maha Ahamkara Namah Om Shri Surya Namah
Om Shri Chandra Namah
Om Shri Tatwa Swamini Namah
Om Shri Vayu Tatwa Swamini Namah
Om Shri Tejas Tatwa Swamini Namah
Om Shri Apa Tatwa Swamini Namah
Om Shri Prithvi Tatwa Swamini
Namah Om Shri Aksha Tatwa Iswari
Namah Om Shri Aneela Tatwa Iswari
Namah Om Shri Tejo Tatwa Iswari
Namah
Om Shri Jala Tatwa Iswari Namah
Om Shri Bhoomi Tatwa Iswari
Namah Om Shri Hiranyagarbhaye
Namah Om Shri Pancha
Tanmatrasye Namah Om Shri Pancha
Bhuteshuye Namah Om Shri Vishwa
Namah
Om Shri Taijasatmika Namah
Om Shri Prajnatmika Namah
Om Shri Turya Namah
Sakshat Shri Adi Shakti Mataji Shri Nirmala Devi Namoh Namah

A PRAYER TO AUM, THE DIVINE ESSENCE

Let our ears hear that which is true; Let
our eyes see that which is pure;
Let our beings praise that which is Divine; And let those
who listen hear not my voice But the wisdom of God.
Let us worship with the same song, the same
strength and the same Knowledge.
And let our meditation enlighten and enrich. Let
there be amongst us compassion and peace.

NOW THE PRAYER

Salutation to Shri Ganesh, Sakshat Shri Jesus
Sakshat Shri Nirmala Devi Namoh Namah.
It is you who is the beginning of all the beginnings.
It is you who is the doer of all deeds which have
been done, are being done and will be done.
It is you who supports all things that are supported. It is you
who protects all things that are protected. It is you who is
the complete, all-pervading Spirit. God's Divine energy.
Think clearly brain. Speak only the Truth.
Let Your presence, awakened in us by Kundalini, speak;
Let Your presence, awakened in us by Kundalini, listen;
Let Your presence, awakened in us by Kundalini, bless;
Let Your presence, awakened in us by Kundalini, pro-
tect; Let Your presence, awakened by Kundalini, in us.
Your disciples, be the disciple.
You are the essence of all the Sacred Literature and Holy Words,
and You are the Energy that understands the Holy Words;
You are the Divine combination of complete Truth,
complete Happiness and complete Energy;
And You are beyond;
You are All Knowledge, and You are the use to which the
Knowledge is put. You exist until the end of all things, and
after the end of all things, You are; You create the end of all
things, and after the end of all things, You remain indifferent;
You are the Earth, You are the Water, You are the Fire,
You are the Air, and You are the space above the Air;
You are the Gunas; and You are beyond the Gunas;
You are the Body; and You are beyond the Body;
You are the Essence of Time; and You are beyond Time;
You and only You exist at the Mooladhar Chakra;
You are the Spirit; and You are beyond the Spirit; And
those who would join God meditate upon You.
You are Brahman, Vishnu, Rudra; You are Indra, Agni, Vayu;

You are the Sun at noon; You are the Full
Moon; Through all of these, and more,
You are the all-pervading energy of innocence and wisdom.
You are the Divine servant who stoops to wash the feet of saints.
You are the tiny core of all things without which the larger
have no purpose; You are the key to the libraries of all
the scriptures, without which the Truth is hidden;
You are the full stop which completes the sentence, and
without which the sentence loses its meaning;
You are the Crescent Moon; You are the Stars; and You are
beyond the Stars; All things, from tiny dot to Universe, are you.
You are where the sounds combine; You are
the silence between the sounds;
You are the rhythm of all music and all prayers;
This is the knowledge of Nirmal Ganesh, and You, Nirmal
Ganesh, are the master of that Knowledge, and all Knowledge.
You are the God; and you are the Goddess.
Aum, Gam Nirmal Ganapataye
To Your powers, Ganesha, let all surrender;

Let the left side of memory and the right side of action surrender to you and let your enlightenment prevail.
Your first tooth you have, and four-hands; one holding a rope, the second a goad, the third is raised in
blessing and the fourth offers sustenance.
Your banner is that of a humble mouse. You
have long ears and are clothed in red;
red decorates You and You are worshipped with red flowers.
You have compassion for those who love You, and it is
for those who love You that You come to this Earth.
You are the force that creates, the energy that pervades and the Spirit that protects.
Those who seek union with God pray through You:
Those who seek union with God worship You.
Aum, Gam Nirmal Jesusye

To Your powers, Aum Jesus, let all surrender;
Let the left side of memory and the right side of action sur-
render to you and let your enlightenment prevail.
You are the Word that was the beginning; You
are the Word that will be the ending.
You are he who was born of a Virgin, and died on the cross;
You are he who absorbs all sins, and who died to live again; You
are God in Man, and you are worshipped with red flowers.
You have compassion for those who love You, and it is
for those who love You that You come to this Earth.
You are the force that creates, the energy that per-
vades and the Spirit that protects.
Those who seek union with God pray through You.
Those who seek union with God worship You.
Shri Ganesha, Salutations to You. Shri Jesus, Salutations to You.
He who is the beginning of all worship, Salutations to You.
He who destroys all the powers of evil, Salutations to You.
Sakshat, Son of Lord Shiva, who is unending blessings, Salutations
to You. Sakshat, Son of Mary Mataji, who is unending Love,
Salutations to You.
Sakshat, Mataji Nirmala Devi, who is unend-
ing Joy, Salutations to You.

Sakshat Shri Adi Shakti Mataji Shri Nirmala Devi Namo Namah

Bibliography

1. Neki, J.S., "Sahaja: an Indian ideal of mental health", *Psychiatry*, Vol. 38, No. 1, Feb 1975, pp. 1-10.
2. Maslow, A., *Religions, Values, and Peak Experiences*, The Viking Press, New York, 1972.
3. Holmes, D.S., "The influence of meditation, versus rest, on physiological arousal", in West, M.A., (ed.), *The Psychology of Meditation*, Clarendon Press, Oxford, 1987.
4. Rai, U.C. et al., "Some effects of Sahaja Yoga and its role in the prevention of stress disorders", *Journal International Medical Sciences Academy*, 1988.
5. Panjwani, U., Selvamurthy, W., Singh, S.H., Gupta, H.L.,Mukhopadhyay, S., Thakur, L., "Effect of Sahaja yoga meditation on auditory evoked potentials (AEP) and visual contrast sensitivity (VCS) in epileptics", *Applied Psychophysiology & Biofeedback*, Vol. 25, No. 1, March 2000, pp. 1-12.
6. Rai, op. cit. (Ref 9).
7. Manocha, R., "Why Meditation?", *Australian Family Physician*, Vol. 29, No. 12, Dec 2000. pp. 1135-1138.
8. References from speeches and writings from sahaja yoga web site www.sahajayoga.org.
9. Pictures collected at various points of time- thanks to all contributors.

The Mystery of Music in Sahaja Yoga

- An article about the musical event for the cancer patients in the Pune Times of the Times of India 18th December 2009.
- Articles appearing under the columns of "The Speaking Tree" in the Times of India, from time to time, on music, by Bindu Chawla, Simanta Mohanty, Madhav Chari, P L Bhola and Anup Taneja.
- Vibrational Medicine by Richard Gerber. M.D.pg. 523-525.
- Notes written down during Dr. Arun Apte's classes and discussions.

The role of Incarnations in Sahaja Yoga

- Chapter on Incarnation of Krishna - H.H. SHRI MATAJI NIRMALA DEVI LORD KRISHNA PUJA (Yogeshwara)
- London, Chesham Road, 15.8.1982 and Shri Virata Pujas 1999
- Chapter on Incarnation of Jesus Christ - C Easter Pujas Turkey, 2001 and Speech by H.H. Shri Mataji Nirmala Devi (Caxton Hall, England, Dec 10, 1979)
- [Footnote 1: Bhagavad-Gita , x. 39.]
- Chapter on the Incarnation of Buddha – excerpts from the speech of Shri Mataji Nirmala Devi on the occasion of SHRI BUDDHA PUJA at SPAIN on 20th May 1989.
- Meta Modern Era-Chapter 9-by Shri Mataji Nirmala Devi
- Chapter 5:
- References:
- [1] Marcia Eliade' The Myth of the Eternal Return, (transl. by Willard R. Track), Bollinger Series XLVI, Princeton University Press' Princeton 1991' p.125.
- [2] The Laws of Manu 1.71 (transl. by G. Buhler), in The Sacred Books of the East, vol.25, book 1, Clarendon Press, Oxford 1886.

[3] The Mahabharata 3.12.826.
[4] Henry Corbin, Spiritual Body and Celestial Earth, From Mazda Iran to Shiite Iran (transl. by Nancy Pearson), Princeton University Press, Princeton 1977, p.49.
[5] Tanner debt Elijah, chi II.
[6] Jean Danni*Lou, Les Symbols char*tines primitive, Sequel, Paris 1961, chi VIII: Les douse palters et le zodiaque.
[7] Eliade' The Myth... ' p.115.
[8] The Rig-Veda 1.164.115 passim; The Atharva-Veda 10.8.4.
[9] Jean Hubaux' Les
•   My Prayer Book

www.ingramcontent.com/pod-product-compliance
Lightning Source LLC
Chambersburg PA
CBHW062113020426
42335CB00013B/948